Canadian Community as Partner

THEORY AND PRACTICE IN NURSING

Canadian Community as Partner

THEORY AND PRACTICE IN NURSING

Ardene Robinson Vollman, RN, PhD
Adjunct Associate Professor
Faculties of Medicine, Nursing and Kinesiology
University of Calgary
Calgary, Alberta

Elizabeth T. Anderson, TN, DrPH, FAAN
Professor
Director
World Health Organization Collaborating Center for Nursing and Midwifery
Development in Primary Health Care
University of Texas Medical Branch
School of Nursing
Galveston, Texas

Judith McFarlane, RN, DrPH, FAAN
Parry Chair in Health Promotion and Disease Prevention
Texas Woman's University
College of Nursing
Houston, Texas

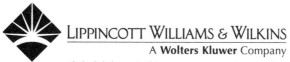

LIPPINCOTT WILLIAMS & WILKINS
A **Wolters Kluwer** Company

Philadelphia • Baltimore • New York • London
Buenos Aires • Hong Kong • Sydney • Tokyo

Acquisitions Editor: Margaret Zuccarini
Managing Editor: Joe Morita
Editorial Assistant: Carol DeVault
Senior Project Editor: Tom Gibbons
Senior Production Manager: Helen Ewan
Managing Editor/Production: Erika Kors
Design Coordinator: Brett MacNaughton

Interior Designer: Joan Wendt
Cover Designer: Melissa Walter
Illustrator: Annelisa Ochoa
Manufacturing Manager: William Alberti
Indexer: Ellen Brennan
Compositor: LWW
Printer: R. R. Donnelley

9 8 7 6 5 4 3 2 1

Library of Congress Cataloging-in-Publication Data

Vollman, Ardene Robinson.
    Canadian community as partner : theory and practice in nursing / Ardene Robinson
Vollman, Elizabeth T. Anderson, Judith McFarlane.
        p. cm.
    Includes bibliographical references and index.
    Canadian version of: Community as partner, by Elizabeth T. Anderson, Judith McFarlane.
    ISBN 0-7817-4162-9 (pbk. : alk. paper)
    1. Community health nursing--Canada. 2. Community health nursing--Canada--Case
studies. I. Anderson, Elizabeth T. II. McFarlane, Judith M. III. Anderson, Elizabeth T.
Community as partner. IV. Title.

RT98.V64 2003
610.73'43'0971--dc22   2003058815

Care has been taken to confirm the accuracy of the information presented and to describe generally accepted practices. However, the authors, editors, and publisher are not responsible for errors or omissions or for any consequences from application of the information in this book and make no warranty, express or implied, with respect to the content of the publication.

The authors, editors, and publisher have exerted every effort to ensure that drug selection and dosage set forth in this text are in accordance with the current recommendations and practice at the time of publication. However, in view of ongoing research, changes in government regulations, and the constant flow of information relating to drug therapy and drug reactions, the reader is urged to check the package insert for each drug for any change in indications and dosage and for added warnings and precautions. This is particularly important when the recommended agent is a new or infrequently employed drug.

Some drugs and medical devices presented in this publication have Food and Drug Administration (FDA) clearance for limited use in restricted research settings. It is the responsibility of the health care provider to ascertain the FDA status of each drug or device planned for use in his or her clinical practice.

Dedicated to
Lillian Robinson, my mother
October 15, 1917–December 13, 2002

Contributors

Lori L. Anderson, RN, MN
Executive Leader Health Services
Headwaters Health Authority — Oilfields
    Hospital
Black Diamond, Alberta
Canada

Sandra A. Cashaw, MPH, RN
Associate Clinical Professor
Texas Woman's University
Houston, Texas
United States

Lynn Corcoran, RN, MN
Counselor
YWCA of Calgary — Family Violence Prevention
    Programs
Calgary, Alberta
Canada

Nina Fredland, MSN, RN-CS, FNP
Assistant Professor
Texas Woman's University
Houston, Texas
United States

Charles Kemp, RN, FNP
Senior Lecturer
Louise Herrington School of Nursing
Baylor University
Dallas, Texas
United States

Jeanne M. Sargent, RN, MN
Project Coordinator, Public Health Nurse
Calgary Health Region
Calgary, Alberta
Canada

Pamela Schultz, PhD, RN
Program Director
University of Texas, MD Anderson Cancer
    Center
Houston, Texas
United States

Catherine M. Scott, PhD
Post-Doctoral Fellow
Department of Community Health Sciences
University of Calgary
Calgary, Alberta
Canada

Wilfreda E. Thurston, PhD
Associate Professor — Department of
    Community Health Sciences
University of Calgary
Calgary, Alberta
Canada

Marlies W. M. van Dijk, RN, MSd
Regional Quality Improvement Consultant
Calgary Health Region
Calgary, Alberta
Canada

Mary Wainwright, RN, MSN
Assistant Director
East Texas Area Health Education Center
Galveston, Texas
United States

Reviewers

Elsa Arbuthnot, MN, RN
Assistant Professor, School of Nursing
Saint Francis Xavier University
Antigonish, Nova Scotia, Canada

Charlene Beynon, BScN, MScN
Director of Research Education, Evaluation
    Development Services
Middlesex-London Health Unit
Associate Professor, School of Nursing
The University of Western Ontario
London, Ontario, Canada

Elizabeth Diem, RN, MSc, PhD
Assistant Professor, School of Nursing
University of Ottawa
Ottawa, Ontario, Canada

Marilyn Evan, RN, MN, PhD(c)
Assistant Professor, Department of Community
    Health Sciences
Brock University
St. Catherines, Ontario, Canada

Joan Evans, RN, PhD
Assistant Professor, School of Nursing
Dalhousie University
Halifax, Nova Scotia, Canada

Adeline R. Falk-Rafael, RN, PhD
Associate Professor of Nursing
York University
Toronto, Ontario, Canada

Sandra E. Flynn, RN, BSN, MEd.
Instructor, Nursing Program
University College of the Fraser Valley
Chilliwack, British Columbia, Canada

Alison Fyfe-Carlson
Nursing Instructor
Red River College
Winnipeg, Manitoba, Canada

Donna Gallant, RN, BScN, MSc, PhD(c)
Assistant Professor
Saint Francis Xavier University
Antigonish, Nova Scotia, Canada

Judith C. Kulig, RN, DNSc
Associate Professor, School of Health Sciences
University of Lethbridge
Lethbridge, Alberta, Canada

Marjorie MacDonald, RN, BN, MSc, PhD
Associate Professor, School of Nursing
University of Victoria
Victoria, British Columbia, Canada

Fran Racher, RN, BA, BScN, MSc
    (Community Health), PhD(c)
Assistant Professor, School of Health Sciences
Brandon University
Brandon, Manitoba, Canada

Dr. Violeta Ribeiro, RN, BNSc, MS, DNSc
Associate Professor, School of Nursing
Memorial University of Newfoundland
St. John's, Newfoundland, Canada

Bonnie Schoenfeld, RN, BSN, MSc
Assistant Professor, College of Nursing
University of Saskatchewan
Saskatoon, Saskatchewan, Canada

Elaine Schow, RN, BScN, MN
Tenure Faculty
Mount Royal College
Calgary, Alberta, Canada

Patricia Seaman, BN, MN
Senior Instructor, Faculty of Nursing
University of New Brunswick
Fredericton, New Brunswick, Canada

Dr. Barbara Thomas, RN, EdD
Professor and Graduate Coordinator, School of
    Nursing
University of Windsor
Windsor, Ontario, Canada

Lynn Van Hofwegen, MS, APRN
Assistant Professor of Nursing
Trinity Western University
Langley, British Columbia, Canada

Lucia Yiu, BSc, BA, MScN
Associate Professor, Faculty of Nursing
University of Windsor
Windsor, Ontario, Canada

Preface

Over the past decade, first as a manager in a rural health unit in Western Canada, then as a professor of nursing at the University of Calgary, I often lamented the lack of "made in Canada" resources for the front-line community worker. Yes, Canada has made, and continues to make, tremendous contributions on the national and international stages, but little trickles down to the grassroots worker. Similarly, little of what the community worker "knows" from his or her practice of community-focused work percolates upward to inform theory. One resource that helped to guide practice was the first edition of *Community as Partner*, written by Elizabeth Anderson and Judith McFarlane; by the time I arrived to teach at the University, the second edition was being published. Still, I dreamed that someone would create a Canadian version of the book that would incorporate a multidisciplinary approach reminiscent of real-life community practice.

At the American Public Health Association conference held in Boston in November 2000, I attended a presentation by Bets Anderson. Then, a Lippincott Williams & Wilkins salesperson said to me "Why don't you do a Canadian version of the book instead of [complaining] about it every year?" Why indeed. With the encouragement of my colleagues, I invited Judith McFarlane to come to Calgary to make a presentation to the Health Promotion Research Group at the University on her work on women's health, and the rest, as they say, is history. With Judith's wonderful encouragement we embarked on a journey that has resulted in this publication. I hope it is the first of many editions, each of them further enriched by the people who read the book, work with the process, and share their experiences and stories.

The book is organised in three sections: a theoretical section that sets the stage for how and why we work with communities as partners; a process section that details the step-by-step activity of community practice; and a case story section where colleagues share their successes in community practice.

Part 1: Theoretical Foundations of Community Practice

In this section, seven chapters detail the philosophical foundations of population health promotion, the scientific foundation of public health practice (demography, epidemiology), the Canadian health system, healthy environments, ethics and advocacy, and healthy public policy. These chapters are presented in such a way as to underscore the importance of public participation and partnerships in community action.

Part 2: The Community as Partner Process

This section begins with the model that guides the process of working with communities. In subsequent chapters the steps of the community process are detailed with the use of examples from five of fifteen downtown Calgary communities. The reader is guided through the steps of the process: assessment; analysis and community diagnosis; planning; implementation of a planned intervention; and evaluation. At all steps in the process the importance of public participation and partnerships is emphasized.

Part 3: Community as Partner in Practice: The Case Studies

In this section, colleagues from across Alberta bring the community-as-partner process to life as they share their experiences. We have also included five chapters that provide strategies to promote health in a variety of settings. Readers will be inspired by the variety of approaches, populations, and issues confronted by the guest contributors.

It is my hope that current readers will turn into future contributors and that future editions of this book will contain a greater variety of successful community-as-partner stories from across this great nation.

Ardene Robinson Vollman, RN, PhD

Acknowledgments

First and foremost, the contributions of the original authors, Judith McFarlane and Elizabeth (Bets) Anderson, must be acknowledged. Without their efforts over the past many years, through four editions of their book, this Canadian edition may never have sprouted roots.

I thank my colleagues and students who generously shared their encouragement, expertise, and stories (some of which are included in this book). My family sustained and nurtured me through the process; I am grateful for their support and apologetic for what were often long hours at the computer.

Two people deserve medals for guiding me through the publication process: Margaret Zuccarini and Joe Morita. They were unfailingly patient and encouraging with a first-time author. Leslie Ann Mosby and Thomas Gibbons marshalled us quickly through the editing, remaining optimistic throughout that we would finish it in good time.

For many reasons I am grateful to Corey Wolfe (Lippincott Williams & Wilkins), Dr. Roxie Thompson Isherwood, Dr. Sandra Tenove, Dr. Wilfreda "Billie" Thurston, and Dr. Lynn Meadows—they exemplify "partnership" in action.

To my colleagues and students, my thanks. This is for you!

Contents

PART III   Community as Partner in Practice/327

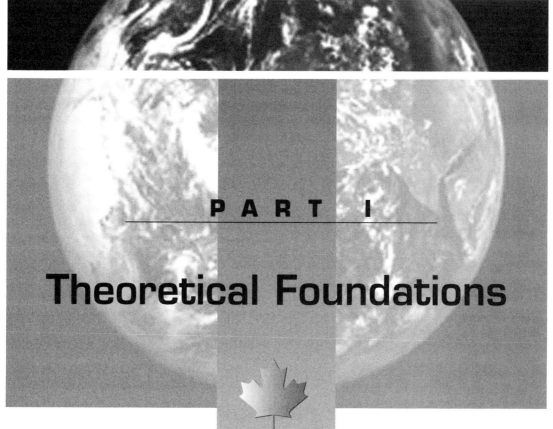

P A R T I

Theoretical Foundations

1

Population Health Promotion

OBJECTIVES

After studying this chapter, you should be able to:

◆ Describe the philosophical foundations of population health promotion

◆ List the five principles and eight essentials of primary health care

◆ Outline the challenges, mechanisms, and strategies of the Canadian framework for health promotion

◆ Detail the prerequisites for health and the action strategies for health promotion as described in the Ottawa Charter for Health Promotion

◆ List the factors that determine health

◆ Understand the evolution of population health promotion

Introduction

In the 20th century many gains in health status among the people of the developed world were achieved. Much was accomplished through four means: (1) advances in knowledge about the causes of disease, (2) development of new technologies and pharmaceuticals to treat and cure many diseases, (3) creation of vaccines and environmental solutions to prevent disease transmission and acquisition, and (4) innovations in surveillance techniques to measure health status. However, it has become increasingly accepted that health is more than the absence of disease—it is a broad manifestation of wellness of body, mind, and environment and is viewed as an essential resource for everyday living. In this chapter the history and the evolution of thought around the concept of health as it relates to individuals, families, groups, and communities is chronicled. Many of the principles and concepts presented in this chapter are discussed more fully in other parts of the book.

In this text, the generic term "health worker" or "health team" is used to connote the multidisciplinary and intersectoral approach that underlies successful community practice. Although initially designed for nurses, this book is intended to be useful to community social workers, nutritionists, health educators, community medicine physicians, pharmacists, and health promoters. It also recognizes that health teams should have members of the public involved in all levels of activities to ensure the foundational principles of community practice are implemented.

As you will see as you progress through this book and learn the processes of community assessment, planning, and evaluation, it will become evident that no single person or agency is capable of addressing the many and complex health problems of communities and populations. Because health is determined by a complex mix of factors, maintaining and creating health requires ongoing action from multiple partners whose mandates support similar goals. Hence, community health workers rely on cooperation with other workers, collaboration among agencies involved in similar work, and partnerships with people, communities, public and private sectors, and business to effect change that has a positive impact on the health of people.

Partnerships may be formed across *sectors* (i.e., broad fields of activity, such as education, health, justice, etc.), and at different *levels*. Levels may be defined by geography, by scope of mandate (e.g., municipal, provincial), or by vertical level within organizations (e.g., senior management, front-line). Action is more effective when it includes vertical as well as horizontal partnerships and collaboration. Horizontal links are created when partnerships are formed at the same level. For instance, to deal with an outbreak of infection in a day care centre, the health district's environmental health officer and community nurse, the school board's preschool education specialist, and the social worker from children's services may be involved in the follow-up action. To illustrate vertical collaboration, to set health policy regarding tobacco, a health region will work with the federal health department, the provincial health ministry, and the municipality, all of whom have different jurisdictions in policy development and enforcement. Horizontally, each partner may also need to work with justice counterparts (e.g., Royal Canadian Mounted Police, provincial police, local by-law enforcement) and other departments to effect change in tobacco policy.

Key to all community practice is the principle of "doing with" not "to" or "for" the people served. This theme is pervasive in all the documents that form the foundation of community practice. The title of this book is "community as partner" meaning that community workers partner not only with professional colleagues to serve the people in communities but also with members of those communities and groups. In the following section, how this principle became the key theme in community practice will be described.

Foundations of Community Practice

Whatever discipline in which community workers are trained, several documents published in the last quarter of the 20th century have been instrumental in the development of guiding principles of ethical community practice. Many of the seminal documents that form this foundation have originated in Canada.

The Lalonde Report

The publication of the report *New Perspectives on the Health of Canadians* in 1974 under the auspices of the then minister of National Health and Welfare, the Honourable Marc Lalonde, heralded a change in the focus of health on disease to a focus on health (Lalonde, 1974). The Lalonde Report, as it has become known, argues that health is not achievable from health care services alone, but from the interaction of health services with human biology, lifestyle, and the environment in which we live. This report suggested that health is tied to overall conditions of living, particularly the environment and the behaviours chosen by people. Lalonde's approach was directed primarily toward the individual and toward individuals taking responsibility for their health. Proponents of the approach tended to focus on behaviours and, when illness or injury resulted, people felt "blamed" for not carrying out the recommended health behav-

iours, or not doing them "enough." Interventions focused on telling people
what the healthy behaviour was, but did not address the social conditions that
militated against its adoption. For instance, mothers were taught to follow
Canada's Food Guide, but for women living in poverty, the means to purchase
wholesome food were not accessible. People wishing to bike to work or school, as
exhorted by ParticipAction advocates, took their lives in their hands as they com-
peted with large vehicles for road space. This emphasis on lifestyle captured the
attention of governments and the social-environmental elements were consequently downplayed in health policy and funding until the next decade when it
became evident that the health education and social marketing approach alone
was not adequate to create the reduction in health expenditures envisioned by
politicians and health planners who initially embraced this new perspective.

Although the Lalonde Report had obvious limitations, it did stimulate
thought in a new direction and led to other important outcomes, not the least
of which was the attention sparked across sectors such as economics, education, social welfare, and justice regarding the environmental imperatives of creating healthy people in healthy nations. As a result, the Lalonde Report
received international attention, and in response to the growing concern about
the disparities in health status between developed and undeveloped countries,
between people with many resources and those with few, the World Health
Organization (WHO) convened a meeting of member countries.

Alma Ata Declaration

The WHO member states met in Alma Ata, Kazakhstan in September 1978 to
develop an action plan to achieve the goal of "Health for All by Year 2000" proposed as the vision by the 30th World Health Assembly (held in 1977). From this
conference came the *Alma Ata Declaration on Primary Health Care* (WHO, 1978),
viewed as the bridge between the Lalonde perspective and the influence of post-
modern thinkers such as Marxists and other critical social activists who critiqued
social structures to better understand and transform the dominant social order. As
historical, cultural, and gendered social constructions were questioned, new ways
of working with people emerged so that the people themselves (not the politicians
or experts) could shape the world in which they live.

The Alma Ata Declaration (Box 1-1) became the philosophy of community
action for health. Its emphasis on social justice, equity, public participation,
appropriate technology, and intersectoral collaboration focused action on the
needs of the population and the root causes of ill health, challenging the system
to move from the traditional biomedical model (disease) to a framework that
promoted health. Influenced by the work of Freire (1970) and others, the Alma

> **BOX 1-1. THE DECLARATION OF ALMA ATA: PRIMARY HEALTH CARE**
>
> Primary health care is essential health care based on practical, scientifically sound, and socially acceptable methods and technology made universally accessible to individuals and families in the community through their full participation and at a cost that the community and country can afford to maintain at every stage of their development in the spirit of self-reliance and self-determination. It forms an integral part both of the country's health system, of which it is the central function and main focus, and of the overall social and economic development of the community. It is the first level of contact of individuals, the family, and community with the national health system bringing health care as close as possible to where people live and work, and constitutes the first element of a continuing health care process. (Article VI)

Ata Declaration called for health providers to work *with* people to assist them in making decisions about their health and how to meet health challenges in ways that are affordable, acceptable, and sustainable in the long term. The Declaration also explicitly stated the elements of a health system that were essential to the achievement of health for all:

◆ Education about the prevailing health problems and their prevention and control
◆ Safe food supply and adequate nutrition
◆ Adequate supply of safe water and basic sanitation
◆ Maternal and child care, including family planning
◆ Immunization against basic infectious diseases
◆ Prevention and control of locally endemic diseases
◆ Appropriate treatment of common diseases and injuries
◆ Essential drugs

Thibaudeau and Fortier (2000) and other authors (Denoncourt et al., 2000; Poirier et al., 2000) describe a primary health care initiative in downtown Montreal. Having identified the homeless as one of the most vulnerable population groups in society, exposed to multiple hazards in a nonsupportive environment, diminishing their ability to stay healthy or to take the necessary steps to seek the services they need to become healthy, an outreach service was initiated. A local community health centre that serves an estimated 8000 homeless people formed an outreach team comprising a general practice physician, a psychiatrist, two nurses, social workers, and support staff. This team works closely with shelter, day centre, hospital, and community professionals to improve the self-care capacities and the use of appropriate services by homeless people. In many instances, homeless people fear and distrust formal health and social services and, as a result, make contact only when their situations are most dire and their health and social conditions have deteriorated extensively. Services available through the combined efforts of the outreach team, soup kitchens, shelters, and churches in Montreal and other Canadian communities are outlined in Table 1-1.

Other services that may be provided include postal facilities, distribution of welfare cheques, legal assistance, job skills education, work placement services, "inn from the cold" shelter in winter, bottled water in the heat of summer, transportation vouchers, and assisted housing. In every community that faces the challenge of homelessness, formal and informal agencies work with tireless volunteers to deliver these services in ways that respect the principles of Alma Ata by:

◆ Ensuring that health and health services are geographically, financially, and culturally within reach of people living in poverty, ethic and cultural minorities, rural residents, stigmatized populations; men and women

TABLE 1-1 ◆ ESSENTIALS OF PRIMARY HEALTH CARE WITH AN APPLICATION TO COMMUNITY PRACTICE

Essentials of Primary Health Care	Services Offered to Homeless People
Education about the prevailing health problems and their prevention and control	Education and counselling for alcohol and drug addictions; needle exchanges and safe havens for injecting drug users; safer sex education; violence prevention
Safe food supply and adequate nutrition	Meals; food bank; collective kitchen
Adequate supply of safe water and basic sanitation	Clothing; laundry and shower facilities and supplies (e.g., soap, shampoo, feminine hygiene products)
Maternal and child care, including family planning	Free male and female condoms; bad date reports for sex trade workers; prenatal care; parenting classes; preschool; respite care for parents (e.g., Calgary Children's Cottage)
Immunization against basic infectious diseases	Hepatitis B vaccination; childhood vaccines; influenza and pneumococcal vaccine
Prevention and control of locally endemic diseases	Directly observed tuberculosis medications; methadone clinics
Appropriate treatment of common diseases and injuries	Wound and foot care; dental care; mental illness treatment; infections; frostbite; fractures; and general health conditions
Essential drugs	HIV medications; prenatal vitamins; lice treatments; antibiotics for communicable diseases

across the life span
◆ Facilitating public participation and empowerment through citizen involvement in service planning, provision, and evaluation
◆ Creating conditions that support intersectoral and interdisciplinary collaborations and private–public–charity partnerships
◆ Adapting technology to the community and population's social, economic, and cultural needs and to its high-risk groups in ways that are sustainable in the long term
◆ Focusing on health promotion and disease and injury prevention within the context of the lives of the people served

Primary health care is more than the first point of contact with the health system. It implies the application of the primary health care philosophy that ensures public participation at all levels of the system, social justice and equity, and a system that balances prevention and promotion with the demands for care, cure, and rehabilitation. Primary health care also extends beyond the health system to the other societal systems that create conditions where health, not disease and injury, can flourish. It can exist not only in community practice but also in other aspects of human services when applied as a pervasive philosophy rather than just as a set of activities. We can see primary health care in action in participatory research, in emancipatory political action, in empowerment education in schools, and in other social movements where social justice, equity and participation are valued.

A Framework for Health Promotion in Canada

In recognition of the social aspects of health promotion and as a signator of the Alma Ata Declaration, the Canadian government in 1986 published the discussion paper *A Framework for Health Promotion* (coined "the Epp Framework" for the Honourable Jake Epp, National Minister of Health and Welfare; Epp, 1986) in preparation for the WHO First International Health Promotion Conference in Ottawa held in that same year (Fig. 1-1).

The times during which the Epp Framework was developed were characterized by rapid and irreversible social change due to shifting family structures, an aging population, and wider participation in the work force by women. These conditions exacerbate certain health problems, create pressure for new kinds of social support, and force community workers to seek new approaches to deal effectively with the impact of these social forces on the future health of Canadians.

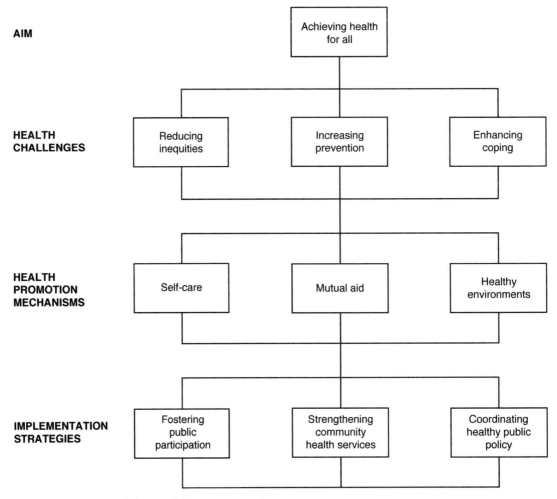

AIM

HEALTH CHALLENGES

HEALTH PROMOTION MECHANISMS

IMPLEMENTATION STRATEGIES

Figure 1-1 ◆ A Framework for Health Promotion in Canada.

The framework defines health as a part of everyday living, an essential dimension of the quality of our lives. In this context, quality of life "implies the opportunities to make choices and gain satisfaction from living." Health is a state that individuals and communities alike strive to achieve, maintain, or regain and is influenced by circumstances, beliefs, culture, and socioeconomic and physical environments. This document reaffirmed the WHO definition of health promotion as "the process of enabling people to increase control over, and to improve, their health."

The **aim** of health promotion is the achievement of health for all. Although the prospects for health of Canadians have improved over recent decades, three major issues remain that are not being adequately addressed by current health policies and practices:

◆ Disadvantaged groups have significantly lower life expectancy, poorer health, and a higher prevalence of disability than the average Canadian.
◆ Various forms of preventable diseases and injuries continue to undermine the health and quality of life of many Canadians.
◆ Many thousands of Canadians suffer from chronic disease, disability, or various forms of emotional stress and lack adequate community support to help them cope and live meaningful, productive, and dignified lives (p. 1).

To achieve the goal of "health for all" ways must be found to overcome three *challenges*: reduce inequities in health status between Canadians with low and high incomes; increase the prevention effort and find new and more effective means to prevent injuries, illness, chronic conditions, and disabilities; and find ways to enhance people's ability to manage and cope with chronic conditions, disabilities, and mental health problems.

In the latter part of the 20th century, chronic conditions and mental health problems replaced communicable diseases as the predominant health problems among Canadians in all age groups. People with disabilities and mental health problems need skills and community support to lead stable and quality lives. Family members, especially women, care for others on a regular basis and also need support. Home support services, home nursing, and respite care services can enhance the coping capacity of both those with disabilities and their care providers.

Three *mechanisms* intrinsic to health promotion are self-care, or the decisions and actions individuals take in the interest of their own health; mutual aid, or the actions people take to help each other; and healthy environments, or the creations of conditions and surroundings conducive to health.

Self-care refers to the decisions made and the behaviours practised by an individual specifically for the preservation of health; encouraging self-care means encouraging healthy choices. An older person using a walking stick when sidewalks are icy, a teenager choosing a fruit for a snack, people engaging in physical activity, choosing not to smoke—these are all examples of self-care. Beliefs, access to appropriate information, and being in surroundings that are supportive are factors that play important roles in making healthy choices.

Mutual aid refers to people's efforts to work together to deal with concerns; it implies people helping each other, supporting each other emotionally, and sharing ideas, information, and experiences. Frequently referred to as social support, mutual aid may arise in the context of the family, the community, a voluntary organization, a self-help group, informal networks, or a special interest association.

Strong evidence indicates that people who have social support are healthier than those who do not; social support enables people to live interdependently within a *healthy environment* while still retaining their independence. A parent with a special-needs child, an older person recovering from a stroke, an adolescent using drugs—these are people who not only need professional services, but also the understanding and the sense of belonging that comes with being in a socially, physically, and economically supportive environment built in a manner that supports interaction and community integration to preserve and enhance health where we live, worship, work, play, and learn. From this perspective, the environment is all encompassing; it includes the buildings in our community, the air we breathe, and the jobs we do. It is also the education, transportation, justice, social services, political, and health systems.

The three leading *strategies* by which we can act in response to the challenges are fostering public participation, strengthening community services, and coordinating healthy public policy. These strategies, in addition to the mechanisms, are mutually reinforcing; one strategy or mechanism on its own will not create significant outcomes.

Public participation is essential to the achievement of health for all Canadians. Encouraging public participation means helping people take part in decisions that influence or control factors that affect health. People (citizens, residents, schools, workplaces, communities) must be equipped and enabled to act, to channel their energy, skills, and creativity to build community capacity and enhance social capital. (Refer to Chapter 6 for more information.)

Community services play a critical role in preserving health particularly if they are expressly oriented toward promoting health and preventing disease/injury. A health promotion and disease/injury prevention orientation means that community services will need to focus more on dealing with the major health challenges we have identified. Greater emphasis will need to be placed on providing services to groups that are disadvantaged, communities will need to become more involved in planning services, and links between communities and their services and institutions will need to be strengthened. In these ways, community health services will assume a key role in fostering self-care, mutual aid, and the creation of healthy environments.

Public policy has considerable potential to influence people's everyday lives; it has the power to provide people with opportunities for health or to deny them such opportunities. All policies, and hence all sectors, have a bearing on health. What we seek is *healthy public policy*. All policies that have direct or indirect bearing on the health of Canadians need to be coordinated. The list is long and includes the broad determinants of health (discussed in greater detail later in this chapter), such as income security, employment, education, housing, economy, agriculture, transportation, justice, and technology. It is not an easy undertaking to coordinate policies among various sectors, all of which obviously have their own priorities, because health is not necessarily a priority for other sectors. Conflicting interests may exist between and among sectors. Take, for example, tobacco. Health promoters are proponents of a smoke-free environment, but some Canadian farmers cultivate this product for their livelihood. Therefore, changes in tobacco policy have broad implications for the economy as well as health. For public policies to be healthy, they must respond to the health needs of people and their communities; this is so whether they are developed in government offices, legislatures, board rooms, church halls, union meetings, schools, workplaces, or seniors' recreation centres.

Global Conferences on Health Promotion

In 1986, the WHO convened the First International Conference on Health Promotion, which resulted in the publication of the *Ottawa Charter for Health Promotion*, jointly with the Canadian Public Health Association and Health and Welfare Canada (WHO, 1986). The Ottawa Charter explicitly identified the *prerequisites for health* as peace, shelter, education, food, income, a stable ecosystem, sustainable resources, and social justice and equity. The health promotion *processes* of enabling, advocating, and mediating were identified. *Advocacy* aims to create the socioenvironmental conditions necessary for health. *Enabling* aims to ensure equal opportunities for achieving health and reducing inequities in health status. *Mediation* between different interests is required to ensure the collaboration needed among disciplines, agencies, and sectors to coordinate action and policy efforts. In the Charter, five *strategies* for health promotion were identified: building healthy public policy, creating supportive environments, strengthening community action, developing personal skills, and reorienting health services (Fig. 1-2). This landmark document built on the Declaration of Alma Ata and Canadian leadership and is considered to be the formal beginning of what is termed "the new public health movement." It was hailed as a signal for change in direction and policy for the reorientation of the health system.

Four International Health Promotion Conferences have followed since 1986: in Adelaide, Australia; Sundsvall, Sweden; Jakarta, Indonesia; and Mexico City, Mexico. At each conference, participants reaffirmed commitment to the Ottawa Charter and extended the discourse by focusing research and discussion on a single Ottawa Charter strategy and making recommendations for action.

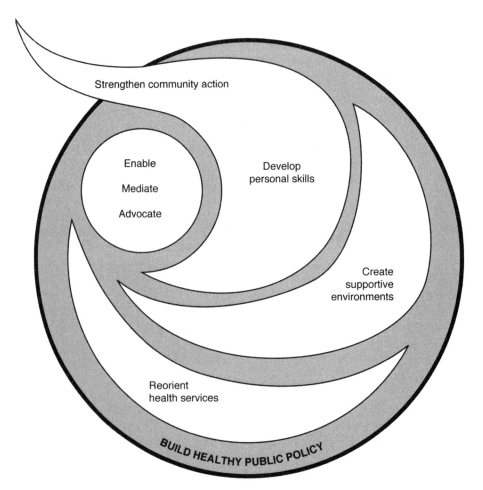

Figure 1-2 ◆ Ottowa Charter for Health Promotion.

In Adelaide, Australia (WHO, 1988) participants called on those who make public policy to examine and be responsive to the health impacts of their policies. Pleas were made for industrialized nations to provide assistance to underdeveloped nations to reduce health disparities. Four priority areas for action were identified: support for the health of women; elimination of hunger and malnutrition; reduction of tobacco growing and alcohol production; and the creation of more supportive environments by aligning with the peace, environmental, and health movements.

The Third International Conference was held in Sundsvall, Sweden in 1991 (WHO, 1991). Here the theme was on supportive environments for health, and the Conference highlighted four aspects of supportive environments: (1) the social dimension, which includes the ways in which norms, customs, and social processes affect health; (2) the political dimension, which requires governments to guarantee democratic participation in decision-making and the decentralization of responsibilities and resources; (3) the economic dimension, which requires a rechannelling of resources for the achievement of "Health for All" and sustainable development, including safe and reliable technology; and (4) the need to recognize and use women's skills and knowledge in all sectors to develop a more positive infrastructure for supportive environments. Conference recommendations for action were to strengthen advocacy through community action, particularly through groups organized by women; enable communities and individuals to take control of their health and environment through education and empowerment; build alliances to strengthen cooperation between health and environment campaigns; and mediate between conflicting interests in society to ensure equitable access to a supportive environment for health.

Six years later, at the Fourth International Conference (and the first to be held in a developing country), the *Jakarta Declaration on Leading Health Promotion into the 21st Century* (WHO, 1997) expanded the conditions (prerequisites) for health to include also social security, social relations, empowerment of women, sustainable resource use, and respect for human rights. "Above all, poverty is the greatest threat to health." The statement noted the need for comprehensive approaches that work on several levels, within various settings, and effective partnerships among all levels of government, nongovernmental organizations (NGOs), and private and public sectors. Five priorities were set: (1) promote social responsibility for health, (2) increase investments for health development, (3) consolidate and expand partnerships for health, (4) increase community capacity and empower the individual, and (5) secure an infrastructure for health promotion.

In 1999, the Fifth Global Health Promotion Conference was held in Mexico City (WHO, 1999); the theme was on bridging the equity gap and recommended strengthening the "art and science" (evidence base) of health promotion and strengthening political skills and actions for health promotion to ensure healthy public policy. Processes suggested to achieve the recommendations were solidarity among practitioners and activists through networks, alliances, and partnerships; mobilization of resources; development of community capacity; development of human resources; and the creation of networks and associations of practitioners for mutual support and personal development.

Population Health

Canadian influence on global health promotion is strong on the international scene; Canadian researchers, policymakers, educators, and practitioners have contributed significantly to each of the WHO conferences. For instance, the Healthy Cities movement began in Canada and has become a dominant force in European countries. Health promotion research, supported by Health Canada through the formation of five funded Canadian Centres for Health Promotion in 1995, has had international impact. Much of the work of these centres has been presented at WHO global conferences. However, on the home front leadership in health promotion has been challenged by traditional biomedical and economic rationalist approaches to policy, care, and research that pervade the Canadian health context. The influence of biostatisticians, epidemiologists, and social demographers is evident by the attraction of policymakers to the population health perspective. Leadership for health promotion at Health Canada has been dispersed, a quarterly journal on the field has been cancelled, funding for the five centres has not been sustained, and none of the 13 Canadian Institutes for Health Research (CIHR) has been dedicated to health promotion research. Instead, the term "population health" has become preeminent. (See Box 1-2.)

CIHR's 13 institutes are Aboriginal Peoples' Health; Aging; Cancer Research; Circulatory and Respiratory Health; Gender and Health; Genetics; Health Services and Policy Research; Human Development, Child and Youth Health; Infection and Immunity; Musculoskeletal Health and Arthritis; Neurosciences, Mental Health and Addiction; Nutrition, Metabolism and Diabetes; and Population and Public Health.

Population health is the term used to describe an approach that is founded on epidemiologic principles, statistical measures, and economic conservatism. Population health provides the data that underscore the importance of factors other than the health care system in determining or influencing the health of large groups (populations). Population health, like health promotion, focuses on the larger scope than the individual. Unlike health promotion, however, it is not rooted in empowerment, community development, qualitative research, social justice, or political advocacy. It purports to be more objective in its stance, citing facts and suggesting causal pathways, without necessarily recommending action. Once the four health fields were articulated in the Lalonde Report (1974), population health scientists stepped up study on the impacts of lifestyle and the environment on health status. This activity led to the identification of a broader range of health determinants, the specification of targets for health promotion, and the description of settings where health promotion can occur.

Although a certain tension exists because of some philosophical differences (Coburn & Poland, 1995), the two perspectives are complementary. Health promoters appreciate the legitimacy population health scientists have given to their longstanding concern about the impact of social forces on health (Labonte, 1995). Population health scientists are now accepting findings from qualitative research and experiential/traditional knowledge as legitimate evidence.

BOX 1-2. DEFINITION OF TERMS

Primary health care: first described in the Declaration of Alma Ata (1978), primary health care refers to the five **principles** on which action on "health for all" must be based: equitable access to health and health services, public participation, appropriate technology, intersectoral collaboration, and reorientation of the health system to promotion of health and prevention of disease and injury. The Declaration further details eight **essentials**—services nations must have in place to create positive conditions for health.

Critical social action theory: attempts to describe and explain oppressive social conditions that limit people from reaching their full potential. In relation to health, its ultimate goal is to liberate (emancipate) people from health-damaging environmental conditions (Stevens & Hall, 1992).This approach involves exposing inequities, empowering citizen engagement, improving health literacy, and creating change.

Health promotion: the process of enabling people to exercise control over those factors and conditions that influence their health. Health promotion is viewed as a collective, rather than individual, activity, and has five key strategies: develop personal skills, create supportive environments, strengthen community action, build healthy public policy, and reorient health services.

Population health: the health of a population as measured by health status indicators and as influenced by social, economic, and physical environments, personal health practices, individual capacity and coping skills, human biology, early childhood development, and health services.

Population health promotion: integration of population health concepts with the principles that guide action on health promotion in efforts to maximize the likelihood of reinforcing and maintaining synergistic effects in health programming.

Population health approach: a strategic administrative focus on the complex interrelated conditions and factors that influence population health, which uses information regarding patterns and trends in health status indicators to create healthy public policy and respond to the needs of Canadians through targeted intervention programs.

Determinants of Health

Central to population health science was the question: "Why are some people healthy and others are not?" (Evans, Barer, & Marmor, 1994). Because health and social services are provincial matters, several provinces commissioned studies to address this concern, leading to the publication of reports that suggested that the impacts of health care services on the health of citizens was far less than expected, and that lifestyles and the social, economic, and physical environments had a potentially larger impact on health status. As technologies improved and extensive databases were created and used to correlate various factors, national population health surveys were carried out, and the scientific community began to create models that suggested causal pathways for health. Canadian Institute for Advanced Research (CIAR) scientists Evans and Stoddard (1990) chronicled the evolution of a model that illustrates feedback loops for human well-being and economic costs (Fig. 1-3).

This model uses the absence of disease as the definition of health because it is more easily operationalized than definitions proposed by health promotion proponents. As well, deaths (and to some extent illness and injury) can be counted, so "absence or presence of disease" became an index to measure health status. In its initial conceptualization, the authors described people getting sick or injured from unspecified reasons and presenting themselves to the health care system, where the diseases or injuries are diagnosed, treatment needs are defined, and the system responds. The level of response is determined by the access to care and technology, and its provision in turn reduces the level of disease/injury and the person returns to health. However, as technology advanced and health care costs rose in response to demands, evidence was growing that interventions and structural changes outside the health sys-

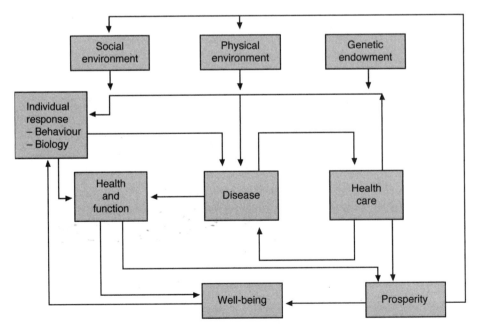

Figure 1-3 ◆ Feedback loop for human well-being and economic costs.

tem were needed to effect further improvements in the health status of the population.

The four-field framework described by Lalonde was incorporated into the CIAR model, so instead of the "unspecified factors" that contributed to illness and injury, human biology, lifestyle, and environment were added to the mix. However, in the years subsequent to the publication of the Lalonde Report, lifestyle choices were increasingly seen to be influenced by social and physical environmental factors, and it was found that underlying conditions influence susceptibility to a whole range of diseases as well as personal sense of well-being and productivity. This complex interaction of factors has provided the foundation for a vast array of research on human behaviour, biologic responses to social and physical environments, and the effects of economic tradeoffs on health and well-being. Research has shown that living and working conditions, such as housing, income, social support, work stress, and education, make a difference in the number and quality of years lived (Frank, 1995).

To further describe the evidence being generated by population health scientists, the Federal/Provincial/Territorial Advisory Committee on Population Health (ACPH) published in 1994 its discussion document *Strategies for Population Health: Investing in the Health of Canadians*. The Canadian Health Network and others have extended the list of health determinants, which now comprises 12 determinants, and researchers are continuing to refine our understanding and will perhaps expand the list further in years to come. The current accepted list of determinants, along with their descriptions, are found in Table 1-2.

Target Populations

By incorporating the determinants, health services and health promotion activities have become targeted to specific groups within the population that had "needs" or deficits that could be addressed to improve health status. This approach rested on the foundation of risk factor assessment; that is, if people will reduce or eliminate risk-taking behaviours, and if risky environments could be fixed, then population health would improve. Therefore, individuals, groups, or aggregates of individuals, families, communities, and society itself became targets for action and intervention.

Many programs were directed toward individuals and aggregates—developing personal skills for healthy behaviours through health education and social marketing. Because, for instance, adolescent pregnancy is viewed as detrimental to health of women and their infants, campaigns to strengthen families, enhance the availability of birth control, delay the onset of sexual activity,

TABLE 1-2 ◆ DETERMINANTS OF HEALTH	
Income and social status	Research shows that poor people in general are less healthy than rich people. Income distribution in a society is also a key element. The greater the gap between the richest and poorest people, the greater the differences in health.
Social support networks	Support from families, friends and communities is linked to better health. This kind of support helps people handle difficult situations.
Employment and working conditions	Unemployment is linked with poor health. Further, those who are employed are healthier when they have more control over their working conditions.
Education	A great deal of research shows that low literacy skills are linked with poor health. Moreover, people with low literacy skills can suffer from stress and reduced self-confidence. This often makes it hard for them to seek employment or social support. So the more education we have, the more likely we are to be healthy.
Physical environments	Clean air and water, healthy workplaces, and safe houses, communities, and roads all contribute to good health.
Social environments	Strength of social networks, social stability, recognition of diversity, safety, good working relationships within a community, region, province or country provide a supportive society that reduces or avoids potential risks to good health.
Biology and genetic endowment	Physical characteristics we inherit play a part in deciding how long we live, how healthy we will be, and how likely we are to get certain illnesses.
Personal health practices and coping skills	Personal practices include whether a person eats well and is physically active, and whether he smokes or drinks. Coping skills refer to the way we relate to the people around us and handle life's stresses and challenges.
Healthy child development	Good evidence indicates that things that happen to us when we are children affect our health and well-being. These experiences affect us not only during childhood, but also through the rest of the life cycle.
Health services	It benefits people's health when they have access to services that prevent disease, as well as maintain and promote health.
Gender	Men and women get different kinds of diseases and conditions at different ages. They also tend to have different income levels and to work at different kinds of jobs. Many of these realities result from the differences in the way society treats men and women.
Culture	People's customs and traditions and the beliefs of their family and community all affect their health. This is because these factors will influence what they think, feel, do and believe to be important.

From: www.canadian-health-network.ca & www.hc-sc.gc.ca/hppb/phdd/approach/e_approach.html

and promote abstinence were mounted across the nation. Motor vehicle mortality was addressed through programs aimed primarily at young men who drive while under the influence of alcohol and programs that exhorted people to use seatbelts in vehicles. The "BreakFree" campaign for youth tobacco reduction is an example of how program planners further categorized the target population through demographics. Youth were surveyed and then described in terms of subpopulations of youth, and messages were targeted accordingly, on the assumption that rural and urban youth, athletes, and honours students would respond to different marketing strategies to reduce tobacco use.

Other programs were directed to creating more supportive family environments for health; for instance, children of families living in poverty were provided educational opportunities in such programs as Head Start that prepared them for school entry, Nobody's Perfect that enhanced parenting skills, and Brighter Futures that supported early childhood development through family nutrition and prenatal support.

At the same time as Canadians' attitudes toward health and wellness were changing, social conventions were being altered, so that behaviours such as tobacco use, substance use, domestic violence, and drinking and driving have become increasingly socially unacceptable. In addition, the move toward self-determination through public participation in policy decision-making has become an imperative rather than a luxury. Canadians now expect to be consulted on matters that relate to health, and health is defined more broadly than the absence of disease.

Settings

Not only have the targets for health interventions expanded from the individual level, but also settings for health service provision and health promotion expanded from health settings (e.g., hospitals, clinics, etc.) to where people live, work, worship, play, and go to school. The WHO Healthy Cities, Comprehensive School Health, and Healthy Workplace movements were attempts to develop strong communities and build social capacity and human capital that would enhance and strengthen the ability of communities, schools, and workplaces to influence the health and well-being of their residents, students and teachers, and employees.

The environment or context provided by various settings also contributes to health. As settings began to change and adapt in response to the needs and preferences of society so, too, did environmental change affect people. That people behave or respond differently in different situations, contexts, and settings has led program planners to view the environment as a predisposing, enabling, and reinforcing factor for individual and collective behaviour (Green, Poland, & Rootman, 2000). Green and Kreuter (1991) state that the effectiveness of a health strategy depends on its fit with the target population, the health issue involved, and the environment in which it is applied. Using the setting as a focus fosters outcomes that are adaptable and sensitive to particular traditions, cultures, and circumstances. A multilevel, multicultural, multisectoral intervention runs the risk of being expensive and perhaps essentially meaningless, as well as not evaluable, because of the breadth of its target, lack of focus, and inability to specify indicators for assessing effectiveness. Hence, we are seeing the implementation of healthy workplace projects, comprehensive school health programs, and parish health initiatives as means of influencing the health of Canadians.

Population Health Promotion

In response to the growing debate and tension among health promotion practitioners and population health scientists, Hamilton and Bhatti (1996), instead of entering the debate, offered for discussion a model they termed *Population Health Promotion* (Fig. 1-4).

In this model the central concepts of the Ottawa Charter for Health Promotion, determinants of health, targets, and settings are integrated with evidence-based decision-making to ensure that policies and programs focus on the right issues, take effective action, and produce sound results. Evidence is derived from three principal sources: research, experience, and evaluation studies. The model is based on the following underlying assumptions and values:

◆ Policy and program decision makers agree that comprehensive action needs to be taken on all the determinants of health using the knowledge gained from research and practice.
◆ It is the role of health organizations to analyze the full range of possibilities for action, to act on those determinants that are within their jurisdiction, and to influence other sectors to ensure their policies and programs have a positive impact on health. This can best be achieved by facilitating collaboration among stakeholders regarding the most appropriate activities to be undertaken by each.
◆ Multiple points of entry to planning and implementation are essential as demonstrated by the examples in the following section. However, there is a need for overall coordination of activity.
◆ Health problems may affect certain groups more than others. However, the solution to these problems involves changing social values and structures. It is the responsibility of the society as a whole to take care of all its members.
◆ The health of individuals and groups is a combined result of their own health practices and the impact of the physical and social environments in which they live, learn, work, pray, and play. There is an interaction among people and their surroundings. Settings, consisting of places and things, have a physical and psychological impact on people's health.

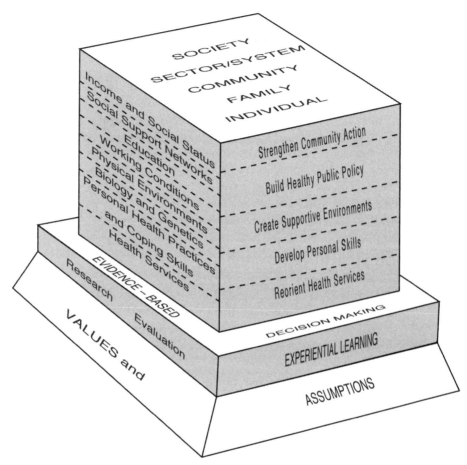

Figure 1-4 ◆ Population health promotion model. (Redrawn from Hamilton, N. & Bhatti, T. [1996]. *Population health promotion: An integrated model of population health and health promotion.* Ottawa: Health Canada.)

◆ To enjoy optimal health, people need opportunities to meet their physical, mental, social and spiritual needs. This is possible in an environment that is based on the principles of social justice and equity and where relationships are built on mutual respect and caring, rather than power and status.

◆ Health care, health protection, and disease prevention initiatives complement health promotion. Comprehensive approaches will include a strategic mix of the different possibilities for action. Meaningful participation of people in the development and operationalization of policies and programs is essential for them to influence the decisions that affect their health. (Hamilton & Bhatti, 1996, p. 3)

Hamilton and Bhatti (1996) make the distinction between risk factors and risk conditions. *Risk factors* are elements, often behaviour patterns, which tend to dispose people to poorer health and are modifiable through strategies that create individual behaviour change. *Risk conditions,* on the other hand, are general circumstances over which people have little or no control that are known to affect health status. Risk conditions are usually a result of public policy and are modified through collective action and social reform.

The population health promotion model allows for the integration of new knowledge from research, experience, and evaluation. It offers an analytic tool to assess situations that put people at risk, to assess populations at risk, and to move away from a victim-blaming approach to a more comprehensive determination of factors that contribute to ill health and injury.

Population Health Approach

Health Canada has adopted the *population health approach* by which it focuses its action toward improved health outcomes, a sustainable and integrated health system, increased national growth and productivity, and strengthened social cohesion. The key elements of this approach are:

◆ Address the determinants of health, recognizing they are complex and interrelated.
◆ Focus on the health of populations.
◆ Invest upstream.
◆ Base decisions on evidence.
◆ Apply multiple strategies to act on the determinants of health.
◆ Collaborate across levels and sectors.
◆ Use mechanisms to engage citizens.
◆ Increase accountability for health outcomes.

More detail on this approach is available from the Health Canada website (http://www.hc-sc.gc.ca/hppb/phdd/approach/). In this chapter the current understanding of the *determinants of health* has been presented; our knowledge will continue to further develop, evolve, and be refined as interventions are implemented and success chronicled. *Investing upstream* means directing attention at the root causes of illness and injury, rather than at the symptoms that are evident. In this way, interventions can be placed earlier in the causal stream and provide greater gains in population health. Traditional and new sources of qualitative and quantitative research and evaluation *evidence* are used to set priorities and identify best practices for influencing health; this is called evidence-based decision-making. A *variety of strategies* applied in a variety of settings are required to create joint action among health and other sectors to effectively influence the factors and improve the health of Canadians. *Collaboration* and horizontal management strategies will require agreement on common goals, coordinated planning, development of related policies, and implementation of integrated programs and services. To do this means that citizens need to be engaged in all aspects of health and social service priority setting, the determination of appropriate interventions, and the review of outcomes. (Chap. 6 discusses *public participation* in detail.) Accountability requires that process, impact, and outcome evaluations be undertaken to assess changes in health status and that the results of evaluations be reported widely not only to the scientific community but also to the public.

In summary, this approach has been articulated by Health Canada as a unifying force for the entire spectrum of health system interventions—from prevention, promotion, and protection to diagnosis, treatment, care, and rehabilitation—that integrates and balances actions among them. As an approach, population health targets factors that influence the health of Canadians across the life span, identifies variations in patterns of health, and uses the resulting knowledge to plan and implement interventions and policies to improve the nation's health status. Even though health and social services are funded by the provinces and territories, Health Canada exercises a strong leadership role in setting direction and standards in its efforts to improve Canadians' health.

Implications of Population Health Promotion for "Community as Partner"

In 1986, the WHO took the lead in providing the scope, definition, and a framework for action to create "Health for All by Year 2000" as mandated by the Declaration of Alma Ata (WHO, 1978). The Ottawa Charter serves to this day as the foundation of health promotion, and as action has taken place, the evidence generated by evaluation and research has expanded. Health Canada has sponsored several population health surveys, created the Canadian Institutes for Health Research (CIHR) and the Canadian Institute of Health Information (CIHI) to gather and report evidence, and has realigned the organization to support and promote a population health approach. Health promotion is a key means of taking action on population health. Consequently, this book is written to be consistent both with the population health approach and the fundamental principles of health promotion. In Chapter 2 the basics of epidemiology are presented as the foundation of understanding patterns of health in populations. Chapter 3 illustrates the Canadian context, patterns of health, and discusses the health system in Canada. Chapter 4 deals with health and the environment and Chapter 5 with ethics and advocacy of population health promotion practice. In Chapter 6, public participation and community development are presented, followed by a discussion of cultural considerations in community practice. In Part Two, the process of working with community is detailed and in Part Three, case studies are presented that offer examples of successful population health promotion interventions in a variety of settings with a range of target groups in Canada.

Summary

In this chapter the history and development of the modern approach to health is chronicled. The Lalonde Report (1974) signalled a paradigm shift in how health was viewed, and the Declaration of Alma Ata (1978) provided the foundational philosophy by which to attain the goal of health for all. Five subsequent International Health Promotion Conferences extended the understanding of the processes (advocacy, enabling, and mediating) and five action strategies for practice. The Canadian Institute of Advanced Research in population health furthered the understanding of the determinants of health, creating conditions for the formation of a population health promotion model (Hamilton & Bhatti, 1996). The policy stance now taken by Health Canada is based on its population health approach to policy and programming. Thus, the stage is set for readers to further investigate key concepts and develop a process for partnering with communities to enhance health and well-being.

References

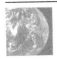Coburn, D., & Poland, B. (1995). The CIAR vision of the determinants of health: A crtitique. *Canadian Journal of Public Health, 87*(5), 308–310.

Denoncourt, H., Desilets, M., Plane, M.-C., et al. (2000). The outreach practice with homeless people sufering from severe and chronic mental illness: Observations, reality and obstacles. *Santé Mentale au Québec, 25*(2), 179–194.

Epp, J. (1986). *Achieving health for all: A framework for health promotion.* Ottawa: National Health and Welfare.

Evans, R., Barer, M., & Marmor, T. (Eds.). (1994). *Why are some people healthy and others not?* New York: Aldine.

Evans, R., & Stoddard, G. (1990). Producing health, consuming health care. *Social Science and Medicine, 31*(12), 1347–1363.

Federal/Provincial/Territorial Advisory Committee on Population Health (1994). *Strategies for population health: Investing in the health of Canadians.* Ottawa: Health Canada.

Frank, J. (1995). Why "population health"? *Canadian Journal of Public Health, 86*(3), 162–164.

Freire, P. (1970). *Pedagogy of the oppressed.* New York: Continuum.

Green, L. W., & Kreuter, M. W. (1991). *Health promotion planning: An educational and envi-ronmental approach*. Mountain View, CA: Mayfield.

Green, L. W., Poland, B., & Rootman, I. (2000). The settings approach to health promo-tion. In B. Poland, L. W. Green, & I. Rootman (Eds.), *Settings for health promotion*. Thousand Oaks, CA: Sage.

Hamilton, N., & Bhatti, T. (1996). *Population health promotion: An integrated model of popu-lation health and health promotion*. Ottawa: Health Canada.

Labonte, R. (1995). Population health and health promotion: What do they have to say to each other? *Canadian Journal of Public Health, 86*(3), 165–168.

Lalonde, M. (1974) *New perspectives on the health of Canadians*. Ottawa: National Health and Welfare.

Poirier, H., Bonin, J.-P., Lesage, A., & Reinhartz, D. (2000). Assessment of quality of life and needs of homeless mentally ill people: Perceptions of an outreach team. *Santé Mentale au Québec 25*(2), 195–215.

Stevens, P. E., & Hall, J. M. (1992). Applying critical theories to nursing in communities. *Public Health Nursing, 9*(1), 2–9.

Thibaudeau, M.-F., & Denoncourt, H. (2000). Nursing practice in outreach clinics for the homeless in Montreal, In M. J. Stewart (Ed.), *Community nursing: Promoting Canadians' health* (2nd ed., pp. 443–460). Toronto: W.B. Saunders.

Thibaudeau, M.-F., & Fortier, J. (2000). Clinical case management of severely mentally ill homeless people. *Santé Mentale au Québec, 25*(2), 155–178.

World Health Organization. (1978). *Alma Ata declaration on primary health care*. Geneva, Switzerland: Author.

World Health Organization. (1986). *Ottawa charter for health promotion*. Geneva, Switzerland: Author.

World Health Organization. (1988). *Adelaide recommendations*. Geneva, Switzerland: Author.

World Health Organization. (1991). *Sundsvall statement on supportive environments for health*. Geneva, Switzerland: Author.

World Health Organization. (1997). *Jakarta declaration on leading health promotion into the 21st century*. Geneva, Switzerland: Author.

World Health Organization. (1999). *Health promotion: Bridging the equity gap*. Geneva, Switzerland: Author.

Internet Resources

Adelaide Recommendations: **www.who.int/hpr/archive/docs/adelaide.html**
Canadian Health Network: **www.canadian-health-network.ca**
Declaration of Alma Ata: **www.who.int/hpr/archive/docs/almaata.html**
Jakarta Declaration: **http://www.who.int/hpr/archive/docs/jakarta/english.html**
Mexico conference report: **http://www.who.int/hpr/conference/index.html**
Ottawa Charter: **www.who.int/hpr/archive/docs/ottawa.html**
Population Health Approach: **http://www.hc-sc.gc.ca/hppb/phdd/approach/e_approach.html**
Sundsvall Statement: **www.who.int/hpr/backgroundhp/sundsvall.htm**

2

Epidemiology, Demography, and Community Health

REVISED FROM THE ORIGINAL CHAPTER
BY MAIJA SELBY-HARRINGTON AND ANITA S. TESH

CHAPTER OUTLINE

Introduction
Demography
Contemporary Community
  Health Practice
Levels of Prevention in
  Community Practice
Descriptive Measures of Health

Analytic Measures of Health
Sources of Community Health Data
Screening for Health Conditions
Epidemiologic Approaches to
   Community Health Research
Summary

OBJECTIVES

To assess community health needs and to plan, implement, and evaluate programs to meet those needs, the community health professional must understand basic concepts in epidemiology and demography.

After studying this chapter, you should be able to:

◆ Interpret and use basic epidemiologic, demographic, and statistical measures of community health

◆ Apply principles of epidemiology and demography to your community practice

Introduction

Epidemiology and demography are sciences for studying population health. To restore, maintain, and promote the health of populations, the community health professional integrates and applies concepts from these fields. In this chapter, we explore the meaning and usefulness of these concepts.

When program planners partner with communities, they bring to the table their expertise supported by the relevant science; in other words, they come armed with the statistics and models that explain patterns in community health. This information might include the current health status of the population according to a number of accepted indicators, allowing local data to be compared with data from other jurisdictions regionally, nationally, and internationally. By being able to see trends and patterns, strengths and risk factors can be identified and, working together, residents and community workers can develop plans and set priorities to address concerns and build on community assets. Epidemiologic and sociodemographic data have traditionally formed the scientific foundation of population health practice, so that comparative and comprehensive evidence is available to inform decision-making. Regardless of what epidemiologic and demographic information reveals, *how* decisions are made at the community level are important to population health practice. That is, the principles of primary health care (public participation, appropriate technology, intersectoral collaboration, accessibility, and a focus on promotion and prevention) must be honoured if efforts to improve the health of Canadians are to be affordable and sustainable in the long term. Hence, the importance of being able to communicate effectively with standard measures of health and wellness is critical to the community health worker.

Demography

Demography (literally, "writing about the people," from the Greek *demos* [people] and *graphos* [writing]) is the science of human populations and is concerned with population size, characteristics, and change. Examples of demographic studies (i.e., demographic research) are descriptions and comparisons of populations according to such characteristics as age, race, sex, socioeconomic status, geographic distribution, and patterns of birth, death, marriage, and divorce. Demographic studies often have health implications that may or may not be addressed by the investigators. The census of the Canadian population is an example of a comprehensive descriptive demographic study that is conducted every 5 years.

Epidemiology ("the study of what is upon the people," from the Greek *logos* [study], *demos* [people], and *epi* [upon]) is the science of population health. Epidemiology investigates the characteristics, distribution, and determinants of health conditions. Epidemiology overlaps with demography. Epidemiologic studies sometimes take on the intrigue of detective stories as the investigators track the factors associated with illness and death. In fact, a number of works concerning epidemiologic studies have become popular classics (e.g., *The Andromeda Strain* [Crichton, 1969]; *The Hot Zone* [Preston, 1994], *Outbreak* [Peterson, 1995]; and *Miss Evers' Boys* [Feldshuh, 1997]).

Early epidemiologic studies were concerned chiefly with the control of epidemics. (An epidemic is an outbreak of an illness beyond the levels expected in a population.) John Snow's study of a cholera epidemic in London in 1853 is a classic in epidemiologic history. At that time, the mode of transmission of cholera was unknown. Snow suspected it was spread by contaminated water. Applying epidemiologic principles, Snow determined that death rates from cholera were highest in areas served by two specific water pumps. He learned that the water from these pumps came from portions of the Thames River into which London sewage was discharged. Thus, this early epidemiologist was able to identify a waterborne mode of transmission of cholera and determine measures to control its spread (Snow, 1936). The handles of the two pumps were removed so people could not draw water from them, and thus that particular cholera outbreak was brought to a halt.

Contemporary Community Health Practice

Today, advanced epidemiologic and demographic measures and research methods are used not only to study disorders such as food poisoning and AIDS but also to investigate environmental conditions, lifestyles, health promotion strategies, and other factors that influence health. This chapter provides an introduction to epidemiologic and demographic concepts that are useful for community practice. If you need more in-depth study, numerous textbooks are available (e.g., Lilienfeld & Stolley, 1994; Mausner & Kramer, 1985).

Levels of Prevention in Community Practice

The concept of prevention is a key component of modern community health. In popular terminology, prevention means warding off an event before it occurs.

In community practice, we consider three levels of prevention: primary, secondary, and tertiary.

Primary prevention involves true avoidance of an illness or adverse health condition through health promotion activities and protective actions. Primary prevention encompasses a vast array of areas, including nutrition, hygiene, sanitation, immunization, environmental protection, and general health education, to name but a few. Research into the causes of health problems provides the basis for primary prevention. For example, just as Snow's 1853 investigation of cholera paved the way for provision of clean water to the residents of London, modern research into motor vehicle injuries has led to the use of seat belts and air bags.

Secondary prevention is the early detection and treatment of adverse conditions. Secondary prevention may result in the cure of illnesses that would be incurable at later stages, the prevention of complications and disability, and confinement of the spread of communicable diseases. An important component of secondary prevention is screening, the examination of asymptomatic people for disorders such as tuberculosis, diabetes, and hypertension. Today, to prevent motor vehicle injuries in populations at the highest risk, some provinces have instituted graduated licences for new drivers.

Tertiary prevention is used after diseases or events have already resulted in damage to individuals. The purpose of tertiary prevention is to limit disability and to rehabilitate or restore the affected people to their maximum possible capacities. Examples of tertiary prevention include provision of "meals on wheels" for the homebound, physical therapy services for stroke victims, and mental health counselling for rape victims. With respect to motor vehicles, the adaptation of vehicles for paraplegic individuals and those with prosthetic lower limbs is an example of tertiary prevention.

To plan appropriate methods of primary, secondary, and tertiary prevention, the community health professional must first assess the health of the community. The following section covers some basic measures used in community health assessment.

Descriptive Measures of Health

Demographic Measures

Certain human characteristics, or demographics, may be associated with wellness or illness. Age, race, sex, ethnicity, income, and educational level are important demographics that may affect health outcomes. For example, men are more likely than women to develop certain heart diseases, aboriginal peoples are more likely to have diabetes than other Canadians, and adolescent women are more likely than adult women to have low-birth-weight infants. To plan interventions for population health, the community health worker must be familiar with the demographic characteristics of the community and with the health problems associated with those characteristics.

Morbidity and Mortality

Although epidemiology encompasses wellness as well as illness, wellness is difficult to measure. Therefore, many measures of "health" are expressed in terms of *morbidity* (illness) and *mortality* (death). An excellent source of U.S. morbidity and mortality data is the Centers for Disease Control and Prevention, *Morbidity and Mortality Weekly Report* (Internet site: http://www.cdc.gov/mmwr). In Canada, Health Canada publications are listed on its website (http://www.hc-sc.gc.ca/pphb-dgspsp/publications_e.html) and include reports on communicable diseases (http://www.hc-sc.gc.ca/pphb-dgspsp/bid-bmi/dsd-dsm/index.html), chronic diseases (http://www.hc-sc.gc.ca/pphb-dgspsp/publicat/cdic-mcc/index.html), as well as other important topics and links to other relevant sites.

Incidence

The *incidence* of a disease or health condition refers to the number of persons in a population who develop the condition during a specified period of time. The calculation of incidence, therefore, generally requires that a population be followed over a period of time in what is called a prospective (forward-looking) study.

Prevalence

The *prevalence* of a disease or condition refers to the total number of persons in the population who have the condition at a particular time. Thus, prevalence may be calculated in a "one-shot" cross-sectional ("slice of time") or retrospective (backward-looking) study.

Interpretation of Incidence and Prevalence

Measures of incidence and prevalence provide different information and have different implications. For example, an increase in the prevalence of cancer means that there are more persons with cancer in the population. This may be because there are more new cases (in other words, increased incidence) or because persons with cancer are living longer. In either case, the community may need to direct resources toward cancer. However, if knowledge of incidence is lacking, it will be difficult to decide whether to target the resources toward primary prevention of cancer or toward secondary prevention (diagnosis and treatment) and tertiary prevention (rehabilitation) services.

Rates

Incidence and prevalence usually are expressed as mathematical measures called rates. Because epidemiology is the study of population health, these measures must relate the occurrence of a health condition to the population base. Rates do exactly this. They express a mathematical relationship in which the numerator is the number of persons experiencing the condition and the denominator is the population at risk, or the total number of persons who have the possibility of experiencing the condition.

Rates must not be confused with other proportions that do not use the population at risk as the denominator. For example, the death rate from cancer is not the same as the proportion of deaths from cancer. In each, the numerator is the number of deaths from cancer. However, the denominators differ. In the death rate, the denominator includes all persons at risk of dying from cancer. Therefore, the cancer death rate is an expression of the risk of dying from cancer. In the proportion of deaths, also called proportionate mortality, the denominator is the total number of deaths from all causes. Therefore, the proportionate cancer mortality simply describes the proportion of deaths attributable to cancer.

CALCULATION OF RATES

Rates are calculated in this general format:

$$\text{Rate} = \frac{\text{number of people experiencing condition}}{\text{population at risk for experiencing condition}} \times K$$

K is a constant (usually 1000, 10,000 or 100,000) that allows the ratio, which may be a very small number, to be expressed in a meaningful way. Let us apply this formula to the calculation of the infant mortality rate, which estimates an infant's risk of dying during the first year of life.

EXAMPLE OF A RATE:
THE INFANT MORTALITY RATE

The infant mortality rate (IMR) usually is calculated on a calendar-year basis: the number of infant deaths (deaths before the age of 1 year) in 1 year is divided by the number of live births (infants born alive) during that year. The numerator represents the number of infants experiencing the "condition" of dying in the first year of life, and the denominator represents the population of infants at risk for dying in the year.

In 1997, there was an average of 5.5 infant deaths for every 1000 live births in Canada. In Alberta in 2000 there were 37,155 live births and 257 infant deaths reported. To compare the infant mortality rate to the Canadian average, we calculate a rate. Applying the formula for a rate, we divide 257 by 37,155 and find that 0.0069 of an infant died during the first year of life. Because it is difficult to relate to 0.0069 of an infant, we multiply by a constant (K), in this case 1000, and find that 6.9 infants per 1000 live births died during the first year of life; that is, the IMR was 6.9 infant deaths per 1000 live births in that year. In comparison to the most recent national data available, we can say that Alberta has a higher IMR than the national average. How does this compare with other provinces and territories? By comparing rates rather than raw numbers, we can then rank parts of the country by infant mortality rate to determine areas of greatest need for intervention. For instance, in 1996 four of the five health regions in the North had IMRs ranging from 10.3 in Burntwood/Churchill health region to 20.9 in Nunavik health region. Within provinces, comparisons can also be made. For example, in 1996 in Saskatchewan, IMRs in the Prince Alberta Service Area had an IMR of 10.6, North Battleford 11.3, Regina 10.1, and Saskatoon 7.8. Each of these areas has very different actual numbers of births, but by comparing rates health program planners are able to determine where need is greatest for programming to improve birth outcomes.

Additionally, trends can become apparent by tracking rates longitudinally over time. In Table 2-1 we can see that the trend in the national IMR over a 5-year period is going down.

For more information on perinatal health (including IMR), see the Health Canada website: http://www.hc-sc.gc.ca/pphb-dgspsp/rhs-ssg/phic-ispc/pdf/indperie.pdf.

INTERPRETATION OF RATES

Rates enable researchers and practitioners to compare different populations in terms of health problems or conditions. To assess whether the population in a

TABLE 2-1 ◆ INFANT MORTALITY (RATE PER 1000 LIVE BIRTHS) IN CANADA, 1993–1997*

Year	IMR
1993	6.3
1994	6.3
1995	6.1
1996	5.6
1997	5.5

*Includes stillbirths of unknown gestational period. Newfoundland, New Brunswick, and Québec do not report fetal death of less than 500 g.

specific community is at greater or lesser risk for the problems or conditions, the rates for the community should be compared with rates from similar communities, from the province or territory, or from Canada as a whole.

The IMRs are considered a key measure of health in a society. In almost all countries, IMRs have declined dramatically over the last century with improvements in sanitation, nutrition, infant feeding, and maternal and child health care, although the decline has been slower in recent years. Nevertheless, disparities in the risk of infant mortality remain, including in Canada. Estimates of preventable infant mortality enable us to better understand the nature of the disparities between population subgroups and the factors that may be responsible and help to direct interventions toward areas where improvement is possible.

Some caution must be taken in interpreting rates. Like most statistical measures, rates are less reliable when based on small numbers. This must be kept in mind when assessing relatively infrequent events or conditions, or communities with small populations.

Many rates are based on data from a calendar year, which may also present some difficulties. When calculating an IMR for a particular year, such as 2002, be aware that some of the infants who die during the 2002 calendar year were actually born in 2001 and thus were not part of the 2002 population at risk (denominator), and some of the infants who were born in 2001 might die in 2002 (numerator) and not be reflected in the 2001 IMR. Also, populations may increase or decrease during a calendar year. In such cases, the midyear population estimate (June 30) is generally used because the population at risk cannot be determined exactly. A study that follows a cohort, or specified group, forward into time (prospectively) can help overcome the limitations of the conventionally calculated calendar-year rate.

Infant mortality can be further divided into three components:

◆ Early neonatal deaths (0–6 days)
◆ Late neonatal deaths (7–27 days)
◆ Postneonatal deaths (28–364 days)

Box 2-1 presents more information regarding causes of infant death.

COMMONLY USED RATES

Table 2-2 summarizes a number of important rates. Note that the measures of natality and mortality are, in essence, measures of incidence of the conditions of "being born" and "dying." Note also the various ways in which the denominator, or population at risk, is determined in different rates.

CRUDE, SPECIFIC, AND ADJUSTED RATES

Rates that are computed for a population as a whole are called *crude rates*. Subgroups of a population may have differences that are not revealed by the crude rates. Rates that are calculated for subgroups are referred to as *specific rates*. Specific rates help identify groups at increased risk within the population

---

BOX 2-1. CAUSES OF INFANT MORTALITY

- Late fetal, neonatal, and postneonatal deaths among babies weighing less than 1500 g may be largely attributable to factors affecting maternal health. Late fetal deaths among babies weighing ≥ 1500 g may result from suboptimal maternal care. For example, regions characterized by relatively high rates of late fetal death among babies with normal birth weight may benefit from better access to caesarean delivery.
- Suboptimal newborn care or lack of access to neonatal intensive care is likely to contribute to early neonatal deaths among babies with birth weight ≥ 1500 g and late neonatal deaths among babies with intermediate birth weight, between 1500 and 2499 g.
- Infant deaths during the late neonatal period for birth weight ≥ 2500 g and postneonatal deaths for birth weight ≥ 1500 g may be largely attributable to factors in the infant environment (e.g., access to immunization, injury prevention and control).

From Health Canada *Perinatal Health Indicators* http://www.hc-sc.gc.ca/ pphb-dgspsp/rhs-ssg/phic-ispc/index.html and *Canadian Perinatal Health Report* http://www.hc-sc.gc.ca/hpb/lcdc/publicat/cphr-rspc00/index.html.

TABLE 2-2 ◆ COMMONLY USED RATES

Measures of Natality

$$\text{Crude birth rate} = \frac{\text{Number of live births during time interval}}{\text{Estimated midinterval population}} \times 1000$$

$$\text{Fertility rate} = \frac{\text{Number of live births during time interval}}{\text{Number of women aged 15–44 at midinterval}} \times 1000$$

Measures of Morbidity and Mortality

$$\text{Incidence rate} = \frac{\text{Number of new cases of specified health conditions during time interval}}{\text{Estimated midinterval population at risk}} \times 1000$$

$$\text{Prevalence rate} = \frac{\text{Number of current cases of specified health condition at a given point in time}}{\text{Estimated population at risk at same point in time}} \times 1000$$

$$\text{Crude death rate} = \frac{\text{Number of deaths during time interval}}{\text{Estimated midinterval population}} \times 1000$$

$$\text{Specific death rate} = \frac{\text{Number of deaths in subgroup during time interval}}{\text{Estimated midinterval population of subgroup}} \times 1000$$

$$\text{Cause-specific death rate} = \frac{\text{Number of deaths from specified cause during time interval}}{\text{Estimated midinterval population}} \times 1000$$

$$\text{Infant mortality rate} = \frac{\text{Number of deaths of infants aged} < 1 \text{ year during time interval}}{\text{Total live births during time interval}} \times 1000$$

$$\text{Neonatal mortality rate} = \frac{\text{Number of deaths of infants aged} < 28 \text{ days during time interval}}{\text{Total live births during time interval}} \times 1000$$

$$\text{Postneonatal mortality rate} = \frac{\text{Number of deaths of infants aged} \geq 28 \text{ days but} < 1 \text{ year during time interval}}{\text{Total live births during time interval}} \times 1000$$

and also facilitate comparisons between populations that have different demographic compositions. Most frequently, specific rates are computed according to demographic factors such as age, race, or sex.

In comparing populations with different distributions of a factor that is known to affect the health condition being studied, the use of *adjusted rates* may be advisable. An adjusted rate is a summary measure that statistically removes the effect of the difference in the distributions of that characteristic. In essence, adjustment produces an estimate of what the crude rate would be if the populations were identical in respect to the factor for which adjustment is made. A rate can be adjusted for age, race, sex, or any factor or combination of factors suspected of affecting the rate. Adjusted rates are helpful in making community comparisons, but they are imaginary rates and so must be interpreted with care.

Analytic Measures of Health

As you have learned, rates are used to describe and compare the risks of dying, becoming ill, or developing other health conditions. It is also desirable to determine if health conditions are associated with, or related to, other factors. The related factors may point the way to preventive actions (e.g., the linking of air pollution to health problems has led to environmental controls). To investigate potential relationships between health conditions and other factors, analytic measures of community health are required. In this section, three analytic measures are discussed: relative risk, odds ratio, and attributable risk.

Relative Risk

To determine if a relationship or association exists between a health condition and a suspected factor, it is necessary to compare the risk of developing the health condition for the population exposed to the factor with the risk for the population not exposed to the factor. The *relative risk* (RR) *ratio* does exactly this by expressing the ratio of the incidence rate of those exposed and those not exposed to the suspected factor:

$$RR = \frac{\text{incidence rate among those exposed}}{\text{incidence rate among those not exposed}}$$

The RR tells us whether the rate in the exposed population is higher than the rate in the nonexposed population and, if so, how many times higher it is. A high RR in the exposed population suggests that the factor is a *risk factor* in the development of the health condition.

Internal and External Risk Factors

The concept of RR is understood readily when one group of people clearly is exposed and another is not exposed to an external agent such as a virus, cigarette smoke, or an industrial pollutant. However, it may be confusing to see RRs applied to internal factors such as age, race, or sex. Nevertheless, as can be seen in the next example, persons are also "exposed" to intrinsic factors that may carry as much risk as extrinsic ones.

EXAMPLE OF RR: DIABETES

Non–insulin-dependent diabetes mellitus (NIDDM) is complicated by conditions such as ischemic heart disease, peripheral vascular disease, cerebral vascular disease, retinopathy, renal vascular disease, and peripheral neuropathy. Complications of NIDDM lead to a poorer quality of life and premature death.

There is general agreement that NIDDM has a genetic basis but that environmental factors, the most important of which is obesity, are also involved in the disease onset. It appears that nongenetic factors may be subject to intervention, and studies of controlling obesity are needed, especially by diet and exercise. Participation in a community-based exercise program can successfully facilitate weight loss in a group of individuals with NIDDM. Participation decreases fasting blood glucose values and decreases the need for insulin or oral hypoglycaemic agents, or both.

CANADIAN PEDIATRIC SOCIETY REPORT: DIABETES AND THE FIRST NATIONS

Health Canada reports that, according to the 1996–1997 National Population Health Survey (NPHS), 3.2% of the Canadian population aged 12 and over have a diagnosis of diabetes. However, among aboriginal people aged 12 and over living on reserve rather than in towns or cities off the reserve to which they belong, the rate was 8.5%. With this information, we can calculate a relative risk. Among on-reserve aboriginals (those "exposed" to the intrinsic condition of being First Nations people living on a reserve), the rate was 8.5/100, and among nonaboriginals living off reserves in Canada (those "not exposed" to the condition) the rate was 3.2/100. Thus, the RR of diabetes for aboriginal people living on reserves compared to Canadians in general can be calculated as follows:

$$RR = \frac{8.5 \text{ per } 100}{3.2 \text{ per } 100} = 2.67$$

In other words, the risk of diabetes is almost three times greater for on-reserve aboriginals than for Canadians in general. Clearly, race is a risk factor. The risk factor itself cannot be altered, but the information provided by this analysis can be used to plan protective services for the population at greatest risk (e.g., Canadian Diabetes Strategy–Aboriginal Initiative).

We must be cautious in making generalizations, however, because further analysis indicates the diabetes rates differ across the country. The prevalence in the Cree-Ojibwa living in North West Ontario and North East Manitoba has been reported as 46/1000 (RR = 1.43). Among the Dogrib Indians in the Northwest Territories, nearly 10% of adults were found to be hyperglycaemic (RR = 3.12). On the Kahnawake reservation near Montreal, 12% of Mohawks aged 45 to 65 were known diabetics, compared to 3.2% of Canadians in the same age group (RR = 3.8). Rates rise in people over age 65, regardless of race, with 23% of senior aboriginals compared with 10.4% of senior Canadians diagnosed with diabetes.

For more information on diabetes in Canada, see:

Health Canada report "Diabetes in Canada" available on-line from
    http://www.hc-sc.gc.ca/pphb-dgspsp/publicat/dic-dac99/index.html
Canadian Pediatric Society report "Diabetes and the First Nations" available on-line from http://www.cps.ca/english/statements/II/
    ii94-02.htm

Odds Ratio

Calculation of the RR is straightforward when incidence rates are available. Unfortunately, not all studies can be carried out prospectively as is required for the computation of incidence rates. In a retrospective study, the RR must be approximated by the *odds ratio* (OR).

As shown in Table 2-3, the OR is a simple mathematical ratio of the odds in favour of having a specific health condition when the suspected factor is present and the odds in favour of having the condition when the factor is absent. The odds of having the condition when the suspected factor is present is represented by *a* divided by *b* in the table (*a/b*). The chance of having the condition when the factor is absent is represented by *c* divided by *d* (*c/d*). The odds ratio is thus:

$$\frac{a/b}{c/d} = \frac{ad}{bc}$$

An example may help. When toxic shock syndrome (TSS), a severe illness involving high fever, vomiting, diarrhea, rash, and hypotension or shock, was first reported, it was neither practical nor ethical to consider cases only on a prospective basis. Therefore, existing cases were compared retrospectively with

TABLE 2-3 ◆ CROSSTABULATION FOR CALCULATION OF ODDS RATIO

	Health Condition		
	Present	Absent	Total
Exposed to factor	a	b	$a + b$
Not exposed to factor	c	d	$c + d$
TOTAL	$a + c$	$b + d$	$a + b + c + d$

controls. Early studies noted an association between TSS and tampon use and suggested that users of a specific brand of superabsorbent tampon might be at especially high risk. To clarify the issue, researchers analyzed data from TSS cases and controls, all of which used tampons. Let's use the TSS data in Table 2-4 to calculate the OR for users of the specific brand of tampon.

$$OR = \frac{ad}{bc} = \frac{30\,(84)}{30\,(12)} = 7$$

Users of the specific brand were seven times more likely to develop TSS than were users of other brands. Based on this and other studies, the brand was voluntarily withdrawn from the market.

RR and OR: Caution in Interpretation

A word of caution: Regard a high OR or RR with appropriate concern, but do not allow the finding to obscure the potential involvement of other factors. Refer to Table 2-4 again and note that 12 persons in the sample had TSS although they did not use the specific brand of tampon. In other words, this product was not the sole cause of TSS. Subsequent research showed that certain

TABLE 2-4 ◆ TOXIC SHOCK SYNDROME CASES AMONG 156 TAMPON USERS

	Toxic Shock Syndrome		
Brand of Tampon Used	Present	Absent	Total
Suspected brand	30	30	60
Other brands	12	84	96
TOTAL	42	114	156

(Data from Centers for Disease Control, 1980.)

superabsorbent materials in tampons or certain aspects of tampon use foster growth of *Staphylococcus aureus*, the probable causal organism in TSS (Centers for Disease Control and Prevention [CDC], 1981, 1983; Davis et al., 1980).

Attributable Risk and Attributable Risk Percent

Another measure of risk is *attributable risk* (AR), or the difference between the incidence rates for those exposed and those not exposed to the risk factor. This measure estimates the excess risk attributable to the factor being studied. It shows the potential reduction in the overall incidence rate if the factor could be eliminated.

AR = incidence rate in exposed group *minus* incidence rate in nonexposed group. AR usually is further quantified into attributable risk percent:

$$\frac{\text{attributable risk}}{\text{incidence rate in exposed group}} \times 100$$

This provides an estimate of the percentage of occurrences of the health condition that could be prevented if the risk factor were eliminated. For example, studies of the relationship between physical inactivity and mortality from coronary heart disease (CHD) showed that the percent of AR associated with physical inactivity was 35% (CDC, 1993). Thus, improved physical activity has the potential to greatly reduce CHD mortality.

Cause and Association

Ultimately, community health professionals hope to determine causes of health conditions so steps can be taken to improve health. In view of the complexity of the human body and human behaviour, establishing causality is difficult. Therefore, investigations of population health generally examine relationships or *associations* between variables. The variables are the characteristics or phenomena (such as age, occupation, or physical exercise) and the health conditions (such as heart disease) being studied.

VARIABLES AND CONSTANTS

An important requirement in any study is that the factors studied must have the potential to vary from person to person. If a factor cannot vary, it is not a variable but a *constant*. It is impossible to establish an association between a constant and a variable because the constant, by definition, cannot change when the variable changes. Thus, a study that looks only at men cannot establish an association between gender and, for example, heart disease; the study has made gender a constant. A study that looks only at persons with heart disease cannot establish an association between heart disease and any other variable; heart disease has become a constant in the study.

CONTROL OR COMPARISON GROUPS

To ensure that associations between variables can be examined, *control groups* or *comparison groups* may be needed. A study of heart disease might compare persons with the disease with a control group of persons without the disease. An investigation of a new treatment would study persons who receive the treatment and a control group of persons who do not receive the treatment.

INDEPENDENT AND DEPENDENT VARIABLES

Frequently variables are referred to as *dependent* or *independent*. The dependent variable is the outcome or result that the investigator is studying. It is a characteristic that conceivably could be altered (e.g., health status, knowledge, or behaviour). The independent variable is the presumed "cause" of or contributor to variation in the dependent variable. For example, in the heart disease study cited earlier (CDC, 1993), physical inactivity, the independent variable, is seen to contribute to heart disease, the dependent variable. An independent variable may be a naturally occurring event or phenomenon such as level of usual physical activity, exposure to ultraviolet radiation, or type of employment, or it might be a planned intervention such as an exercise regimen, a medical treatment, or an educational program. An independent variable might also be an intrinsic quality such as age, race, or sex. (Note that these intrinsic qualities, although they cannot vary within an individual, can vary from person to person; thus, they can be studied as independent variables.)

CONFOUNDING VARIABLES

When an association is identified between variables, it is tempting—but incorrect—to assume that one variable causes the other. If, for example, a study found that communities with lower salaries for public health workers had higher crime rates, we could not conclude that low public health salaries led to high crime rates. Common sense suggests that economic conditions might influence both salaries and crime; that is, economic conditions intervene in the study and confound the results. Any factor that may influence a study's results is referred to as an extraneous, intervening, or confounding variable.

CRITERIA FOR DETERMINING CAUSATION

If an association is found between variables, it means the variables tend to occur or change together, but it does not prove that one variable causes the other. Because of the possibility of confounded results, very strict criteria for determining causation have been established. An association must be evaluated against all of these criteria; the more criteria that are met, the more likely it is that the association is causal. However, an association may meet all the criteria for causation and later be shown to be spurious because of factors that were not known at the time the study was done. For this reason, investigators must interpret their results with great caution; they rarely consider a cause "proven." Six widely used criteria for evaluating causation are listed below.

1. The association is strong. The strength of the relationship may be evaluated statistically by a variety of measures. For example, the higher the RR or OR, the stronger the association.
2. The association is consistent. The same association must be found repeatedly in other studies, in other settings, and with other methods.
3. The association is temporally correct. The hypothesized cause of the health condition must occur before the onset of the condition.
4. The association is specific. The hypothesized cause should be associated with relatively few health conditions. For example, speaking English may be associated with many health conditions, but it is a cause for none. This criterion must be tempered by the knowledge that certain factors, such as cigarette smoking, have been shown to have multiple effects.
5. The association cannot be explained as being the result of a confounding variable. Not all potential intervening variables can be explored, of course, but alternate explanations for the association must be examined carefully before considering an association to be causal.
6. The association is plausible and consistent with current knowledge. An association that contradicts current scientific views must be evaluated very carefully. However, associations may be inconsistent with current knowledge simply because current knowledge is not as advanced as a new discovery.

The usefulness of information to a community depends on its accuracy, completeness, and reliability. If data are to provide a realistic profile of a community, identify issues placing people at risk, and assess areas of strength on which to build programs, then planners must have confidence in the information they gather and in the interpretations made by residents and community workers.

Hence, data must be from credible sources, collected by ethical and valid methods, appropriate to the issues involved, and detailed enough to allow quality interventions to be developed. In the next section common sources of data are identified and, when combined with assessment strategies presented in Chapter 10, can form a solid foundation for community action.

Sources of Community Health Data

To be an effective community health professional, you will also need to interpret and use data from various sources. In this section, we present the use of several important sources of data.

Census

The census is the most comprehensive source of population data for Canada. Every 5 years, under the Statistics Act, the government of Canada enumerates the population and surveys it for basic demographics such as age, race, marital status, and sex as well as numerous other factors such as employment, housing, income, migration, religion, language, and education.

Canada's first census was in 1666 when Jean Talon counted the 3215 inhabitants of the Colony of New France, noting their age, sex, marital status, and occupation. Approximately 98 colonial and regional censuses took place between then and Canada's first official census in 1871. The Census Act (1870) required that enumeration of the population take place every 10 years, providing the cornerstone for representative government. Since 1951, Canada has conducted a census every 5 years. Refinements have been made to methods of data collection as technology has advanced; questions have changed as information needs have developed with changing populations, immigration, wars, and social trends. An overview of the history of the census is located at http://www12.statcan.ca/english/census01/Info/history.cfm.

The 2001 Census took place May 1–12; 11.8 million households received a Census of Population questionnaire, and 276,000 farm operations received a Census of Agriculture form at the same time. An adult in each household is required to complete the questionnaires and return them to Statistics Canada. There is a short form of the questionnaire, containing seven questions, that will be completed by 80% of households, and a long form of the questionnaire that will go to every 20th household and contains the original 7 plus 52 additional questions. In remote or rural areas, a census representative conducts household interviews.

Census reports are available in public libraries, in municipal, provincial, and federal government offices, and on the Internet. Although census data are comprehensive, bias does occur. For example, people may answer personal questions dishonestly. Perhaps more significantly, the census is believed to underrepresent low-income residents, residents of First Nations reserves, and transients. These people are more difficult to locate and enumerate and tend to be less likely to respond to census surveys. However, efforts are made to capture information on as many people as possible; forms are available in more than 50 languages, in Braille, and in large print. Forms are also available in electronic formats, and a census representative is available to collect the data in person if necessary. People are required by law to complete census forms every 5 years, and there are penalties for those who refuse or who do not tell the truth.

Vital Statistics

Vital statistics are the data on legally registered events (such as births, deaths, marriages, and divorces) collected on an ongoing basis by government agencies. Provincial health departments usually publish vital statistics annually. Health Canada also gathers data from the provinces and publishes annual volumes as well as periodic reports on specific topics.

To view your provincial or territorial vital statistics, see the following website and follow the links or locate the addresses (Box 2-2): http://www3. gov.ab.ca/gs/information/vs/canada_offices.cfm

Beginning researchers tend to consider vital statistics "hallowed" because they are, after all, legal data. However, legality does not guarantee validity. For example, the manner in which cause of death is recorded on death certificates is inconsistent. The numbers of unmarried but cohabitating couples—and the occasional news reports of newly discovered bigamists—also demonstrate that marriage and divorce records are also not completely valid measures of reality. Despite their limitations, vital statistics are often the best available data and much useful information can be gained from them.

Notifiable Disease Reports

Health Canada reports data collected by provincial and local health departments on legally reportable diseases and also periodically requests voluntary reporting of nonnotifiable health conditions of special interest. Canada Communicable Disease Report (CCDR), formerly called Canada Diseases Weekly Report (CDWR), is available on the Internet at http://www.hc-sc.gc.ca/pphb-

BOX 2-2. OFFICES OF VITAL STATISTICS

Alberta
Government Services
Alberta Registries, Vital Statistics
Box 2023
Edmonton, Alberta T5J 4W7
Telephone: (780) 427-7013 (recording)
http://www3.gov.ab.ca/gs/
   information/vs/statistical_info.
   cfm

British Columbia
British Columbia Vital Statistics
   Agency
PO Box 9657 STN PROV GOVT
Victoria, BC V8W 9P3
Telephone: In the Vancouver Area:
   660-2937
In the Victoria Area: 952-2681
or elsewhere in BC toll free at:
   1-800-663-8328
Outside of BC call 1-250-952-2681
Fax: (250) 952-2527
www.vs.gov.bc.ca/index.html
   (off-site)

Manitoba
Division of Vital Statistics
Community Services
254 Portage Avenue
Winnipeg, MB R3C 0B6
Telephone: (204) 945-3701
(204) 945-2034 (recording)
www.gov.mb.ca/cca/vital/index.
   html (off-site)

New Brunswick
Registrar General
Division of Vital Statistics
Department of Gov't Services and
   Lands
Centennial Building
Box 6000
Fredericton, NB E3B 5H1
Telephone: (506) 453-2385
www.gnb.ca/0379/en/index.htm
   (off-site)

Newfoundland
Vital Statistics Division
Department of Government Services
   & Lands
P.O. Box 8700
5 Mews Place
St. John's, NF A1B 4J6
Telephone: (709) 729-3308
Fax: (709) 729-0946
www.gov.nf.ca/gsl/gs/vs/ (off-site)

Northwest Territories
Registrar General
Vital Statistics
Department of Health and Social
   Services
Government of NWT
Bag 9
Inuvik, NT X0E 0T0
Telephone: (867) 777-7420
Fax: (867) 777-3197
www.hlthss.gov.nt.ca/ (off-site)

Nova Scotia
Deputy Registrar General
1723 Hollis Street
Box 157
Halifax, NS B3J 2M9
Telephone: (902) 424-4381
(902) 424-4380 (recording)
www.gov.ns.ca/snsmr/vstat/
   default.asp (off-site)

Nunavut
Registrar General of Vital Statistics
Nunavut Health and Social Services
Bag #3
Rankin Inlet, NT X0C 0G0
Telephone: (867) 645-5002
Toll-free (800) 661-0833
Fax: (867) 645-2997
www.gov.nu.ca/gnmain.htm
   (off-site)

(continued)

BOX 2-2. OFFICES OF VITAL STATISTICS (*Continued*)

Ontario
Office of the Registrar General
Box 4600
189 Red River Road
Thunder Bay, ON P7B 6L8
Telephone: (416) 325-8305
In Ontario call: 1-800-461-2156
www.cbs.gov.on.ca:80/mcbs/
english/4VYSS5.htm (off-site)

Prince Edward Island
Division of Vital Statistics
Department of Health & Community
Services
35 Douses Road, Box 3000,
Montague, PE C0A 1R0
Telephone: (902) 838-0880 or (902)
838-0881
Fax: (902) 838-0883
www.gov.pe.ca/vitalstatistics
(off-site)

Quebec
Ministère des Relations avec les
citoyens et de l'Immigration
Le Directeur de l'etat civil

Quebec (continued)
Service a la clientele
205, rue Montmagny
Quebec, QC G1N 2Z9
Telephone: (418) 643-3900
www.etatcivil.gouv.qc.ca/
ENGLISH/Default.htm
(off-site)

Saskatchewan
Division of Vital Statistics
Department of Health
1942 Hamilton Street
Regina, SK S4P 3V7
Telephone: (306) 787-3092
www.health.gov.sk.ca/ps_vital_
statistics.html (off-site)

Yukon Territories
Registrar of Vital Statistics
Box 2703
Whitehorse, YT Y1A 2C6
Telephone: (403) 667-5207
www.hss.gov.yk.ca/vsaframe.html
(off-site)

---

dgspsp/publicat/ccdr-rmtc/. Other reports on chronic diseases and special topics are also available from Health Canada Publications, which also archives past reports.

Even legally mandated disease reports may not be representative of all cases of the disease. Thus, they may not provide valid descriptions of a disease as it exists in the community. In practice, health care providers may fail to report diseases that should be reported; for instance chickenpox (varicella) is consistently underreported.

Medical and Hospital Records

Medical and hospital records are used extensively in community health research. These records, however, do not provide a completely representative or valid picture of community health. In the first place, not all persons with health problems receive medical attention, so medical records are obviously biased. Second, medical documentation is not always complete. Finally, hospitalized patients are also more likely to have another illness along with the one being studied. This phenomenon, called Berkson's bias, creates the likelihood of finding a false association between the two illnesses.

Social Welfare Reports

Statistics Canada and Human Resources Development Canada (HRDC) publish regular reports on current issues about the social situation experienced by Canadians. A survey of the websites of these organizations can offer the community professional insight into social conditions such as homelessness, poverty, education, and the economy.

HRDC publications:
http://www.ncwcnbes.net/htmdocument/principales/onlinepub.htm
Poverty Profile: http://www.ncwcnbes.net/htmdocument/
   reportpovertypro99/Introduction.html

Other national Internet sites offer opinion and analysis of social and economic conditions, such as:

Canada's Social History: http://www.socialpolicy.ca/cush/index.htm
Conference Board of Canada: http://www.conferenceboard.ca
The Canadian Institute of Advanced Research: http://www.ciar.ca
The Fraser Institute: http://www.fraserinstitute.ca

There are also regional "think tanks" that offer comment on issues specific to people in groups of provinces, such as:

The Parkland Institute: http://www.ualberta.ca/~parkland
Canada West Foundation:
   http://www.cwf.ca/abcalcwf/doc.nsf/doc/News

Various national and provincial professional associations also offer publications on issues relevant to their disciplines. As with any site, you must be cautious in interpreting the opinions and analysis because they will come from a particular perspective and are trying to make an argument that supports their specific viewpoint. Seeking information from several sites will provide the community health professional with a broad perspective on issues.

Screening for Health Conditions

Thus far, we have focused on methods for studying community health problems and assessing health risks for populations. In this section, we discuss screening, a method of secondary prevention. Screening is an effort to detect unrecognized or preclinical illness among individuals. Screening tests are not intended to be diagnostic. Their purpose is to rapidly and economically identify persons who have a high probability of having (or developing) a particular illness so they can be referred for definitive diagnosis and treatment.

Considerations in Deciding to Screen

Screening goes further than identifying groups at risk for illness; it identifies individuals who may actually have an illness. Screening carries an ethical commitment to continue working with these individuals and provide them access to diagnostic and treatment services. In general, screening should be conducted only if:

◆ Early diagnosis and treatment can favourably alter the course of the illness.
◆ Definitive diagnosis and treatment facilities are available, either through the screening agency or through referral.
◆ A group being screened is at risk for the illness (in other words, the group is likely to have a high prevalence of the illness).
◆ Screening procedures are reliable and valid.

Screening Test Reliability and Validity

Reliability refers to the consistency or repeatability of test results; *validity* refers to the ability of the test to measure what it is supposed to measure. A few considerations specific to screening tests are discussed below.

SCREENING TEST RELIABILITY

A reliable screening test yields the same result even when administered by different screeners. Training for all screening personnel in use of the test is essential. Lack of reliability may suggest that the screeners are administering the test in an inconsistent manner.

Screening Test Validity: Sensitivity and Specificity

To be valid, a screening test must distinguish correctly between those individuals who have the condition and those who do not. This is measured by the test's sensitivity and specificity, as shown in Table 2-5.

Sensitivity is the ability to correctly identify individuals who have the disease, that is, to call a true positive "positive." A test with high sensitivity will have few false negatives.

Specificity is the ability to correctly identify individuals who do not have the disease, or to call a true negative "negative." A test with high specificity has few false positives.

Relationship Between Sensitivity and Specificity

Ideally, a screening test's sensitivity and specificity should be 100%; in practice, however, screening tests vary in this regard. As shown in Table 2-5, sensitivity, or the true positive rate, is the complement of the false-negative rate, and specificity, or the true negative rate, is the complement of the false-positive rate. Thus, as sensitivity increases, specificity decreases. Therefore, decisions regarding screening test validity may require uncomfortable compromises, as you will see from the following examples.

TABLE 2-5 ◆ SENSITIVITY AND SPECIFICITY OF A SCREENING TEST

Screening Test Results	Reality	
	Diseased	Not Diseased
Positive	True positive	False positive
Negative	False negative	True negative
Total	Total diseased	Total not diseased

$$\text{Sensitivity (true-positive rate)} = \frac{\text{True positives}}{\text{Total diseased}}$$

$$\text{Specificity (true-negative rate)} = \frac{\text{True negatives}}{\text{Total not diseased}}$$

$$\text{False-negative rate} = \frac{\text{False negatives}}{\text{Total diseased}} \quad or \; 1 - \text{Sensitivity}$$

$$\text{False-positive rate} = \frac{\text{False positives}}{\text{Total not diseased}} \quad or \; 1 - \text{Sensitivity}$$

Decision-Making in Screening: Practical and Ethical Considerations

Suppose you are screening for a deadly disease that is curable only if detected early and you have a choice between a test with high sensitivity and low specificity or one with high specificity and low sensitivity. To save the most lives, you need high sensitivity; that is, a low rate of false negatives (people who *have* the disease but are not detected by the screening test). However, if you select the test with high sensitivity, its low specificity means that you will have a high rate of false positives (people who do *not* have the disease but whom the test identifies as having it). That is, you will alarm many people needlessly and will cause unnecessary expenses by overreferring them for nonexistent disease. Which test would you choose?

Now, suppose you are screening for the same disease, but the diagnostic and treatment facilities in the community are already overloaded, and further budget cuts are projected. To minimize unnecessary referrals of false positives, you would want the test with high specificity. However, because of the low sensitivity of this test, you will have to weigh the benefits of a low false-positive rate against the ethics of a high false-negative rate. Is it justifiable to lull the undetected diseased persons into a false—and potentially fatal—sense of security? Which test would you choose now?

Decisions regarding screening involve seeking the most favourable balance of sensitivity and specificity. Sometimes, sensitivity and specificity can be improved by adjusting the screening process (e.g., adding another test or changing the level at which the test is considered positive). At other times, evaluating sensitivity and specificity may result in a decision not to conduct a screening program because the economic costs of overreferral or the ethical considerations of underreferral outweigh the usefulness of screening. An understanding of the principles discussed in this section will help you make informed decisions regarding community screening. You also are encouraged to pursue further study regarding screening.

Epidemiologic Approaches to Community Health Research

In studying the determinants of population health, investigators may be guided by epidemiologic models. This section describes three models and explains how each might guide the approach to the same problem.

The problem to be considered is an increase in the IMR in a hypothetical community. The IMR is a particularly important health index that should be understood even by health professionals whose main concern is not maternal or child health. Because infant mortality is influenced by a variety of biologic and environmental factors affecting the infant and mother, the IMR is both a direct measure of infant health and an indirect measure of community health as a whole.

The Epidemiologic Triad

The epidemiologic triad or agent-host-environment model is a traditional view of health and disease, developed when epidemiology was concerned chiefly with communicable disease. As you will see, however, the model is applicable to other conditions as well. In the model, the *agent* is an organism capable of causing disease. The *host* is the population at risk for developing the disease. The *environment* is a combination of physical, biologic, and social factors that surround and influence both the agent and the host. According to this model, by examining the characteristics of, changes in, and interactions among the agent, host, and environment, health (and illness) can be more holistically understood.

Figure 2-1 shows the triad in its normal state of equilibrium. Equilibrium does not signify optimum health but simply the usual pattern of illness and health in a population. Any change in one of the sides (agent, host, or environment) will result in disequilibrium, in other words, a change in the usual pattern.

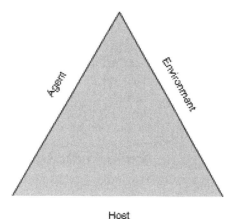

Figure 2-1 ◆ The epidemiologic triangle is the traditional view, showing health and disease as a composite state of three variables.

How would this model guide the investigation of an increased IMR? To understand this, let us consider the three facets of the model.

AGENT

At first glance, it might be concluded that the investigation should focus on types of infections as agents that cause infant deaths. However, major causes of infant mortality in Canada and the United States include prematurity and low birth weight, birth injuries, congenital malformations, sudden infant death syndrome (SIDS), accidents, and homicides. Therefore, the investigation will try to determine whether there has been a change in any of these other agents.

HOST

The investigators also will want to know the characteristics of the host; that is, the infant population. This involves examining infant birth and death patterns in terms of age, ethnicity, sex, and birth weight. These characteristics have been shown to be important risk factors for infant mortality. By studying these factors, it may be possible to identify groups of infants who are at particularly increased risk of dying.

ENVIRONMENT

Finally, the environment must be assessed. The mother is a significant part of the infant's prenatal and postnatal environment. Therefore, the investigators will analyze birth and infant mortality patterns according to factors such as maternal age, ethnicity, parity (number of previous live births), prenatal care, and education or socioeconomic status (SES). Analysis of these factors, which are also related to infant mortality, will help provide further identification of at-risk groups. Other conditions in the environment also need to be considered. For instance, has migration into the community from other areas increased? Has adult morbidity or mortality, particularly among pregnant women, increased? Have there been changes in health services, policies, personnel, funding, or other factors that could affect infant health?

PRACTICAL APPLICATION

The analysis of these three areas—the agent, host, and environment—should provide information regarding groups at risk for increased infant mortality and may point the way toward a program aimed at reducing that risk. Thus, the epidemiologic triangle, although it was designed with a communicable disease orientation, can provide a useful guide for studying the multifaceted problem of infant mortality, as well as other health problems.

The Person-Place-Time Model

An approach similar to the epidemiologic triangle is one that guides the investigators to consider the health problem in terms of person, place, and time (Mausner & Kramer, 1985). The investigators examine characteristics of the persons affected (the host in the triangle model), the place (environment) or location, and the time period involved (which could relate to the agent, host, or environment). In studying infant mortality according to the person-place-time model, infant and maternal factors are considered traits of "person." Aspects of "place" are such factors as whether the community is rural or urban, affluent or poor. Aspects of "time" include seasonal or age-specific patterns or trends in mortality.

The Web of Causation

The web of causation (MacMahon & Pugh, 1970) views a health condition not as the result of individual factors but of complex interactions among multiple factors. One factor may lead to others, which, in turn, lead to others, all of which may interact with one another to produce the health condition. Factors can be at the *macro* (multisystem, societal) level, *meso* (familial, local) level, or *micro* (individual) level.

Central to this model is the concept of synergism, wherein the whole is more than the sum of its separate parts. For example, the effects of a *Shigella* infection on the infant, combined with the effects of poverty, youth, and low educational level of the mother, are more deleterious to infant health than the sum of the effects of the individual risk factors.

Use of the web of causation may result in a more expansive study of infant mortality than one guided by other models. Ideally, investigators using this model first identify all factors related to infant mortality. Next, they identify factors that are related to each of these factors. These two comprehensive steps provide the outline for the web of causation for infant mortality. Finally, the investigators examine the relationships among all the identified components of the web and attempt to determine the most feasible point of intervention to improve infant mortality in the community. Figure 2-2 depicts a web of causation for infant mortality. Other webs are proposed in literature related to specific issues (e.g., myocardial infarction, adolescent pregnancy, addiction).

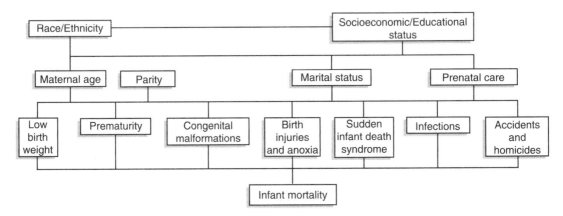

Figure 2-2 ◆ A web of causation for infant mortality based on information available from birth and death certificates.

PRACTICAL APPLICATION

This multifaceted approach addresses the concept of causation in a manner consistent with current knowledge of human health. However, it may be overwhelming to carry out in everyday practice. In fact, it is more usual to examine only a portion of the web, acknowledging that other relationships exist. Thorough examination of one portion of the web may provide sufficient information for initiation of useful actions to improve community health.

Models: Guides to Investigation and Practice

In this section, we showed how three models each provide a slightly different approach to a community issue. Community issues can be related to "problems" or "wellness," and in future chapters you will see how the models can apply to both situations. As you continue to study community health, you will find other models that can guide your practice and investigation. There is no one "correct" model; as you gain experience, you will be able to choose or adapt those that are most appropriate for your work.

Summary

In this chapter, you have been introduced to demography, the broad science of populations, and epidemiology, the specific science of population health. Examples have been offered as to how these two sciences can be used to guide community practice. For more detailed information on epidemiology and demography, you may wish to consult the reference list.

References

Centers for Disease Control and Prevention. (1980, September 19). Follow up on toxic shock syndrome. *Morbidity and Mortality Weekly Report, 29*, 441–445.

Centers for Disease Control and Prevention. (1981, June 30). Toxic shock syndrome— United States, 1970–1980. *Morbidity and Mortality Weekly Report, 30*, 25–33.

Centers for Disease Control and Prevention. (1983, August 5). Update: Toxic shock syndrome—United States. *Morbidity and Mortality Weekly Report, 32*, 398–400.

Centers for Disease Control and Prevention. (1993, September 10). Public health focus: Physical activity and the prevention of coronary heart disease. *Morbidity and Mortality Weekly Report, 42*, 398–400.

Crichton, M. (1969). *The Andromeda strain.* New York: Alfred A. Knopf.

Davis, J. P., Chesney, P. J., Ward, P. J., LaVenture, M., & the Investigation and Laboratory Team. (1980). Toxic shock syndrome: Epidemiologic features, recurrence, risk factors, and prevention. *New England Journal of Medicine, 303*, 1429–1435.

Feldshuh, D. (1997). *Miss Ever's boys.* New York: Home Box Office Production with Anasazi Productions.

Lilienfeld, D. E., & Stolley, P. D. (1994). *Foundations of epidemiology* (3rd ed.). New York: Oxford University Press.

MacMahon, B., & Pugh, T. F. (1970). *Epidemiology: Principles and methods.* Boston: Little, Brown.

Mausner, J. S., & Kramer, S. (1985). *Epidemiology: An introductory text.* Philadelphia: Saunders.

Petersen, W. (1995). *Outbreak.* Warner Brothers Entertainment, Los Angeles, CA.

Preston, P. (1994). *The hot zone.* New York: Random House.

Snow, J. (1936). Snow on cholera, being a reprint of two papers by John Snow, M.D., together with a biographical memoir by B.W. Richardson, M.D., and an introduction by Wade Hampton Frost, M.D. New York: Commonwealth Fund.

3

Canadians and the Health System

OBJECTIVES

Community practitioners need to know the characteristics of the population and understand the various human service systems that provide support to the citizens of Canada.

After studying this chapter, you should be able to:

◆ Describe the jurisdictional responsibilities of the federal, provincial, and municipal governments for health, education, and social services

◆ Describe the health status of Canadians from the determinants of health perspective

◆ Note critical issues that place certain population groups at risk

Introduction

Canada is a federation of ten provinces and three territories where bilingualism and multiculturalism are encouraged and supported. Canada's vast land area is geographically varied, whereas its increasingly diverse population is concentrated in certain parts of the country, with large parts very sparsely populated. The Canadian economy is broadly based and offers many opportunities for employment and economic growth: there are fisheries inland and on both coasts; agricultural enterprises are present in every province; manufacturing operations are many, particularly in Ontario; and it is an international tourist destination. The country has abundant natural resources such as forests, minerals, water, oil, and gas that support a variety of industries. As Canadians we also pride (and frequently identify) ourselves by the social safety net that has been developed and supported since Confederation (Vollman & Tenove, 2001).

Jurisdictions for Health and Social Services

The British North America Act (BNA Act) of 1867 established Canada as a federation and delineated the jurisdictional powers of the federal and provincial governments. Over the years, judicial interpretations, new legislation, emerging needs of the population, and the changing scopes of the various stages of government have substantially amended the relative influence of federal powers on the lives of Canadians.

Provinces are responsible for policies in relation to education, excepting military and on-reserve schools. With its role in employment insurance, however, the federal government plays a key role with the provinces in manpower training. Additionally, the federal government provides financial aid to students through a student loan program, second language training grants, second official language instruction programs, and postsecondary education for Aboriginal students. As well, federal grants support universities through a variety of granting councils (e.g., Social Sciences and Humanities Research Council, National Science and Engineering Research Council, Canadian Institutes for Health Research).

With respect to health, the provinces were granted jurisdiction over hospitals under the BNA Act (1867) and have gained regulatory authority over local occupational health and safety, licensing of professionals, and health and hospital insurance plans (including Workers' Compensation Boards). The federal government regulates food and drugs, inspects medical devices, provides health information services, regulates health and safety in federally regulated economic sectors, and operates a national network of public health laboratories. The provision of health services to the military, First Nations and Inuit peoples, immigrants, civil aviation personnel, and public service employees is the responsibility of the federal government. Medical research is supported through a variety of granting councils and initiatives. The Canada Health Act (1984) sets the standards for public funding of health services and imposes penalties on provinces that contravene the five principles of the Act (Box 3-1). The principles of the Canada Health Act began as simple conditions attached to federal funding for Medicare. Over time, they became much more than that. Today, they represent both the values underlying the health care system and the conditions that governments attach to funding a national system of public health care. The five principles have stood the test of time and continue to reflect the values of Canadians (Romanow, 2002).

BOX 3-1. CRITERIA OF THE CANADA HEALTH ACT (1984)

1. **Public administration:** This criterion applies to the health insurance plans of the provinces and territories (not to hospitals or the services hospitals provide). The health care insurance plans are to be administered and operated on a nonprofit basis by a public authority, responsible to the provincial/territorial governments and subject to audits of their accounts and financial transactions.

2. **Comprehensiveness:** The health insurance plans of the provinces and territories must ensure all insured health services (hospital, physician, surgical-dental) and, where permitted, services rendered by other health care practitioners.

3. **Universality:** One hundred percent of the insured residents of a province or territory must be entitled to the insured health services provided by the plans on uniform terms and conditions. Provinces and territories generally require that residents register with the plans to establish entitlement.

4. **Portability:** Residents moving from one province or territory to another must continue to be covered for insured health care services by the "home" province during any minimum waiting period, not to exceed 3 months, imposed by the new province of residence. After the waiting period, the new province or territory of residence assumes health care coverage. Accommodations are made for travellers if they need urgent or emergency services when temporarily away from home.

5. **Accessibility:** The health insurance plans of the provinces and territories must adhere to three provisions. The first is reasonable access to insured health care services on uniform terms and conditions without charges (user charges or extra-billing) or other conditions (age, health status, or financial circumstances). This has been interpreted to mean that residents of a province or territory are entitled to have access to insured health care services at the setting "where" the services are provided and "as" the services are available in that setting. Second, physicians and dentists must be given reasonable compensation for all the insured health care services they provide, and, third, hospitals are paid to cover the cost of insured health care services delivered.

Social services and the provision of welfare are in the jurisdiction of the provinces. However, the Canadian government administers universal programs such as family allowances, old age pensions, and certain supplementary programs (e.g., survivors' and disability benefits, guaranteed income supplement, and employment insurance).

Financing the Social Safety Net

Education, health, and social services are supported by federal fund transfers (Canada Health and Social Transfer, 1995; Established Programs Financing Act, 1977), special grants, incentive programs, and cost-sharing initiatives. For instance, through the Heart Health, Brighter Futures, Canada Prenatal Nutrition Program, and other such initiatives, community agencies and non-profit organizations have been able to undertake community development programs aimed directly at those factors that contribute to the health and well-being of the nation's population. Community workers are ever vigilant for new provincial, municipal, or federal programs that can support the development of local capacity to address social conditions that affect health.

Costs of Health and Social Services in Canada

Approximately half of Canada's gross domestic product (GDP) is spent on social security, welfare, education, and health. When private expenditures are added to public costs, the proportion of GDP spent on health in 2000 was 9.6%. Figure 3-1 illustrates the trend in public expenditures over the 25 years from 1972 to 1997 as percent of GDP.

Costs for health and social services are considerable in Canada (Table 3-1). Efforts have been made over recent years by the provinces to reduce expenditures through regionalization and amalgamation of service providers. Recent reports from several provinces call for the reorientation of services from institutions to the community (Table 3-2). Two national reports, *The Health of Canadians—The Federal Role* of the Standing Senate Committee on Social Affairs, Science and Technology (Kirby Report, 2002) and *Building on Values: The Future of Health Care in Canada* (Romanow Report, 2002), have also been published that deal with health care in Canada. There is a common message in all reports: Canadians value the health care system and Medicare, but changes are needed to make service delivery more efficient, effective, and affordable. To do this, the various reports recommend sweeping changes in how services are organized, funded, and resourced (in terms of personnel and technology). In most

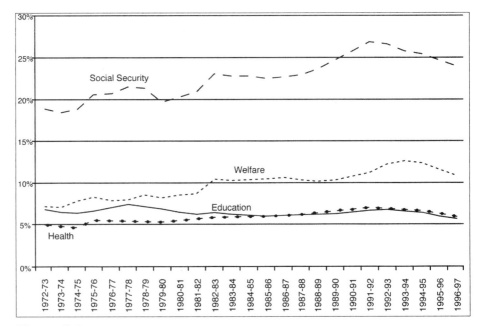

Figure 3-1 ◆ Social security, welfare, health, and education expenditures as a percentage of gross domestic product (GDP) 1972–73 to 1996–97.

TABLE 3-1 ◆ HEALTH AND SOCIAL SERVICES EXPENDITURES IN CANADA—ACTUAL DOLLARS					
	1995/96	2000/01	2001/02	1995/96–2001/02	2000/01–2001/02
	\$ Millions			% Change	
Consolidated provincial, territorial and local governments	89,818	112,043	117,245	30.5	4.6
Newfoundland and Labrador	1,515	2,005	2,165	42.9	8.0
Prince Edward Island	264	416	443	67.8	6.5
Nova Scotia	2,400	2,878	2,950	22.9	2.5
New Brunswick	1,994	2,222	2,351	17.9	5.8
Quebec	25,147	30,473	31,848	26.6	4.5
Ontario	34,794	42,282	43,463	24.9	2.8
Manitoba	2,994	4,126	4,338	44.9	5.1
Saskatchewan	2,409	3,439	3,538	46.9	2.9
Alberta	6,202	9,089	10,207	64.6	12.3
British Columbia	11,826	14,734	15,510	31.2	5.3
Yukon	130	149	160	23.1	7.4
Northwest Territories	—	291	352	—	21.0
Nunavut	—	212	212	—	0.0

TABLE 3-2 ◆ RECENT ROYAL COMMISSION AND TASK FORCE REPORTS ON HEALTH CARE IN CANADA

Jurisdiction	Title (Lead Author)	Report Date	Website
New Brunswick	Health care renewal: Discussion paper New Vision— New Brunswick	January 2002	http://www.gnb.ca/0089/cpqs/pdfs/ health.pdf http://www.gnb.ca/0051/pub/pdf/ hrepcard-e.pdf(pages 4-8)
Quebec	Commission d'etude sur les services de sante et les services sociaux "Emerging solutions" (Michel Clair)	January 2001	http://www.cessss.gouv.qc.ca/pdf/en/ 01-109-01a.pdf
Saskatchewan	Commission on medicare (Ken Fyke)	April 2001	http://www.health.gov.sk.ca/hplan_ health_care_plan.pdf
Alberta	A framework for reform (Don Mazankowski)	December 2001	http://healthreform.ca/maz_report_1.html
British Columbia	Patients first: Renewal and reform of BC's health system	December 2001	http://www.legis.gov.bc.ca/cmt/37thparl/ session%2D2/health/reports/healthtoc.htm
Northwest Territories	It's time to act: A report on the health and social services system of the NT	June 2001	http://www.hlthss.gov.nt.ca/content/ Publications/reports/cuff/cuffreportfinal.pdf
Federal	Commission on the future of health care in Canada (Roy Romanow)	November 2002	http://www.healthcarecommission.ca/ Suite247/Common/GetMedia_WO.asp? MediaID=1162&Filename=HCC_Final_ Report.pdf
Federal	The health of Canadians— the federal role (Michael Kirby)	June 2002	http://www.altapharm.org/ims/client/upload/ Senator_Kirby_HIGHLIGHTS__ FINAL__-_Oct_25-02.pdf

instances, people, and keeping people well, are the highest priorities and competition, choice, and accountability are key concerns in service delivery to maintain health and care for those who need care. Improving access to services, shortening waiting lists, maintaining an adequate number and variety of health care staff, supporting health promotion, and increasing the prevention effort are the means suggested for achieving the results needed to sustain the Canadian health care system. It is also clear from the reports that the health system cannot be held solely responsible for the health of the nation's people; cooperation and collaboration are required with other sectors and governments to align services, policies, and programming.

Hence, we see increasing examples of education, health, and social service sectors collaborating to address gaps and reduce duplication of population health services. In addition, community involvement in making policy decisions around education, health, and social services is increasingly more apparent as agencies deal with lower levels of funding, high consumer expectations, and changing demographics. For this purpose, community-based professionals are interested in building skills that foster community capacity. These skills are outlined in detail in Part Two of this book: community assessment, problem analysis and asset identification, program planning and intervention, and evaluation using the principles and processes of public participation, partnership, and health promotion.

Education, health, and social services departments are organized differently from province to province. For this reason, community workers from all disciplines must be knowledgeable about the multiple service sectors that influence community health and well-being. In addition to those sectors mentioned previously, local and provincial government ministries that address justice, housing, transportation, and economic development are also important to the community worker. Several nonprofit or charitable institutions (e.g., Boys and Girls Clubs of Canada) or special interest associations (e.g., Lung, Heart and Stroke, Cancer, Mental Health) are involved also at the local level. To enhance the health of communities and the people who live in them, community workers must be aware of the multiplicity of programs and services available—a daunting task indeed.

How Healthy and Well Are Canadians?

A variety of factors affect health, including gender, age, culture, genetics, personal health practices, coping skills, social support, working conditions, socioeconomic status, education, physical environment, and early childhood experience. These factors are referred to as the determinants of health, and the most powerful of these is socioeconomic status. By whatever measure we apply (e.g., infant mortality, premature death, chronic disease incidence, or self-reported wellbeing), socioeconomic status remains strongly related to health status. The health of the Canadian population improves as income and education levels increase, and persistent differences in health status exist between those Canadians with the lowest and highest income levels. Hence, the equitable distribution of income and educational opportunity is a stronger determinant of the overall health of Canadians than the provision of illness care services. In Chapter 1, the evolution of population health and the population health promotion approach were presented. In this chapter, some of the highlights from the *Second Report on the Health of Canadians* (1999) will be excerpted to illustrate the determinants of health and their impact on the population (Boxes 3-2 and 3-3).

BOX 3-2. REPORT ON THE HEALTH OF CANADIANS

Toward a Healthy Future: Second Report on the Health of Canadians helps us take stock of where we are and measure our progress by looking at changes over time. This is an essential first step in addressing the challenges to Canadians' health and well-being in the next millennium. It also identifies priorities for action for policymakers, practitioners, and researchers. The full text of the report can be accessed on the web: http://www.hc-sc.gc.ca. Printed copies of the Report are available from Provincial and Territorial Ministries of Health or from: Publications, Health Canada, Tunney's Pasture (AL 0900C2), Ottawa, ON K1A 0K9 Telephone: (613) 954-5995; Fax: (613) 941-5366; e-mail: Info@www.hc-sc.gc.ca.

BOX 3-3. JASON'S STORY

"Why is Jason in the hospital?
  Because he has a bad infection in his leg.
But why does he have an infection?
  Because he has a cut in his leg and it got infected.
But why does he have a cut on his leg?
  Because he was playing in the junk yard next to his apartment building and there was some sharp, jagged steel there that he fell on.
But why was he playing in a junk yard?
  Because his neighbourhood is kind of run down. A lot of kids play there and there is no one to supervise them.
But why does he live in that neighbourhood?
  Because his parents can't afford a nicer place to live.
But why can't his parents afford a nicer place to live?
  Because his Dad is unemployed and his Mom is sick.
But why is his Dad unemployed?
  Because he doesn't have much education and he can't find a job.
But why...?"

From: Federal, Provincial, Territorial Advisory Committee on Population Health. (1999). *Toward a healthy future.* Ottawa: Health Canada.

By almost any measure, Canada is a highly desirable, healthy place to live. An overall high standard of health, however, is not shared equitably by all sectors of society. Sixty-three percent of adult Canadians say that their health is excellent or very good, and only 9% rate their health as fair or poor. Canada ranks in the top three developed countries in the world in measures of life expectancy, self-rated health, and mortality rates. Life expectancy in Canada has reached a new high at 75.7 years for men and 81.4 years for women. Most recent immigrants to Canada are in good health and the majority of our older citizens enjoy independence and good health. In 1996, Canada's infant mortality rate dropped below the level of six infant deaths per 1000 live births for the first time. The United Nations (U.N.) in 2002 ranked Canada third in the world (behind Norway and Sweden) on its Human Development Index, down from its first place ranking in 2001. This index measures a country's achievements in terms of life expectancy, educational attainment, and income (United Nations Development Programme, 2002) and also assesses factors such as human dignity, freedom, and the role of the people in development. That standing drops to 10th place, however, when the U.N. Human Poverty Index for industrialized countries is applied. The U.N. report suggests that this drop is because "Canada has significant problems of poverty and their progress in human development has not been evenly distributed."

Human Biology and Age

Sex and age have varying effects on health status. Men are more likely than women to die prematurely, largely as a result of heart disease, fatal unintentional injuries, cancer, and suicide. Men are almost twice as likely as women to die before age 70. Although women live longer than men, they are more likely to suffer depression, stress overload (often due to efforts to balance work and family life), chronic conditions such as arthritis and osteoporosis, and injuries and death resulting from family violence. Although overall cancer death rates have declined in men, they have remained persistently stubborn among women, mainly due to increases in lung cancer mortality. Teenage girls are now more likely than adolescent boys to smoke. If increased rates of smoking among young women are not reversed, lung cancer rates among women will continue to climb.

Rates of physical activity drop quickly as age increases, and boys/men are more active than girls/women in every age group. Older Canadians are far more likely than younger Canadians to have physical illnesses; however, youths aged 12 to 19 report the lowest levels of psychological well-being. Despite a 50% reduction in mortality over a generation, unintentional injuries are still the leading cause of death of children and youth, as well as a tragic and costly cause of disability. Boys and young men experience more unintentional injuries and more severe injuries than girls and young women. Suicide rates among young men (especially in Aboriginal communities) are high in Canada compared to other countries. Young children, especially those who live in poor neighbourhoods, are most likely to suffer illnesses related to environmental toxins and second-hand smoke. Asthma has dramatically increased among young children in the last decade.

Early Childhood Development

Experiences from conception to age 6 have the most important influence of any time in the life cycle on the connecting and sculpting of the brain's neurons. Positive stimulation early in life improves learning, behaviour, and health right into adulthood. A loving, secure attachment between parents, caregivers, and babies in the first 18 months of life helps children develop trust, self-esteem, emotional control, and the ability to have positive relationships with others in later life. However, some families are dysfunctional and their impact on young family members does not enhance health. In 1996, family members were responsible for one fifth of physical assaults and one third of sexual assaults on children. Infants and children who are neglected or abused are denied the stimulation and nurturing they need in the early years. This puts them at higher risk for behavioural, social, and learning problems throughout the life cycle. Readiness for school is an important indicator of developmental maturity and future success in school. In 1996–1997, approximately 15% of preschoolers arrived at school with low cognitive scores and 14% had high scores in behavioural problems. Children from safe, more economically secure neighbourhoods and whose mothers had higher levels of education were most likely to have better scores.

A healthy childhood begins before conception. Positive prenatal nutrition and other personal health practices, as well as social support to pregnant mothers, can help reduce low birth weight and other problems associated with birth. In 1996, 5.8% of all live births in Canada resulted in low-birth-weight babies (a total of 21,025 babies). Despite a parliamentary resolution in 1989 to eliminate child poverty by the year 2000, the number of young children who lived in low-income families increased from one in five in 1990 to one in four in 1995. These proportions are higher in Aboriginal and recently arrived immigrant communities and in families headed by very young parents and women who are single parents. Children in low-income families and neighbourhoods are at higher risk than children who grow up in families with higher incomes for infant death and low birth weight. They are more likely to experience developmental delays and injuries and to be exposed to environmental contaminants that have a negative effect on health. Research shows that even families with higher income sometimes have children who experience difficulties. The greatest proportion of children who experience difficulties are found in the bottom 20% of the socioeconomic scale. However, due to the large size of the middle class in Canada, the number of children not doing as well as they might is greatest in the middle socioeconomic group. Many parents, especially mothers, are highly stressed by time pressures as they try to balance work and family responsibilities. Low wages, part-time work without benefits, and shift work make it particularly difficult for young parents to spend time with their children and to obtain high-quality childcare when they are at work—without compromising their ability to provide the financial means required to support and raise healthy children.

With nurturing and consistent support in later years, many children can overcome early disadvantages. However, the preferred strategy is to prevent problems by providing all children with the social and physical environments they need to thrive. Traditionally, communities, governments, and the private sector have invested more time and money in the later years of childhood than they have in the first 6 years of life. Given the importance of this stage of development on future health and well-being, and the current time and economic pressures on young parents, we need to make at least the same investment in the early years. Supporting optimal child development in the early years will require direct action by the health sector, as well as collaboration with other public sectors (e.g., education, social services, and finance) and the many people and institutions that affect child development (e.g., families, schools, communities, workplaces, other governments, and the media). Ensuring a continuum of early stimulation and learning opportunities will need to be coordinated with entry to school at the junior or senior kindergarten level. Over time, investing in our youngest citizens will bring major benefits to Canadian society by raising a healthy population that is optimally prepared to deal with the challenges of a global economy and a changing society.

Community workers have long been involved in preserving and protecting the health of children; indeed, this focus was largely responsible for the advent of community nurses and social workers. Many policies have been legislated and many programs are in place at local, provincial, and federal levels to address this health determinant. Community-based nonprofit agencies and charitable organizations (such as faith-based institutions) have also exercised considerable leadership in this regard. Collaboration among communities, health agencies, schools, recreation services, and clubs dedicated to creating healthy children in healthy communities has been effective in creating supportive environments for children and strengthening community action to promote healthy child development.

Socioeconomic Environment

How does the socioeconomic environment influence health? Numerous studies from around the world have shown that social and economic conditions (often called the socioeconomic environment) affect both individual and collective health. There are a number of factors in the socioeconomic environment: employment and unemployment, working conditions, factors in the social environment (such as social support, civic participation, and violence), income and income distribution, and education and literacy. Although the links between income, income distribution, and health are clear, our understanding of how these links work is still evolving. A number of researchers have shown that small gaps in income in a population give individuals and groups of people a better sense of control, trust, and well-being. Large income gaps contribute to increases in crime and violence, deteriorating health and education delivery systems, and other social problems. Thus, middle- and high-income Canadians, as well as low-income Canadians (those who live below the Statistics Canada low-income cutoff [LICO]), stand to benefit from increases in income equality (Box 3-4).

BOX 3-4. LOW INCOME CUTOFF (LICO) DEFINITION

Poverty has a relative definition rather than an absolute one. Statistics Canada frequently updates its poverty lines based on changes in the proportion of average income devoted to essentials.

To create a method of defining and measuring poverty, the Working Group on Social Development Research and Information was created by Human Resources Development Canada, supported by social services ministers in the provinces and territories. It proposed a preliminary market basket measure of poverty—a "basket" of market-priced goods and services. The poverty line is based on the income needed to purchase the items in the basket. It can be adapted to the unique conditions of each province and settings within the provinces.

LICO defines as low-income those families that spend a significantly higher proportion of their income on food, shelter, and clothing than an average Canadian family of comparable size and community of residence. To be considered low income under the LICO definition, a family must spend more than 54.7% of its gross income on these necessities.

Wealth and Its Distribution

Canadians with low incomes are more likely than Canadians with high incomes to suffer illnesses and to die early. Canadians who live in the poorest neighbourhoods are more likely than residents of the richest neighbourhoods to die at an early age. As previously stated, children in low-income families and neighbourhoods are at higher risk than children who grow up in families with higher incomes for infant death and low birth weight. They are more likely to experience developmental delays and injuries. The number of young children who lived in low-income families increased from one in five in 1990 to one in four in 1995. These proportions are higher in Aboriginal and recently arrived immigrant communities and in families headed by very young parents and women who are single parents.

Only 47% of Canadians in the lowest income bracket rate their health as very good or excellent, compared with 73% of Canadians in the highest income group. Low-income Canadians are more likely to die earlier and to suffer more illnesses than Canadians with higher incomes, regardless of age, sex, place of residence, or cause of death. At each rung up the income ladder, Canadians have less sickness, longer life expectancies, and improved health. In 1995, children and unattached seniors (mostly women) were most likely to be living in low-income situations. In 1995, almost 50% of lone-parent, mother-led families were in low-income situations. However, poverty was not restricted to single-parent families. From 1990 to 1995, the percentage of married couples with children in low-income situations rose from 9.5% to 13% (a total of almost 460,000 families). In 1996, many Canadians faced housing affordability problems. At this time, some 58% of lone-parent families and 59% of older Canadians living in one-person households were spending more than 30% of their income on housing. Anecdotal evidence suggests that an increasing number of Canadians are homeless, including families with children, Aboriginal people, adolescents, and people with mental illness. Overall, inequalities in income distribution remained relatively constant in Canada between 1985 and 1995. This was largely due to the effect of redistributive taxes (e.g., child tax benefits) and transfer payments (GST rebates) that helped to offset a growing income gap between the 10% of Canadians with the lowest incomes and the 10% of Canadians with the highest incomes. Changes in income distribution are closely related to changes in employment and wages. In recent years, some workers have been gaining higher income levels, most notably older workers and those who are highly skilled. Others, especially young workers and lower paid, lower skilled men have experienced declines. Although women are making progress in the workplace, they still earn less than men, mainly because they hold the majority of the lowest paying jobs.

Education, Literacy, and Health

Canadians with low literacy skills and low levels of education are more likely than Canadians with high levels of literacy and education to be unemployed and poor and, subsequently, to suffer poorer health and to die earlier. In 1994–1995, about 17% of Canadians scored in the lowest prose literacy category; another 26% achieved the second level, which means that they can read, but not well. In 1995, Canada had twice the proportion of citizens who lacked adequate literacy skills as Sweden, the number one ranked country on this index. People with higher levels of education have better access to healthy physical environments and are better able to prepare their children for school than people with low levels of education. They also tend to smoke less, to be more physically active, and to have access to healthier foods.

In 1996, more young Canadians (especially women) were gaining advanced degrees than ever before. However, a core of young people leaves high school early. Most often, they are young men who are having difficulty in school and have limited emotional and financial support for staying in school. Young women who leave school early tend to do so because of pregnancy or other family problems. Lifelong learning opportunities in the later years may be particularly important for maintaining mental health and learning capacity in old age. The demand for workers with advanced knowledge and skills will continue to increase in the new millennium. Thus, addressing the challenges of literacy and education must be a priority for all parts of society: schools, workplaces, communities, governments, and families. Because of the important links between education, literacy, and health, the health sector needs to collaborate with other sectors to prevent teen pregnancies, to help young people stay in school, and to support learning opportunities in early childhood and later life, and to upgrade literacy programs for people of all ages.

The Physical Environment

The prevalence of childhood asthma has increased sharply over the last two decades, especially from birth to age 6. Children, especially poor children, are more vulnerable to airborne contaminants and other environmental toxins than adults. In 1995, at least 1.4 million Canadian children were exposed to environmental tobacco smoke in their homes. As we learned from the Walkerton, Ontario and North Battleford, Saskatchewan experiences, the hazards of contaminated water are significant for children and the elderly. In both instances deaths due to water contamination were in these population groups. The Sydney, Nova Scotia tar pond situation has also illustrated the impact of environmental contamination on health. Children's health has been adversely affected through high blood lead levels from industrial contamination of the soil. Climate change and environmental hazards in the food supply may have a particularly negative impact on Aboriginal people who depend on the land and water for their food supply.

Health Services

One of the challenges facing Canadians is how to renew and reorient the health sector to increase accountability and effectively improve the health of all Canadians. Canadians value their health care system and want to maintain high-quality care. But health services are among many factors that influence health. Factors in the socioeconomic and physical environments, as well as healthy child development, personal health practices, and biology have a major impact on health. These factors operate independently of whether or not we spend more money on health care.

Disease and injury prevention activities in areas such as immunization, seat belt use, and mammography, as well as health promotion efforts in areas such as early child development, are showing positive results. These activities must continue if progress is to be maintained.

The annual growth rate of Canada's insured health care expenditures fell from 11.1% between 1975 and 1991 to 2.5% between 1991 and 1996. Despite these spending slowdowns, Canadians did not report a significant increase in unmet health care needs in 1996–1997, and most measures of population health (such as life expectancy) continued to improve. At the same time, little information on the quality of care or the impact of restructuring was available.

However, some evidence suggests that the public's assessment of the overall quality of the health care system, although still largely favourable, has declined to some extent since the beginning of the 1990s. Although overall access to universally insured care remains largely unrelated to income, low- and moderate-income Canadians are less likely than high-income Canadians to have insurance for health services such as eye care, dentistry, mental health counselling, and prescription drugs, and they tend to report lower rates of use of such services. There has been a substantial decline in the average length of stay in hospital. Shifting care into the community and the home raises concerns about the increased financial, physical, and emotional burdens placed on families, especially women. The demand for home care has increased in several jurisdictions and there is a concern about equitable access to these services. Expenditures on medications and the use of prescription drugs have increased dramatically since 1975. In 1996–1997, 30% of

Canadians aged 12 and over and 46% of Canadians aged 75 and over used three or more medications.

Personal Health Practices

Rates of physical activity drop quickly as age increases and there are large differences between boys/men and girls/women. In the 12 to 14 age group, 54% of boys and 33% of girls were active in their leisure time. By age 20 to 24, the percentage of people who were active dropped to 39% among men and 22% among women. The proportion of overweight men and women in Canada increased steadily between 1985 and 1996–1997, from 22% to 34% among men and 14% to 23% among women. In 1994–1995, 51% of sexually active 15- to 19-year-old women who had more than one sex partner and 29% of sexually active young men in the same age group reported that they had had sex without a condom in the past year. Among 20- to 24-year-olds, 53% of sexually active women and 44% of men reported having had sex without a condom during the previous year. Injection drug use (IDU) and its relationship to HIV infection and hepatitis C is a major concern. In 1997, 20% of adult AIDS cases were attributed to IDU, compared with less than 2% prior to 1990 and 5% in 1993.

Populations at Risk

ABORIGINAL CANADIANS

Many Aboriginal communities and groups have made impressive improvements in education levels and equally impressive reductions in infant mortality rates and substance use. Despite these successes, Aboriginal people remain at higher risk for illness and earlier death than the Canadian population as a whole. Despite major improvements since 1979, infant mortality rates among First Nations and Inuit people in 1997 were still twice to three times as high as among the Canadian population as a whole. Life expectancy is significantly lower among Aboriginal people than the overall Canadian population (e.g., 7-9 years for Inuit). High rates of suicide and fatal unintentional injuries among First Nations and Inuit young people partly account for this difference. The prevalence of major chronic diseases, including diabetes, heart problems, cancer, hypertension, and arthritis/rheumatism, is significantly higher in Aboriginal communities and appears to be increasing.

Aboriginal people face a number of disadvantages in the underlying factors or "determinants" of health. Compared to Canadian families as a whole, a greater proportion of Aboriginal families are experiencing problems with housing and food affordability. These problems are likely linked to high levels of unemployment and pervasive low incomes. Aboriginal leaders have identified low incomes as a critical factor in their health status and have called for a better understanding of the links between income, social factors, and the health of their people.

In 1995, at least 44% of the Aboriginal population and a full 60% of Aboriginal children under the age of 6 lived below Statistics Canada's LICO rates. In 1996, the unemployment rate among First Nations people on-reserve was 29%; off-reserve it was 26%. Statistically, unemployed people have a reduced life expectancy and suffer more health problems than people who have a job. Inadequate housing and crowded living conditions are factors in the higher rates of respiratory problems and other infectious diseases among Aboriginal children, compared with non-Aboriginal children. Children in Aboriginal families also have high rates of unintentional injuries and early deaths from drowning and other causes. Young men (particularly in Inuit communities) are far more likely to commit suicide than their peers in Canada as a whole. Aboriginal children in some communities are more likely than children in the general population to begin adult behaviours such as smoking, drinking, and drug use at a young age.

CANADA'S YOUTH

A number of things are going well for young Canadians. For example, youth volunteering has increased dramatically and the number of young women completing postsecondary levels of education is at its highest point ever. At the same time, *Toward a Healthy Future* alerts to us some conditions affecting the psychosocial well-being of Canada's youth.

In contrast to the high levels of physical health enjoyed by most young Canadians, psychological well-being is, on average, lowest among this age group. Canadians aged 18 and 19 were the most likely to report high stress levels (37%) and to report being depressed. Women aged 15 to 19 were the most likely of any age-sex group to show signs of depression (9%). The 1996 suicide rate of 19/100,000 among young men aged 15 to 19 was almost twice as high as the 1970 rate. Suicide rates among young men aged 20 to 24 were even higher (29/100,000). The suicide rate for Aboriginal youth is much higher than for their peers in the general population. As in the case of the population at large, young men are the most likely to commit suicide.

Despite some recent improvements, youth unemployment and underemployment rates remain high. Between 1990 and 1995, the proportion of young people aged 18 to 24 (with their families or alone) who lived in low-income situations (i.e., below Statistics Canada LICOs) increased from 21% to 26%. Education is often an important factor in determining whether young people obtain jobs that enable them to support themselves and their families. Young people who leave school before high school graduation (22% of young men and 14% of young women in 1995) are more likely to dislike school, to have failed a grade in the past, to come from low socioeconomic backgrounds, and to be young parents. Young women aged 12 to 17 are particularly vulnerable to sexual abuse by a family member or date. Young women aged 18 to 24 are most likely of all age groups to report being assaulted by an intimate partner. Despite recent high-profile events of youth violence, in 1997, the percentage of young people aged 12 to 17 charged with Criminal Code offences dropped 7% from the previous year. The 1997 rate, however, was still more than double that of a decade ago. Over the last 10 years, the rate of young women charged with violent crimes has increased twice as fast as that of young men; however, young men are still three times more likely than young women to be charged with violent crimes.

Increased risk taking among young people may be a reflection of reduced opportunities and increased pressures to succeed. Unintentional injuries, most often due to motor vehicle collisions, are the leading cause of death and disability among young people. Teenagers are the only age group in which smoking levels continue to increase. Young women aged 12 to 17 are more likely than young men the same age to smoke. Many of them report that they smoke to manage stress and control their weight. Underage drinking and the combined use of alcohol, tobacco, and cannabis increased dramatically between 1991 and 1998 in several provinces. In 1996–1997, almost 50% of sexually active young people aged 20 to 24 and 40% of young people aged 15 to 19 reported an inconsistent or no use of condoms.

A Call to Action: The Population Health Promotion Approach

A population health promotion approach focuses on the conditions that underlie health, and then uses what is learned to suggest policies and actions that will improve the well-being of all Canadians. A population health approach uses both short- and long-term strategies to:

◆ Improve the underlying and interrelated conditions in the environment that enable all Canadians to be healthy

◆ Reduce inequities in the underlying conditions that put some Canadians at a disadvantage for attaining and maintaining optimal health

How can the health sector, whose traditional role is treating the sick, influence the root causes of health and help to reduce disparities in health status? The answer lies in a collaborative effort to renew and reorient the health sector so that it can:

◆ Take action to meet the emerging challenges in health promotion, injury and disease prevention and health protection, as well as in treatment services
◆ Increase the accountability of health services through improved reporting on the quality of health services, and improving access to all needed services
◆ Increase our understanding of how the basic determinants of health influence collective and personal well-being
◆ Evaluate and identify policy and program strategies that work
◆ Influence sectors outside of health that can significantly affect health status

Obviously, the health sector has a key direct role in improving health. But, because many of the determinants of health are outside the traditional system, building alliances with other sectors is a primary strategy for improving the health of the population. Other health-determining sectors that need to be involved include finance, justice, housing, education, recreation, the physical environment, employment, transportation, and social services. The ideal outcome of these collaborations will be healthy public policies in a variety of sectors, as well as in the health sector itself. The health sector cannot do it all nor can it impose its agenda on other sectors. It can, however, initiate dialogue and partnerships with others and act as a collaborator for change. All sectors stand to benefit from improvements in health and the conditions that influence health. Healthy, well-educated, productive citizens who nurture their young people and live in a civic, egalitarian, sustainable society feel in control of their destiny. They are better prepared to address the local, provincial/territorial, national, and global challenges of the new millennium. Improving health is everyone's business. Collaboration in the pursuit of the public's health needs to occur at all levels—families, neighbourhoods, communities, provinces and territories, regions, and in the country as a whole. Partners need to include voluntary, professional, business, consumer, and labour organizations, private industry, governments, and representatives of communities of faith, various cultures, population groups, and disadvantaged groups.

References

Federal Provincial Territorial Advisory Committee on Population Health. (1999). *Intersectoral action . . . Towards population health.* Ottawa: Health Canada.

Health Canada. (1999). *Second report on the health of Canadians.* Ottawa: Author.

Human Resources and Development Canada: http://www.hrdc-drhc.gc.ca/common/home.shtml.

Statistics Canada Home Page: http://www.statcan.ca/start.html.

United Nations Development Programme. (2002). *Human development report 2002.* Cary, NC: Oxford University Press.

Vollman, A. R., & Tenove, S. C. (2001). The Canadian health care system. In J. Ross Kerr and M. Wood (Canadian Eds.), *Canadian fundamentals of nursing.* St. Louis, MO: Mosby-Year Book.

4

Healthy Environments

OBJECTIVES

The community health practitioner needs to understand the principles and applications of human ecology as they affect health.

After studying this chapter you should be able to:

◆ Understand the mechanisms by which contaminants enter the human populations

◆ Apply this understanding to the promotion of health by the reciprocal adaptation of human behaviour and the physical and social environments

Introduction

Public health has embraced an ecological perspective on health with its roots in biology, epidemiology, and communicable disease control. Demography as a subdiscipline of sociology and geography emerged in the 1800s as scientists investigated population movement and settlement growth in relation to the environment's ability to support human populations. Further interest in human behaviour in different contexts was fuelled by the

---

*Contributions from the original chapter by Robert W. McFarlane and Judith McFarlane.

emergence of social psychology, social learning theory, and the interest in community practice by nursing and social work. In this chapter, the environmental determinants of health are examined, first from a traditional ecology perspective on which the field of health protection is based, and then from a social ecological foundation on which health promotion is based.

The Ecological Perspective

Physical and social environments play an important role in people's health and well-being. In virtually every physical setting in Canada—homes, schools, workplaces, and public places, whether built or natural—major health and safety issues must be considered. Environmental health issues are different for each person; people who differ by age, sex, family or household type, race, culture, level of health, degree of mobility, sexual orientation, and lifestyle vary also with respect to the environmental issues they encounter. Each physical setting, social situation, and economic condition creates a unique interaction between the person and the environment (Small, 1990).

Canadians are among the healthiest people in the world, but Health Canada (1997) asserts that constant vigilance and effort are required, not only by government and industry but also by individual Canadians, to keep ourselves healthy and to protect the nation's environment. We cannot afford to be complacent; the environment is under constant global, as well as local, pressure. Despite the fact that Canada compares very favourably with other countries, the nation still faces a variety of potential threats to health from the environment:

◆ Issues related to air quality (e.g., asthma, environmental tobacco smoke, indoor and outdoor air pollution, ultraviolet [UV] radiation, and global warming)
◆ Water contamination (e.g., microorganisms, chemicals)
◆ Food contaminants (e.g., bacteria and endocrine disruptors)
◆ Lead in the soil
◆ The impact of the built environment (e.g., automobile traffic injuries, stress, noise, housing)

To assess and manage environmental risks (whether they result from personal choice or substances, processes, or products in the environment) involves a process that identifies the specific hazards, estimates the associated level of risk, develops and analyzes potential options for managing that risk, selects and implements a risk management strategy, and monitors and evaluates the impact of the strategy chosen.

How people judge risks, that is, our *risk perception*, affects how we act and the decisions we make about avoidance, control, or protection. Risk perception is affected by many factors (e.g., age, sex, level of education, region of the country, values, previous exposure) and it changes over time as new information becomes available. Risk communication must take these factors into account. *Risk communication* involves the exchange of information about the existence, nature, form, severity, or acceptability of health or environmental risks (Health Canada, 1997). Some examples of risk communication include the provision of information to the public to assist people with making decisions (e.g., food product labels), alert the public to a significant risk (e.g., weather alerts, smog warnings) or calm concerns, and put certain public concerns in perspective (e.g., more risk of getting struck by lightning than being infected by the West Nile virus in Alberta in the summer of 2002).

Health Canada reports that over 90% of Canadians surveyed in 1996 believe our air, water, and land are more contaminated now than in 1989, and two of three people said their health had been affected by pollution. Nevertheless, despite several years of rising economic uncertainty and unemployment, three of four Canadians surveyed want current strict environmental regulation to continue (1997), affirming that the future health of the environment is more important than today's economic conditions.

Over the past century the environment has been used as a convenient disposal site for all sorts of wastes—biologic, radioactive, physical, and chemical (Fig. 4-1). Some parts of the country, in fact, display the results of these abuses, and many Canadians now have detectable levels of many contaminants in our blood, hair, and body tissues (e.g., polychlorinated biphenyls [PCBs], mercury, and lead), particularly if we live near manufacturing and processing plants or in remote areas. Fortunately, since reaching a peak in the 1970s, levels of many hazardous contaminants in the environment have declined dramatically. For instance, with the ban on leaded gasoline, air lead levels dropped to trace levels. Contaminants of both natural and human origin are still found in the air, water, food, and soil and have many adverse effects on human health (e.g., cancer, birth defects, respiratory diseases, and gastrointestinal illness). Built environment housing, urban planning, and the design of transportation systems affect psychological health and well-being. People's emotional health is affected by the extent to which our natural resources are preserved for recreation and leisure. Indeed, how well we conserve our resources has a direct impact on Canada's future economic health.

There are three broad categories of environmental contaminants:

1. Biologic agents—bacteria, protozoa, viruses, fungi, algae and their products, insects, pollens, and so forth

Source of contamination	Environmental media	Route of exposure	Receptor person or population at point of exposure

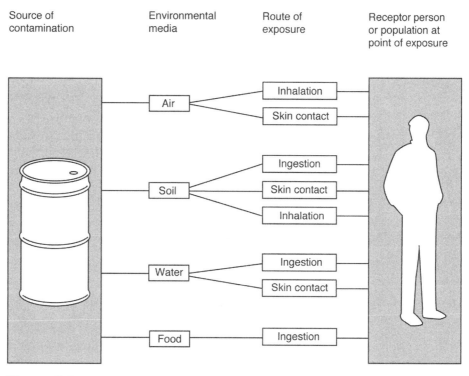

Figure 4-1 ◆ Major pathways and routes of human exposure to environmental contaminants. (From *Investigating human exposure to contaminants in the environment: A handbook for exposure calculations, Draft,* Health Canada, 1994, p. 7.)

2. Chemical agents—organic (carbon-containing) and inorganic compounds of human and natural origin
3. Radiation—natural or artificial sources of wave or particle energy that are ionizing (high energy, e.g., x-rays, radioactive substances) or non-ionizing (low energy, e.g., microwaves, UV light, electromagnetic fields, sound)

Ecological Interactions and Health

Interactions between organisms are particularly important in the cause, transmission, and persistence of disease. Infectious diseases fall into several broad categories, depending on the number of organisms involved. The simplest consists of only two members, a pathogen and its host. Smallpox is such a system; the virus is the pathogen and a human is the host. Infected individuals who recover are no longer susceptible to reinfection. The immune mechanisms can be stimulated with a vaccine, and, through this action, the host becomes immune to the pathogen. As the potential host population is reduced (by way of vaccination), the pathogen is unable to persist and will eventually become extinct.

Many diseases include a third party—a vector that transmits the pathogen from host to host without becoming infected itself. For example, the pathogen that causes the bubonic plague is a bacterium that is transmitted to humans (and other animals) through the bite of a flea. The bacterium is maintained in populations of rodents of various kinds. The rodents provide the reservoir wherein the bacillus persists; the fleas are merely vectors of transmission from an infected rodent to an uninfected rodent or to a human being. Humans are secondary hosts, but when the bacillus is introduced into a crowded human population, the results can be devastating, as has been demonstrated by the epidemics that occur every few centuries. These epidemics have disappeared on their own, not as the result of human countermeasures.

Pollution

Pollutants are the residues of things humans make, use, and throw away. Nondegradable pollutants either do not degrade or degrade very slowly in the natural environment. Biodegradable pollutants are rapidly decomposed by natural processes unless input exceeds decomposition or dispersal capacity. Degradable pollutants that provide energy or nutrients may increase the productivity of an ecosystem by providing a subsidy when the rate of input is moderate. However, high rates of input can cause productivity to oscillate, whereas additional input may poison the system completely.

When any pollutant is introduced into the environment, we must be concerned about both the fate of the pollutant (where it goes and how it gets there) and its effect on humans or any of the ecosystems on which we depend. We must always keep in mind that any effects that pollutants have on other species are early warning symptoms that something is amiss in the ecosystem and that humans may well be the next to be affected. There are five mechanisms of particular concern.

Major Pollutant Mechanisms

TRANSPORT

Transport of the pollutant, once it is introduced into the environment, is generally accomplished via wind patterns or aquatic systems. Pollutants can be dispersed aerially as particulates or in a gaseous state; they can travel long distances before falling to earth as dust or being carried in rain. Ironically, the construction of taller smokestacks to relieve local pollution generally results in greater dispersal, thus enlarging the area affected without diminishing the amount of pollutant released. Once air pollutants have settled to earth, they frequently continue their movement by travelling along waterways. Following a single heavy rainfall, runoff of storm water can mobilize more suspended particulates than may be transported during the rest of the year. Dissolved pollutants may be transported long distances before settling onto the bottom sediments through some precipitatory mechanism.

Pollutants generally exert greater influence on aquatic ecosystems than on terrestrial environments. Air pollutants may enter a person's lungs or settle on vegetation and then be eaten with the plants. Water, though, is nature's best solvent, and many pollutants go into solution in aquatic ecosystems, with the result that aquatic animals and plants live in a weakly polluted "soup." Many chemicals enter the biota directly through the skin or across gill surfaces because there is no escape from a dissolved pollutant. The effects of a given one-time polluting event, such as an accidental spill, are therefore exerted for a longer time in aquatic ecosystems. Not only is a greater portion of the pollution incorporated into and cycled within the biotic nutrient pool, but material that settles into the sediment can also be resuspended and redistributed with every major storm event. The dispersion of pollutants is also more restricted in aquatic systems than in terrestrial ones because movement is always downstream, until the pollutants reach the ocean. The efficacy of ocean transport has been demonstrated by the ubiquitous spread of several insecticides throughout the world; their area of distribution even includes the Antarctic continent.

TRANSFORMATION

Transformation of a pollutant within an ecosystem occurs in many ways. Harmful substances can be rendered innocuous or even helpful during the biodegradation process. But, occasionally, a relatively harmless substance is transformed into a noxious form. A classic example is the transformation of metallic or inorganic mercury, which is relatively immobile, into methylmercury by microorganisms living in aquatic sediments. Methylmercury is readily incorporated into detrital food chains, which may terminate with human consumption of contaminated fish and shellfish, producing the neurologic disorder known as Minamata disease. Nonbiogenic chemical transformations are more common in the environment (e.g., one such transformation is the conversion of sulphur dioxide and nitrous oxides in the atmosphere to form sulphuric and nitric acids and create acid rain).

BIOACCUMULATION

Bioaccumulation refers to the introduction of substances into ecological food webs. Chemicals that behave in a manner similar to essential elements are most susceptible to rapid uptake and retention. Chiefly because of human beings and their activities, the ecologist must now be concerned with the cycling of nonessential elements. For example, the radionuclides of strontium and cesium, whose chemical behaviour is analogous to calcium and potassium, respectively, are introduced into the environment by nuclear reactors and represent a potential health hazard.

BIOMAGNIFICATION

Biomagnification results when the accumulation of a pollutant greatly exceeds the rate at which an organism eliminates it. The pollutant is concentrated in organisms at a low trophic level, where it is further concentrated and passed to the third level, and so forth. For example, PCBs are a large class of 209 separate chemical compounds that held many industrial applications before 1978, when they were banned in Canada. Each of these compounds has a different type and degree of toxicity, bioaccumulates at different rates, and behaves differently when free in the environment. In the 1970s, these PCB compounds were associated with adverse health effects in people eating fish from the Great Lakes. The PCBs were acquired by phytoplankton that innocuously acted as tiny scavengers of the pollutant, reaching levels of only 2.5 parts PCB per billion parts of phytoplankton. These were then eaten by zooplankton, which, in turn, were eaten by larger zooplankton, in which PCB concentrations increased nearly 50-fold, reaching 123 parts per billion. The zooplankton were eaten by small fish, rainbow smelt, with PCBs increasing 9-fold to 1 part per million (ppm). Next, the smelt were eaten by lake trout, which reached 5 ppm PCB, and finally consumed by humans (or other end-chain carnivores). At each step, the PCBs were sequestered in the fatty tissue of the carrier and stored. The final concentration of PCBs in herring gull eggs, which are rich in stored fat and sometimes consumed by humans, was 124 ppm, or 50,000 times greater than the original concentration in the phytoplankton.

SYNERGISM

Synergism is the simultaneous action of separate substances or agencies that together produce a greater total effect than the sum of their individual effects. It is common to discover that a given substance behaves in one fashion in a controlled laboratory environment and quite another when introduced into a natural ecosystem, where it interacts with a number of physical and chemical properties of the environment.

TOXIC SUBSTANCES

In recent years, toxic substances have received a great deal of attention in governmental regulations and the news media. Any chemical can be toxic, including table salt, sugar, and the chlorine in drinking water. Toxic substances are generally considered to be any chemicals or mixtures of chemicals, either synthetic or natural, that are poisonous to humans or plants or animals under expected conditions of use and exposure. There are four major categories of toxic substances. Pesticides are lethal chemicals specifically designed to kill weeds, fungi, insects, mites, rodents, and other pests. Four pesticides have been banned from further use in Canada: DDT (1974) and aldrin, dieldrin, and chlordane (1984). Industrial chemicals are particularly numerous and a few have proven especially dangerous (e.g., asbestos, benzene, vinyl chloride, and PCBs). A number of metals, such as arsenic, lead, cadmium, and mercury, have also proven to be very toxic in the environment. The fourth category includes those substances with isotopes that emit various types of radiation, such as strontium, cesium, iodine, and so forth.

Approximately 60,000 different chemical substances are used in commercial activities in Canada and the United States today, and 98% of these chemicals are safe. In 1988, the baseline year for the U.S. Environmental Protection Agency (EPA) Toxics Release Inventory, 20,458 manufacturing facilities released 2.18 billion pounds of toxic wastes directly into the air and 164 million pounds were discharged to surface waters. By 1997, these releases had been reduced to 982 million pounds into the air and 61 million pounds to surface waters from 19,597 facilities.

Chemical toxicity occurs when a chemical agent produces detrimental effects in living organisms. The effects of a toxic substance can be immediate or long term and can harm selected tissues or the entire organism. Both the toxicity of the substance and the expected exposure to the organism must be considered to define the anticipated risk. Neurotoxins are likely the most significant toxic substances in both prevalence and severity that pose a risk to human health. Epidemiologically, a relatively small fraction of major neurologic disorders are inherited; most neurologic diseases appear to be associated with environmental factors. Many commercial chemicals used in very large amounts and known to persist in the environment have neurotoxic properties. In fact, insecticides, designed to have neurotoxic properties, are manufactured for deliberate release into the environment.

Pollutants and Human Population Size

All of the environmental processes described so far can influence human health. Any pollutant or toxic substance introduced into the environment is subjected to these processes, many of which lead directly to human beings. Pollution of the environment occurs when these pollutants overwhelm the capacity of the environment to assimilate them without being thrown out of balance. Thus, pollution is a rate function involving a quantity of pollutant introduced over a period of time. This rate is directly correlated to population size.

It can be said that all pollution is the result of population growth. A single family, living on a subsistence level in the wild, burning wood as their fuel and discarding rubbish and human wastes on the landscape, would seldom be a polluting factor in their environment. The population of a small village would denude the landscape of wood fuel, pollute the air with smoke from numerous wood fires, and litter the ground with rubbish and human wastes randomly dispersed. Cities, with more numerous inhabitants, totally overwhelm the environment with rubbish and human wastes, fostering the development of sewage and garbage disposal systems. Industrial development increases the number of pollutants and environmental insults. Our past practice for handling pollutants has been to just dump them, taking further action only when the natural systems have been overwhelmed. We need to reverse this practice and remove the bulk of pollutants before inflicting them on nature. Then the natural ecosystem can work for us by removing the final bit of pollution that always proves so difficult and expensive to neutralize.

Demographic changes can rapidly alter the stress inflicted on the environment. As population grows, the stress increases. If the population moves, both the nature and the intensity of an environmental problem can shift. For example, the recent decline of industrial productivity in the northeastern United States has resulted in a shift in the population caused by the exodus of workers (particularly younger families) and an improvement in the surface water quality. The growth of population in the south, especially the arid southwest, is both increasing water pollution and straining the overall water supply.

The solution to one environmental problem may be the creation of another. Pollutants do not disappear. Sulphur that is scrubbed out of power plant smokestack gases ends up as sludge stored on the ground, where it may threaten water quality. Pollutants removed from wastewaters by precipitation end up in the bottom sludge, which also requires disposal. Unfortunately, if the sludge is burned, the pollutants may be released into the air, to settle and become incorporated into the water or land once again. If the sludge is buried in a landfill, it may threaten surface water or groundwater supplies. Sewage treatment plants that aerate water as part of the process may discharge substantial amounts of volatile toxic substances to the air. Everything has to go someplace.

In summary, virtually any pollutant that is introduced into the environment will subsequently be transported away from its point of entry. It may be transformed into another chemical form, either less or more hazardous. It will probably be accumulated by biologic organisms, possibly becoming magnified in its concentration. It is likely to react with other chemicals or physical processes and to produce unanticipated effects. Distinct and efficient chemical cycles and pathways that have evolved over millions of years ensure that toxicants will enter biologic systems and eventually reach humans or other organisms on which they depend. Everything is connected to everything else, and everything has to go someplace. There is nowhere to hide. The only solution is to stop the pollution.

Health and the Environment— Partners for Life

In the next section, the findings from the Health Canada Report (1997) "Health and the Environment—Partners for Life" are summarized. The full text is available from the Health Canada website: http://www.hc-sc.gc.ca/ehp/ehd/ catalogue/general/97ehd215/ex_sum.pdf.

This report gives a comprehensive view of the contaminants that are of greatest concern to the health of Canadians. In the next section we explore the relationship between health and the quality of the air we breathe, the water we drink, the food we ingest, and the soil on which we live.

Air Quality

Air is a mixture of gases that surrounds the planet and makes up the atmosphere. Pure air consists of 21% oxygen and 78% nitrogen by volume, plus traces of other gases and water vapour. However, the composition of air can vary significantly both from one location to another and between indoors and outdoors because of the contaminants it contains. Contaminants in the air pose health risks to Canadians either directly through inhalation or indirectly through their effects on the environment. When inhaled, air pollutants can cause a variety of health effects, depending on their physical properties, concentration in the air, the rate and depth of breathing, and the health of those exposed. Young children, the elderly, and people with existing respiratory disease are more susceptible to the health effects of air pollution.

Asthma is a respiratory disease that affects more than one million Canadians. It is a chronic disease among children and is the leading cause for school absence. The costs to the health system from asthma are enormous—an estimated $500 million in 1990 and up to 100 deaths annually. Asthma can be triggered by a variety of airborne contaminants (e.g., dust, pollen, pets, tobacco smoke) and often requires hospitalization.

Natural sources of outdoor contaminants include smoke from forest fires, windblown dust particles from soil and volcanoes, fungi, bacteria, plants, and animals. Pollutants are also released from human sources such as motor vehicles, industrial processes, burning fuels, and so forth. The level of contamination in outdoor air is influenced by population density, degree of industrialization, local pollution emission standards, season, climate, and daily weather conditions. Air pollutants may originate from both local sources and remote locations, travelling thousands of kilometres from one part of the world to another through the phenomenon called "long-range atmospheric transport."

Indoor air quality is an increasingly important issue in Canada. Canadians spend nearly 90% of their time indoors and as a result of the natural flow of air inside and outside buildings, outside air quality can affect the quality of indoor air. Pollutants can arise from poor ventilation that allows contaminants from building materials, furnishings, heating, cooking, consumer products (e.g., tobacco), and the soil to build up indoors. This often results in "sick buildings." Air quality in Canada has improved as a result of the reduction in levels of the most common air pollutants through regulation of lead in fuel and paint, bans on chlorofluorocarbons (CFCs) that had been used in cooling systems, and emission controls on industry and agriculture. For instance, the oil and gas industry has taken measures over the past two decades to control emissions and reduce the gas well flaring (i.e., burning off the small amounts of natural gas that is found in the oil pumped from gas wells) that has been a cause of concern for Western Canadians (Petroleum Communication Foundation, 2000a, 2000b).

Since 1895, average global temperatures have increased by 0.5°C, a trend termed "global warming" caused by increasing levels of greenhouse gases in the atmosphere (Health Canada, 2001). Environmental experts predict the pace of global warming will increase markedly over the next few decades, causing natural disasters such as flooding, severe weather, and the migration of tropical diseases to the north. (See Table 4-1.)

UV radiation is one of the main causes of skin cancer in Canada. Some exposure to UV radiation is beneficial because it helps produce vitamin D, although dietary sources are also available. However, UV rays pose a health hazard to anyone who is exposed for long periods of time; in 1995 more than 55,000

TABLE 4-1 ◆ CANADA'S HEALTH IMPACTS FROM CLIMATE CHANGE AND VARIABILITY

Health Concerns	Examples of Health Vulnerabilities
Temperature-related morbidity and mortality	• Cold- and heat-related illnesses • Respiratory and cardiovascular illnesses • Increased occupational health risks
Health effects of extreme weather events	• Damaged public health infrastructure • Injuries and illnesses • Social and mental health stress due to disasters • Occupational health hazards • Preparedness and population displacement
Air pollution-related health effects	• Changed exposure to outdoor and indoor air pollutants and allergens • Asthma and other respiratory diseases • Heart attacks, strokes, and other cardiovascular diseases • Cancer
Water- and foodborne contamination	• Enteric diseases
Vector-borne infectious diseases	• Changed patterns of diseases caused by bacteria, viruses and other pathogens carried by mosquitos, ticks and other vectors
Stratospheric ozone depletion and increased exposure to UV radiation	• Skin damage and skin cancer • Cataracts • Disturbed immune function
Population vulnerabilities in rural and urban communities	• Disturbed immune function • Seniors • Children • Poor health • Low income and homeless • Traditional populations • Disabled • Immigrant populations
Health and socioeconomic impacts on community health and well-being	• Changed determinants of health and well-being • Global burden of disease • Vulnerability of community economies • Health cobenefits and risks of greenhouse gas reduction technologies

Canadians developed various forms of skin cancer and the incidence for malignant melanoma has doubled. Sun tanning is considered to be the primary cause for the present incidence because skin cancers can take years to appear, but future cases may well be influenced by the depletion of the earth's ozone layer that prevents UV radiation from penetrating the atmosphere.

Did You Know?

In 1992, Environment Canada scientists developed a method to predict the strength of the sun's UV rays based on day-to-day changes in the ozone layer. In the same year, Canada became the first country to issue nation-wide daily predictions of UV radiation levels. The UV rating is now a common feature of daily weather forecasts.

These and other issues associated with airborne contaminants to which Canadians are directly exposed through inhalation are discussed in the full report and include tobacco smoke; commonly measured air pollutants, such as ground-level ozone (smog), carbon monoxide, and particulates; biologic agents, such as fungi, bacteria, and dust mites; hazardous organic compounds, such as benzene; metals, such as lead, cadmium, chromium, and nickel; and radon and other natural or artificial radionuclides in the air.

Water Quality

Health Canada reports that this country contains 15% of the earth's fresh water supply. However, 60% of our water exists far from heavily populated areas, where it is needed for human use. The proportion that is accessible, although generally of high quality, often contains small amounts of environmental contaminants. Compared with other media, such as food and air, drinking water is a minor source of most pollutants—although it is our principal source of exposure to some microorganisms and to water disinfection by-products. The estimated health care costs related to water pollution are $300 million per year.

About 87% of Canadians receive treated municipal tap water. With a few exceptions, the most potentially serious contamination problems involve tap water from untreated sources, such as private wells. Recent outbreaks of waterborne disease (e.g., *Escherichia coli*, cryptosporidium) in Ontario (Kitchener-Waterloo, Collingwood, Walkerton), Kelowna, British Columbia, and North Battleford, Saskatchewan have affected thousands of people and have been responsible for several deaths. Chlorine is a simple, effective, yet relatively inexpensive agent for destroying harmful microorganisms in tap water, although it can generate potentially harmful by-products that have been linked to certain cancers. A recent Health Canada study found that long-term consumption of chlorinated surface water with elevated levels of such by-products is associated with an increased risk of bladder cancer and possibly colon cancer. The health risks associated with drinking unchlorinated water, however, are much higher than the risks posed by chlorination by-products, as is evident in developing countries with inadequate water treatment systems.

Did You Know?

Many Canadians believe that bottled water is safer to drink than municipal tap water, although this is not necessarily the case.

Water fluoridation helps prevent tooth decay in children without endangering their health. However, even at optimal levels, fluoride may cause dental fluorosis in some children, a generally mild condition involving tooth discolouration. Despite claims to the contrary, there is no evidence that fluoridated water causes heart disease, cancer, thyroid problems, birth defects, miscarriages, or hearing or vision problems. About 100,000 home water treatment devices are sold annually in Canada. When not used properly, some devices can become health hazards. Studies have shown that levels of bacteria present in water that has passed through an improperly maintained home filtration device may be up to 2000 times higher than levels in unfiltered water.

Did You Know?

In the world as a whole, diarrhea due to infectious (waterborne) microbes is responsible for more deaths each year than AIDS and cancer combined. Globally, about 34,000 deaths occur daily from water-related diseases. This is equivalent to 100 jumbo jets crashing daily.

The section on water in the full report "Health and the Environment—Partners for Life" describes in more depth the health issues associated with contaminants in the water supply, including biologic agents, such as bacteria and protozoa; water disinfection by-products; pesticides and other organic pollutants; metals, such as aluminum, arsenic, and uranium; fluoride; nitrates; and radionuclides.

Food Safety

Health Canada (1997) reports that Canadians are exposed to environmental contaminants primarily through food, although the levels of many pollutants found in commercial foods are kept very low by strict control through federal and provincial legislation and by voluntary actions taken by food producers, processors, and packagers. Microbial food-borne diseases, which cost, in health care terms, an estimated $1 billion per year in Canada, appear to pose a significant risk to our health. However, proper food handling and cooking practices could probably prevent most adverse incidents.

Did You Know?

Thorough cooking kills parasites in fish and meat. Cooking fish to an internal temperature of 60°C for several minutes usually kills any parasites present in the flesh. Beef should be heated to 65°–75°C and pork requires temperatures of 70°–75°C.

Contaminants can enter the food supply through a number of different routes and sources. Most contamination arises from natural processes or from the normal operation or use of various human technologies and products. Contamination may occur at the site of production, in the processing plant, at the distribution centre, in the retail outlet, and in your refrigerator or even on your kitchen counter. For example, crops may become contaminated as a result of the atmospheric deposition of pollutants or through the uptake of contaminated water that is used in the growth or processing. Food may become contaminated through contact with microorganisms (and the toxins they produce) during processing and packaging, during handling and storage, or through the improper preparation of foods in restaurants or homes.

Many food contaminants pose a risk to human health, although the length of time before health effects appear can vary. For example, bacteria typically produce adverse effects within hours or days of exposure when ingested at sufficiently high levels. By contrast, some chemical contaminants may produce noticeable health effects only after decades of continuous exposure to elevated levels, or they may ultimately have no impact on our health at all. Our exposure to food-borne contaminants is affected by many factors: food availability, the preparation method, the amount and type eaten, age, occupation, sex, health status, culture, religion, socioeconomic factors, geography, and the nature of the contaminant. People who have high intakes of wild game, birds, fish, and shellfish are exposed to higher levels of contamination. Some groups are more susceptible than the general population to the effects of food-borne contaminants (e.g., unborn babies, breast-fed infants, the elderly, and people with weakened immune systems).

Food accounts for 80% to 95% of our total daily intake of persistent organic pollutants and pesticides. As a result of stringent controls placed on these substances, levels in the environment and in human breast milk have fallen significantly. For example, PCB concentrations in some species of Great Lakes fish are about 10 times lower than they were in the 1960s. Certain organic pesticides that are no longer registered in Canada may persist in soil or enter our environment through long-range atmospheric transport from countries where they are still in use.

> **Did You Know?**
>
> The quarter of the population with the lowest dietary intake of fruits and vegetables compared to the quarter with the highest intake has roughly twice the cancer rate for most types of cancer.

Fruits and vegetables may contain natural substances that have been shown to cause cancer in laboratory animals. However, studies have shown that individuals with diets rich in fruits and vegetables have a significantly reduced risk of cancer, possibly because of the presence of "anticarcinogens"— substances that may reverse or inhibit the development of cancer.

Since the 1970s when mercury contamination was first reported in Canada, mercury levels in the blood and hair of First Nations and Inuit peoples have dropped significantly. However, the mercury threat has disrupted severely the social and cultural practices in Aboriginal communities; in many instances fishing enterprises, hunting, and gathering food from the land has been restricted as a result of environmental contaminants forcing communities to import food at high cost, impose new diets on residents that have contributed to obesity and the diabetic epidemic, and find new ways to support the economy. Further, without the availability of outdoor cultural and social pursuits that hunting and fishing offer, social ills such as violence and substance abuse have developed because of inactivity and boredom.

Workplace exposure to high levels of some endocrine disruptors is associated with lower sperm counts, decreased fertility, and altered development of the reproductive tract. It is not known, however, whether such substances can cause adverse effects at the levels found in our environment.

For a more complete discussion of the health issues associated with contaminants in our food supply, including biologic agents, such as microorganisms, parasites, and natural toxins; persistent organic pollutants (POPs), such as chlorinated dioxins and furans; heavy metals; and radionuclides, as well as an examination of the potential health impact of pesticides and food additives—substances that, by definition, are not considered "contaminants" because they are intentionally used to grow or enhance the value of foods, please refer to the text for the full report of the section on food, located on the Health Canada website:http://www.hc-sc.gc.ca/ehp/ehd/catalogue/general/97ehd215/food.pdf.

Soil Safety

As a cornerstone of our environment, soil plays a central role in our planet's life support system. Soil stores and recycles essential nutrients such as nitrogen and thus supports the plant and animal life that forms the basis of our food chain. To a limited extent, soil also serves as a natural waste treatment plant. Microorganisms found in soil break down and recycle dead plant and animal matter, and they even feed on chemical contaminants, gradually breaking them down into (generally) less harmful substances. However, when soil is heavily contaminated, it can endanger our health. Soil contaminants may pose a human health risk as a result of the accidental ingestion of soil particles or as a result of their migration into air, water, and food. Few soils exist that have not been contaminated to some degree, however small, although the extent of contamination varies widely from place to place.

The ancient Greeks labelled *soil* (or earth) one of the four fundamental elements of the environment, along with water, air, and fire. Today, soil is defined as a complex mixture of crumbled rock, organic matter, moisture, and gases that varies in texture and composition. Soil contamination was a common occurrence long before humans began to alter their surroundings.

Soil contaminants may pose a health risk to Canadians either directly or indirectly. For example, soil quality affects the quality of crops, which in turn affects human health. Additionally, people may ingest small amounts of soil, particularly when produce has not been adequately washed, or they may inhale airborne soil particles during outdoor activities. Infants and toddlers may consume soil (or house dust) directly by sucking their fingers. Tiny amounts of soil may also enter our bodies through skin absorption or may be ingested from dirty hands. In addition, pollutants present in soil may reach us through more indirect routes. Soil gases such as radon may seep into our houses, offices, and other buildings, contaminating the air we breathe.

Crops grown in contaminated soils may take up various pollutants and be eaten by people or by livestock, which are, in turn, consumed by humans. Soil pollutants may also leach into water bodies, particularly groundwater (approximately 26% of Canadians rely on groundwater for domestic use). Population increases, urban sprawl, agricultural chemicals, and unsound waste management practices have adversely affected soil quality in many areas of the country.

Natural catastrophes (e.g., volcanoes, floods, forest fires) as well as every day phenomena (e.g., weather, combustion, and erosion) release contaminants into the soil. Some microorganisms, plants, and animals release harmful substances into their surroundings. Soil contaminants released by natural sources include metals, radioactive elements, and microbial toxins.

Various human activities, such as agriculture, manufacturing, mining, and waste disposal, are also responsible for vast amounts of pollutants entering our soil each year. Contaminants released by human sources include organic compounds, such as pesticides, chemicals, petroleum and its by-products, and inorganic compounds such as heavy metals. From the soil, these substances may ultimately end up contaminating our food, air, or water.

In sheer numbers, as well as their potential to cause harm, old or inadequate waste disposal sites are among the principal sources of soil (and groundwater) contamination today. The majority of waste disposal sites in Canada are rather primitive facilities in which garbage is piled in layers, and few precautions are taken to prevent contaminants from leaking into the surrounding soil. Across the country, more than 10,000 active, closed, or abandoned public waste disposal sites have been identified, excluding privately owned landfills. Approximately 10% of these sites are believed to pose a potential risk to human health or the environment, including contaminated industrial sites, municipal waste dumps, and locations where large chemical spills have occurred.

Older homes are a potential source of lead-based paint dust and contaminated soil. Young children are at highest risk of exposure because of their habit of placing objects or dirt into their mouths. Elevated lead levels in blood are associated with behavioural and developmental problems in children and with adverse reproductive effects in adults. Average blood lead levels in Canadian children are significantly lower today than in the 1970s. To estimate the number of children for whom a concern may exist, it is assumed that 5% to 10% of urban children have more lead in their bloodstream than the lowest level (10 µg/dL) at which adverse effects have been identified.

Wood preservatives can migrate out of treated wood and waste materials into soil and may contaminate groundwater supplies. Treatments are added to products to prevent decay, rot, and insect infestation.

Leaking motor fuels and oils, lead, and pesticides are other soil contaminants that affect the health of Canadians. Other contaminants commonly found in soil were addressed in the air, food, or water sections of this chapter. For a more complete discussion, refer to the Health Canada website: http://www.hc-sc.gc.ca/ehp/ehd/catalogue/general/97ehd215/soil.pdf. Waste management issues are discussed in the section on the built environment.

The Built Environment

According to the Health Canada report (1997), most Canadians spend more time indoors than outdoors and live in or near cities. We are as much a part of our fabricated or *built* environment as we are part of our natural environment. The built environment encompasses all of the buildings, spaces, and products that are created or significantly modified by humans. It includes our homes, schools, workplaces, parks, business areas, and roads. It extends overhead in the form of electric transmission lines, underground in the form of waste disposal sites and subway trains, and across the country in the form of highways.

In Canada, the built environment is generally cleaner and healthier today than it was 100 years ago. Although it still has an impact on our health, the magnitude of the effects is minor compared with what it once was. In the 1800s and early 1900s, many health problems plagued the towns and cities that developed in Canada. For example, overcrowding and improper sanitation fostered the spread of communicable diseases. Uncontrolled pollution affected air and water quality. Political leaders responded by introducing piped water, sewers, and garbage disposal services. Zoning was used to ensure that most new residential areas were kept away from industrial areas. Building and fire codes raised housing standards. Such legislation, along with advances in medical treatment and nutrition, resulted in significant improvements in the health of Canadians.

During World War II and the postwar years, the accelerated industrialization of the Canadian economy led to a relative increase in incomes, which was accompanied by further improvements in health status. Notable demographic changes included a population migration from the country to the city, the "baby boom," in which Canada's birth rate soared, and foreign immigration to urban areas. As the prosperity and growth continued, suburbs zoned for residential uses were built further from urban centres. Industries moved to new industrial parks located along major roads, often at the edge of town. In large urban areas, expressways were cut through older residential areas to provide faster access from the suburbs to the downtown area. This contributed to the decline of inner-city housing areas, which were increasingly populated by low-income families. One of the main impacts of segregating land according to residential, commercial, and industrial uses is an increase in commuting. Vehicular travel is a significant source of air pollution, stress on the driver, and preventable injuries. In areas where public transit is inadequate, people who do not own cars face mobility problems because walking and cycling are not always feasible alternatives.

Many aspects of the built environment can affect our health, including the design and construction of our homes, schools, and workplaces, as well as the products we buy, how we use them, and the waste products they generate. For example, the fertilizers and pesticides we put on our lawns, gardens, and crops can run off into rivers and lakes or seep into ground water, where they may contaminate drinking water supplies or the waters we use for recreational activities. Similarly, motor vehicle emissions can affect our air quality and respiratory health. The way our communities are planned and built can also affect our health, including such aspects as the availability of affordable housing, public transportation and bicycle paths, and the design of public spaces. For example, people are more likely to exercise when facilities are located near their homes. Commuting can have a negative impact on the psychological state of commuters and the quality of social life. And the parks we build can provide opportunities for reducing stress and meeting our spiritual needs. On an international scale, the cumulative impact of the way we live in our urban and rural areas can affect the health of the environment, which in turn can affect our health.

In Canada, urban land is generally segregated according to residential, commercial, and industrial uses. Canadian cities are spread out over a large area, which discourages walking and cycling, and the construction and maintenance of services, such as public transit, are expensive. Studies have shown that suburban residents drive twice as far, walk and cycle one third as often, consume double the energy, and produce twice the air pollution as their downtown neighbours.

Did You Know?

One in four Canadians feels unsafe walking in their own neighborhood at night: 10% of men and 42% of women.

Did You Know?

Reducing the fear of crime is an important part of the job of protecting communities. To reassure the public, many police forces are increasing their community presence by reinstating foot patrols.

Noise pollution can come from a number of sources, including road, rail, and air traffic, construction and industrial activities, motorboats, snowmobiles, and loud music. Environmental noise is stressful, interfering with sleep, communication, and relaxation. It is not known whether its effects on our well-being increase the risk of illness.

Limited access to affordable housing is a common problem in First Nations communities, especially in northern Canada. Overcrowding as a result of housing shortages can accelerate the spread of communicable diseases.

Injury, not disease, is the leading cause of death in infants and children under the age of 14. Each year, approximately 1000 children die from causes related to unintentional injuries. Motor vehicle traffic accidents are the leading injury-related cause of death in this age group.

Insufficient lighting in buildings can cause headaches and eyestrain. In the workplace, excessive heat and humidity can make employees feel lethargic, whereas insufficient heat and humidity can make them restless and easily distracted.

In 1993, there were more than 12 million cars in Canada, almost one for every two Canadians—one of the highest ratios of car ownership in the world. Engine exhaust from motor vehicles is the largest single source of outdoor air pollution; automobiles alone account for 10% of all carbon dioxide emissions in Canada. However, federal regulations controlling automobile emissions have led to a significant decline in the concentrations of several common air pollutants over the past two decades.

The health impact of low-level exposure to electromagnetic fields (EMFs) is unknown. Most studies have failed to establish a clear association between exposure to EMFs from common household electric appliances or from living in proximity to high-tension electricity lines and adverse health effects. However, there is enough anecdotal evidence to cause a level of anxiety among some members of the community to cause scientists at Health Canada to assess the potential cancer risks associated with extremely low-frequency EMFs and prepare safety guidelines for radio-frequency emissions.

More than 32 million tonnes of solid wastes are generated in Canada each year, including residential, commercial, institutional, light industrial, and construction wastes. More than 90% of the Canadian population now has access to recycling programs, either curbside or depot, for one or more household products.

The full report (Health Canada, 1997) discusses in detail urban systems, housing and the home environment, work and school environments, transportation, waste management, human-made sources of radiation, and environmental emergencies. The report is located on the Health Canada website: http://www.hc-sc.gc.ca/ehp/ehd/catalogue/general/97ehd215/built.pdf.

Future Challenges: Sustainable Development and Environmental Health

Because Canada is taking a population approach to health and development, it is imperative that we recognize the impact the environment has on people as it interacts with other health determinants—personal health practices, genetics, gender, culture, early child development, income, employment, education, health services, and social support.

Did You Know?

"Perhaps the greatest challenge we face to ensure our long-term health and the health of our environment is to create a more sustainable society—or, in other words, to embrace the concept of *sustainable development*. Sustainable development is development that meets the needs of the present without compromising the ability of future generations to meet their own needs. Sustainable development involves the integration of economic, social, and environmental goals, taking into account effects on health. It reflects the fact that development is essential to satisfy human needs and to improve the quality of human life, but it must be based on the efficient and environmentally responsible use of all of society's scarce resources: natural, human, and economic." (Health Canada, 1997, p. 164)

The Complex Human Environment

The preceding section has described humans interacting with the physical world and other species in a simplistic fashion. The complete human environment is difficult to comprehend because of the multiplicity of interrelated elements. The delivery of health care sometimes goes awry because the influence of certain elements is underestimated or unappreciated. A conceptual model of the human environment from an ecological viewpoint can often illuminate the problem and guide efficient intervention.

An ecological model (Fig. 4-2), like most models, proposes a framework from which to study and understand a phenomenon. A complete enumeration of all salient components of human health would be too complex to illustrate; therefore, this model is limited to environmental variables. The environment is the world that surrounds people wherever they go, whatever they do. An ecological approach to the study of human health relates the biologic, physical, sociocultural, and politicoeconomic components of our environments to any deviation in our state of health. The model can be applied to study the health of any defined subpopulation (e.g., infants, children, adolescents, and the elderly) as well.

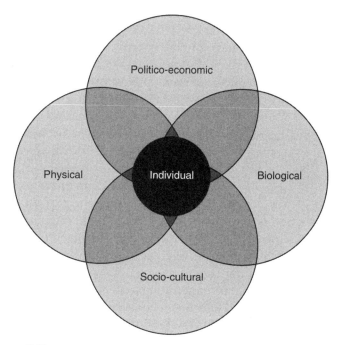

Figure 4-2 ◆ The environmental subsystems that affect each individual.

Environmental systems not only act on the individual person but also inter-act with one another, and a change occurring in one system will frequently affect others. Each system consists of components that act with and on other systems to bring about equilibrium or disequilibrium within the system.

Change occurs within a system when one variable acts on a second variable to force alteration. Climate and topography are variables within the physical system that can act separately or in unison to cause change within the other systems. For example, food distribution (determined by a set of politicoeco-nomic variables) depends on the production ability of the land (determined by physical variables such as climate and topography), which, in turn, influences the selection and consumption of food (determined by sociocultural variables); all of these affect human growth (a biologic variable).

The environmental systems show both interdependence and intradepen-dence in function and effect. The systems (depicted as circles in Fig. 4-2) inter-face with each other and overlap to form a network that encases the individual (the inner circle of Fig. 4-2). At any time, all systems may impinge on the indi-vidual simultaneously.

Layered within the systems is a hierarchy of four subsystems: the individual, the family unit, the community (ecologically speaking, the human population), and the nation (Fig. 4-3). Each subsystem is conditioned for the occurrence of illness by the environmental systems. When acted on, the subsystems interact both intradynamically and interdynamically to mitigate or reinforce the condi-tioning influences of the systems' variables; in this way, the subsystems modi-fy the systems. Each subsystem is also influenced by its developmental stage. For instance, an individual may react to an external perturbation differently as an infant, child, adolescent, adult, or elder. A family may be small or extended, with young or school-age children, semi-independent adolescents, or elderly parents to accommodate. A community may be small, homogeneous, and cohe-sive or large, diverse, and divisive. A nation may be agrarian, industrial, and poor or rich in human and natural resources.

To explain, a family with inadequate access to the basic needs of food and shelter (conditioned by politicoeconomic production and accompanying distri-bution policies) may act to change these impediments by migrating to an area of improved access to basic needs. Migration, in turn, can force change in the intrafamily physical, biologic, sociocultural, and politicoeconomic composition of the community and nation.

Conceptually, both the subsystems and environmental systems are in a con-stant state of interaction (everything is connected to everything else and is con-stantly changing). Enumerating the variables within the systems and measur-ing the interaction among them is the key to operating the model. In Figure 4-3, the environmental systems and subsystems are displayed in a tabular

ENVIRONMENTAL SYSTEMS

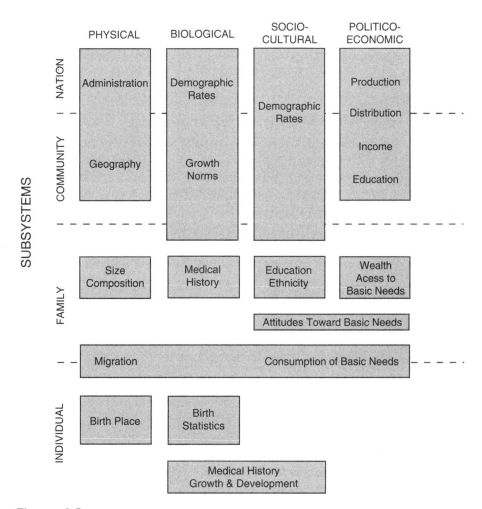

Figure 4-3 ◆ The environmental systems and subsystems affecting human health.

arrangement, with variables boxed according to the systems most acutely affected by their interaction. Certain variables, such as migration and consumption of basic needs, equally interact with all systems as they affect the family and individual's functioning. Other variables, such as birth statistics (age at birth, sex, birth order, and condition), are primarily within one system, affecting one developmental stage (the child) of one subsystem (the individual). Lines encasing variables are not set boundaries; rather, they serve as a guide to identify the system and subsystem most affected by variable manipulation.

The purpose of the conceptual model is to offer a framework from which to select significant variables related to the health status of a chosen individual. The variables that appear in Figure 4-3 are a synthesis of the epidemiologic, demographic, and social health indicators consistently proposed, tested, and recommended as valid and reliable indices of child health.

Social Ecology

The field of social ecology has evolved over recent decades to take the ecological perspective a step further in considering how humans interact mutually and reciprocally with the environment, constructing and being shaped by it at the same time. *Social ecology* is defined as a reconstructive, ecological, communitarian, and ethical approach to society. It is an interdisciplinary field informed by and contributing to knowledge in the social, behavioural, legal, environmental, and health sciences. Social ecologists apply scientific methods to the study of a wide array of recurring social, behavioural, and environmental problems. Among issues of interest are crime and justice in society, social influences on human development over the life cycle, and the effects of the physical and social environments on health and human behaviour. Although the field of ecology focuses on the relationships between organisms and their environments, social ecology is concerned with the relationships between human populations and their environments. The interdisciplinary nature of social ecology is based on the core belief that the analysis and amelioration of complex societal problems requires interdisciplinary and intersectoral effort.

An ecological model of population health promotion acknowledges health as a product of the interdependence of person with the ecosystem. The ecosystem comprises subsystems such as family and community, culture, physical environment, and social context. The ecosystem must offer the following to promote the health of the population (Fig. 4-4): physical, economic, and social environments conducive to health and healthy lifestyles; education and information so that people can make health-enhancing choices; and available goods and services that are health promoting (Green, Richard, & Potvin, 1996).

Population health promotion is drawn to social ecology because it offers a broader perspective to understanding health behaviours and attitudes; individuals are not solely responsible for their actions because the environment exerts an effect on their perceptions and choices. Ecology also offers lessons for health practitioners against tampering with any part of the system without considering the consequences on other parts. For instance, urban planning decisions had a huge impact on the pace of inner city decay and the quality of life of the people living there. As a consequence, when fitness proponents used the

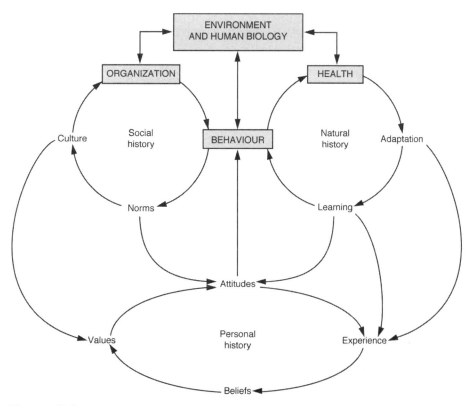

Figure 4-4 ◆ The place of social and personal histories in the development of lifestyle (behavior) and health shows the interaction of biological, environmental, social, and other determinants of coummunity health. (Green, L. W., & Ottoson, J. M. [1995]. *Community health* [7th ed.]. St. Louis: Mosby-Year Book.)

Lalonde Report (1974) to promote healthy lifestyles without considering social context, it created the unanticipated effect of victim blaming when people who lived in inner-city neighbourhoods were found to be less fit than their suburban counterparts that lived in aesthetically pleasant surroundings removed from traffic, smog, and crime. Now, however, the stress generated by urban sprawl is forcing governments to examine transportation issues, location of industries and business, and means to strengthen local communities as self-sustaining entities.

Social ecology is built on the philosophy of reciprocal determinism that states that human behaviour is mediated by interaction with the environment. The environment controls or sets limits on the behaviour that occurs within it, and changing the environment results in the change of behaviour. Population health promotion seeks to enhance people's ability to exercise control over the conditions (environmental or behavioural) that affect health and quality of life.

The environment is a factor that predisposes, enables, and reinforces individual and collective behaviour. People will behave differently when observed in different environments; witness the hockey fan at a game and when at worship. Thus, to be most effective, health promotion interventions depend on the fit between people, the health issue, and the environment. Because of the complexity of this ecology, population health promotion must be interdisciplinary and multisectoral to address the organizational levels, social sectors, and political systems involved in creating the environment in which people live, work, play, and go to school.

Summary

Social and economic conditions affect people's health. Unemployment, poverty, work pressures, stress, family problems, prejudice, victimization, isolation, and lack of control over their lives all have an adverse effect on people's physical and mental health (Small, 1990).

There is a wide range of vulnerability in the population; each individual is unique in the response to factors in the physical environment. There appear to be limits to people's ability to adapt to changing environmental conditions; some people seem to be unable, whether temporarily or otherwise, to adapt to changing conditions (McFarlane & McFarlane, 2000).

Many of the environments in which we live do not accommodate the full range of human needs. When public places (e.g., buildings, schools, workplaces) are accessible to people who are disabled, less mobile than others, or chemically hypersensitive, society benefits—physically, from safety features, and socially, from their presence (Small, 1990).

Many groups of Canadians are in situations that expose them to unhealthy environments. The devaluing or undervaluing of certain groups of people (e.g., the poor, women, immigrants, elderly, gays and lesbians, Aboriginals, homeless, unemployed, and disabled people) has produced widespread disparities between their social and physical environmental conditions and those in which other Canadians live (Advisory Committee on Population Health [ACPH], 1999).

It is becoming increasingly evident in the literature that having strong personal and social support networks is an important determinant of health. People who are isolated are more susceptible than others to ill health, recover more slowly, and suffer from decreased quality of life.

Population health promotion practitioners seek to find ways of enabling individuals and groups of Canadians to have greater control over where and how they live, work, play, pray and go to school. Creative effort is needed at every system level (individual, family, community), in every portfolio of government, by every human service discipline, and in every social institution (schools, churches) to create conditions that ensure that every Canadian has control over his or her life and access to a diversity of choice. Deciding how or where to live, what work to do, what education or lifestyle to pursue is impossible if you lack resources or experience conditions that limit opportunity and choice.

References

Federal, Provincial and Territorial Advisory Committee on Population Health (ACPH). (1999). *Toward a healthy future: Second report on the health of Canadians*. (Cat. H39-468/1999E, ISBN 0-662-27625-6). Ottawa: Health Canada.

Green, L. W., Richard, L., & Potvin, L. (1996). Ecological foundations of health promotion. *American Journal of Public Health, 10*(4), 270–281.

Health Canada. (1997). *Health and environment—Partners for life*. (Cat. H49-112/1997E, ISBN 00662-26149-6). Ottawa: Public Works and Government Services Canada.

Health Canada. (2001). *Climate change and health and well-being: A policy primer*. (Cat. H/46-2/01-260, ISBN 0-662-66266-0). Ottawa: Public Works and Government Services Canada.

McFarlane, R. W., & McFarlane, J. (2000). Ecologic connections. In E. T. Anderson & J. McFarlane (Eds.), *Community as partner: Theory and practice in nursing* (3rd ed., pp. 49–77). Philadelphia: Lippincott Williams & Wilkins.

Petroleum Communication Foundation. (2000a). *Flaring: Questions and answers*. Calgary: Author.

Petroleum Communication Foundation. (2000b). *Sour gas: Questions and answers*. Calgary: Author.

Small, B. (1990). Healthy environments for Canadians: Making the vision a reality. *AEHA Quarterly*, Winter. Retrieved from: http://www.environmentalhealth.ca/w90vision.html.

Ethics and Advocacy in Community Practice

OBJECTIVES

After studying this chapter, you should be able to:

◆ State the ethical principles on which community practice is founded

◆ Describe the rights of people in the community

◆ Outline the key sources of ethical problems in community practice

◆ Understand the roles of advocacy and public participation in social justice and how they affect empowerment at the community level

Introduction

Traditionally, health care and human services ethics have focused on the individual client/patient. Defining the community as partner, however, offers a different ethical approach, that of advocacy (Schroeder & Gallow, 2000). An ethic of advocacy calls for formation of partnerships among professionals and community members to enhance community self-determination. The aim of such partnerships is to improve community health and well-being *as defined by the members of the community* rather than as defined by professionals (Schroeder & Gallow, 2000, p. 79). Taking an advocacy approach to community practice dictates that the views of all groups in the community be incorporated in the community processes of assessment, analysis, intervention, and evaluation. This makes each community, population, or aggregate profile unique to the community that develops it. Diversity is embraced, people take part in decision-making, and resultant program planning efforts are aimed at implementing initiatives that are tailored to the situation, setting, and target population.

Ethics in Community Practice

Ethics is defined as the "philosophic analysis of morality, the systematic endeavour to understand moral concepts, and justify moral principles and theories" (Pojman [1992] as cited in Clark, 2000, p. 304). A discussion of ethics can assist in the prevention of harm and the reduction of wrongs visited on people in the community by professional "helpers" and the implementation of community interventions. We are provided general guides to ethical action by principles. In this section, those principles that guide community practice are presented.

There are four ethical principles key to community practice: beneficence, nonmaleficence, justice, and autonomy. The ethical principle of *beneficence* "requires that potential benefits to individuals and to society be maximized, and that potential harms be minimized" (Coughlin, Soskolne, & Goodman, 1997, p. 4). The promotion of the common good as well as the protection of individuals is considered.

The principle of *nonmaleficence* requires that harmful acts not be committed—*Primum non nocere*—first, do no harm. Balancing potential benefits and potential harms, however, are not precluded by this principle.

The principle of *justice* requires the equitable distribution of potential benefits and burdens (Coughlin et al., 1997). Three perspectives on distributive justice are:

◆ Egalitarian: each person/group should receive an equal share of potential benefits
◆ Libertarian: resources are best distributed by individual choice and enterprise
◆ Utilitarian: maximization of potential benefits and fair distribution to all who are affected

Community practice is traditionally based on the third perspective and supports the position that maximizing benefits to socially disadvantaged groups ultimately benefits society as a whole.

The principle of *autonomy* is focused on the right of self-determination that grants importance to individual freedom. Associated with autonomy are privacy, free choice, and self-responsibility. Coughlin and coworkers (1997) list 10 moral rules: "Don't kill; don't cause pain; don't disable; don't deprive of freedom; don't deprive of pleasure; don't deceive; keep your promise; don't cheat; obey the law, and do your duty" (p. 12). An ethical dilemma arises when two possible courses of action in a given situation are in conflict. Clark (2000) identifies four societal factors that can place values in conflict (p. 306), as shown in Table 5-1.

People's Rights and Community Practice

People have several critical rights related to community practice: protection of privacy and confidentiality, informed consent, protection from scientific misconduct, and protection from conflicts of interest. These rights allow clients (individuals, families, or communities) the freedom to choose among options and to find meaning in their chosen experiences. Community practitioners strive to avoid *paternalism* (imposing choices and meanings on others) and *consumerism* (remaining indifferent to people's choices and the meaning of their experiences) in efforts to reach mutuality in their relationship with clients (Schroeder & Gallow, 2000).

TABLE 5-1 ◆ SOCIETAL FACTORS THAT CAN CONFLICT WITH VALUES

Factors	Questions	Examples
Society's choice of some values over others emphasizes certain goals and minimizes others.	Which is more important— quality or quantity of life?	Focus on curative care minimizes ability to focus on prevention
The choice of target groups to benefit from a service places those groups at an advantage over others not chosen.	What are the rights of one group compared with another?	Free needles and equipment for people who use intravenous street drugs, but not for diabetics who must pay for their materials
The means chosen to achieve a goal may benefit a majority but infringe on the rights of a minority.	Does responsibility for health rest with society or with individuals?	Tobacco-free family restaurants discriminate against those parents who smoke in the interests of protecting the health of children.
Consequences of social change can influence policy and service decisions.	How are scarce resources allocated?	A declining economy results in a copayment arrangement for seniors' rugs when they were provided previously at no cost.

Clark, M. J. (2000) *Nursing in the community* (3rd ed., pp. 303–316). Norwalk, CT: Appleton & Lange.

Protection of Privacy and Confidentiality

Coughlin and colleagues (1997) note that what constitutes personal or private information varies over time and between cultures. Reasons people may want to have their personal information kept private include fear of discrimination, social ostracism, or marginalization. Community practitioners must be diligent in protecting privacy and ensuring confidentiality by keeping records locked, limiting access to confidential records to those who need to know, protecting electronic records or removing personal identifiers, reinforcing the importance of confidentiality, and releasing information in aggregated form to avoid personal identification. Researchers may be allowed access to large databases on approval from research ethics boards for studies that identify disease and risk factor association, analyze the costs and benefits of interventions, and assess the quality and effectiveness of services.

Informed Consent

Community professionals, to act responsibly with their community participants, can use the informed consent process to ensure free choice with full information about the risks and benefits of participation. Participants should understand what their participation means in terms of time and other commitments and should not feel coerced into taking part in planned activities. Whether people are participating in providing information, collecting data, interpreting findings, or generating ideas for interventions and evaluation, they should be fully informed. In a hepatitis/HIV prevention project for street-involved sex trade workers, staff explained in clear and simple language the benefits of becoming involved with the project (e.g., anonymous blood tests, free access to condoms and clean needles, vaccination, treatment if infected), the risks (e.g., staff had to report anyone who revealed they were under age 16 to the child welfare authorities), and how they would protect their privacy. In this instance, clients chose a pseudonym by which they would be named on project records. If staff contacted them by phone, they would be asked to call "Emily," the code name chosen for the project office, thus retaining privacy by not revealing they were calling from the project office.

Additionally, professionals should remember that any information collected belongs to the community and, if they are planning to publish reports, the community should be informed and have the opportunity to review manuscripts before publication. Professionals should be sensitive to the community in any published reports because ultimately, it is the client (community) whose story is being narrated in the report.

Protection From Misconduct

Scientific or professional misconduct is not unknown in the field of human services. In particular, communities are often in vulnerable positions and therefore issues of due process must be considered because professionals, in their positions of authority and their enthusiasm to "help," may act overzealously. An example of misconduct might be coercing an ethnic community to take part in a new project by creating an impression that regular services may be disrupted if the community does not participate, even though the planned project is not culturally sensitive or appropriate to community values. It may be in the interests of the community worker to get communities "signed on" the project, but not in the interests of the community. Good collegial relations rest on the moral foundations of integrity and mutual trust (Coughlin et al., 1997), and when eroded by lack of objectivity or inappropriate behaviour can have a negative impact on projects, team and community relationships, and reputations of those involved. As well, extreme amounts of energy and other resources can be expended in attempting to resolve conflicts, mend fences, and repair relationships, at the expense of project work. Clear agreements on expectations and responsibilities, oversight by arm's length review boards, and open communication can minimize opportunities for misunderstanding.

Conflict of Interest

Conflicting interests occur when one's self-interest is at odds with one's obligations to others (Coughlin et al., 1997). For instance, tobacco companies are involved in businesses that have retail chains or services related to pharmaceuticals, food, and agricultural products. When a community practitioner accepts donations and agrees to allow those businesses to sponsor health-related events, there is the appearance that the event endorses the tobacco product. In another instance, an infant formula company's posters of babies decorated the waiting room of a service that promoted the "Breast is Best" campaign to increase breastfeeding by new mothers. The breastfeeding message was simultaneously provided with the formula product name on the posters, sending mixed messages to the public! Community workers must act to prevent actual, potential, and the appearance of conflicts in their activities. Disclosures of funding sources and partnership agreements, policies against incentive funding, advertisement of products, and transparent decision-making processes serve to maintain objectivity and independence.

Ethical Problems in Community Practice

Oberle and Tenove (2000) describe five themes of ethical problems that face community nurses: relationships with health care professionals, systems issues, character of relationships with the community client/partner, respect for persons, and putting self at risk.

Relationships With Health Care Professionals

Because teamwork is the hallmark of community practice, interprofessional and intraprofessional tensions can develop. Because community practice is a small component of the helping professions, compared with those who work with individuals in health and social services institutions, it is not uncommon for misunderstandings to occur. Also, long-standing traditions of power and control can place practitioners from one discipline higher in authority than others, particularly in health care institutions. However, community roles are often more collegial and equal, and those making the transition to community practice may be uncomfortable initially with this shift. Community workers advocate for community members, giving voice to their concerns, while also taking steps to build the capacity of the community to act on its own behalf; this is an empowerment process that equalizes the power distribution among partners.

Systems Issues

Systems issues such as the just distribution of resources, policy and legislation that requires, prohibits, or permits certain actions, and system support for community practice can cause ethical dilemmas for community practitioners. Does the community have access to needed resources and are they of high quality and provided by the right mix of professionals? For instance, in a low-income neighbourhood with many single parents, immigrant groups, little social cohesion, and fragmented services, residents were faced with municipal policy proposals that would have a profound effect on quality of life in that community. Staff of a local community health and social services centre arranged a central place for residents to meet to talk about how they would be affected by proposed zoning changes, school closures, and industrial traffic. Car pools and childcare availability were arranged in partnership with the local high school. The people who attended were vocal and enthusiastic in their opposition to the proposal, of a single mind in their feelings of discrimination on the basis of the community's "reputation," and eager to lobby their local alderman to take action on the community's behalf. They wanted appropriate services allocated to the neighbourhood or at least the opportunity to have their voices heard regarding their needs, capacities, and alternative solutions to the problems at hand. In this example, community workers (as employees of the municipality) were not able to personally lobby for the community; their professional recommendations had been dismissed, but they were able to create an environment that brought people together to strengthen community action.

Relationships With the Community Client/Partner

When the community is client or partner, issues such as the *context and nature of the relationship*, empowerment versus dependency, and setting boundaries are issues of concern. Oberle and Tenove (2000) point out that community clients have the freedom to choose whether or not they avail themselves of the services of community practitioners. As a result, the establishment of good communication, the building of trust and rapport, maintenance of confidentiality, and gaining respect are uppermost in the minds of community professionals. On the other hand, they walk a fine line between creating dependency (doing "to" or "for") and fostering empowerment (doing "with") of the community. In this instance, professionals sometimes have to set boundaries between their personal and professional lives, circumscribing their interactions with the client in the interests of maintaining a healthy balance for both parties. Professionals working in small communities often feel they are never "off duty" and are constantly under scrutiny by members of the community they serve. Advice is often solicited in public places, for instance, and they risk offending people if they refuse to respond. In another example, a worker crossed professional lines and "did for" a family when, after referring a family to the food bank, the family did not go. The social worker then purchased food out of her own pocket and took it to the family outside of work hours. Doing "to" or doing "for" people is patriarchal and oppressive and risks increasing dependency on the community worker, care provider, or the agency. Allowing the client family to make its own decisions and take actions with which it is most comfortable would have been more empowering; the social worker has facilitated access to services so that when the client is ready to use the resources, they will be available. This is doing "with" the client—at the client's own pace, in the way the client wants, and under the circumstances the client deems appropriate.

Protecting Self From Risk

Respect for persons underscores the earlier discussion on informed consent and respect for autonomy. In addition, the notion of protecting the vulnerable and advocating or "giving voice" to those who are marginalized or disenfranchised is a key to community practice. For instance, the actions of community social workers, police, and nurses in large urban centres have made a difference to how homelessness is viewed and the services that have become available to members of this community. Nevertheless, community workers are not required to place themselves at physical *risk* in assisting a community client, but sometimes feel they are abandoning their client when they cannot interact without fear for their own safety or the safety of vulnerable others. Context (e.g., street, correctional facility, shelter) and the situation (e.g., the support of others, the trust of the client) are important considerations to community teams, and often the decisions made are not linear, but "are highly relational in nature; they require an exquisite sense of balance and a finely developed sensitivity to the many factors that play into each situation" (Oberle & Tenove, 2000, p. 436).

Advocacy

It is from the above ethical tenets that the notion of advocacy was born. *Advocacy*, in general terms, can be defined as the act of disseminating information intended to influence opinion, conduct, public policy, or legislation. It is the pursuit of influencing outcomes, including public policy and resource allocation decisions within political, economic, and social systems and institutions, which directly affect people's lives. Advocacy consists of organized efforts and actions to highlight critical issues that have been ignored and submerged, to influence public attitudes, and to enact and implement laws and public policies so that vision of "what should be" in a just, decent society becomes a reality. Human rights—political, economic, and social—is the overarching framework for this vision (Advocacy Institute, 2001).

Community workers, as advocates, represent the interests of the people in the community, intervene to investigate problems and resolve conflicts, develop the capacity of the community to advocate on its own behalf, review and comment on public policy, and disseminate information to the community, political leaders, and the media. As employees, political action is often not supported, but social action through professional organizations is an acceptable form of advocacy.

The goal of advocacy is to promote social justice and equity. At the end of the 19th century, when the term "social justice" came to prominence, it was first used as an appeal to the ruling classes to attend to the needs of the new masses of uprooted peasants who had become urban workers (Novak, 2000). It is "social" in two senses. "First, the skills it requires are those of inspiring, working with, and organizing others to accomplish together a work of justice. These are the elementary skills of civil society, through which free citizens exercise self-government by doing for themselves (that is, without turning to government) what needs to be done. " Not only do people want to "give back" to society, activities are carried out *with* others in the interests of free choice and autonomy, thus demanding a broad range of social skills. Social justice is aimed at the common good, not individual benefit. Citizens may come together in efforts to make a difference in their community. For instance, people from all over the city gather to clean the riverbank every spring on the Saturday of the long weekend in May. Businesses sponsor refreshments and provide equipment, community associations organize work groups, and the event is given a festive atmosphere by the presence of local celebrities and the media.

An example of advocacy by a community agency is illustrated in Box 5-1. The Calgary Urban Project Society (CUPS) has attracted the attention of the Governor-General, Her Excellency Adrienne Clarkson, and the Canadian Public Health Association who awarded it the 2003 Ron Draper Health Promotion Award. There are examples of agencies doing similar advocacy work in every part of Canada.

Social Justice

Novak (2000) points out that social justice is ideologically neutral. It is open to people of all political and religious affiliations, all socioeconomic brackets, all cultures and ethnic groups, and both genders, and all ages. The field of activity may be literary, scientific, religious, political, economic, cultural, athletic, and so on, across the whole spectrum of human social activities. The virtue of social justice allows for people of good will to reach different, even opposing, practical judgments about the material content of the common good (ends) and how to get there (means). Social justice is based on the application of equity, rights, access, and participation principles (Box 5-2).

Without social justice there is oppression and powerlessness. People are made dependent; they are silenced and victimized by those who are more influential or in positions of authority. Vulnerability is increased for those who are not part of the majority. The role of community workers is to ensure the marginalized are as empowered as the majority so that they are capable of freely

BOX 5-1. ADVOCACY IN THE INNER CITY

In the late 1980s, downtown churches met to develop an ecumenical project to provide service to people in need who were coming to their doors. There appeared to be few resources available for needy people in the downtown core; referral services were required and a coordinator was needed to help guide people needing help to health and social services agencies. At the same time some physicians were interested in providing medical care to the inner-city population, many of them unemployed, homeless, and destitute. The Calgary Urban Projects Society (CUPS) began in 1988 with two services staffed by volunteers in a building provided by Central United Church. CUPS, funded now by government grants and charitable donations, currently provides health care, social services, and educational services to an inner-city population that continues to struggle with poverty, addiction, marginalization, mental illness, hunger, and homelessness. Programs have developed over time based on the needs and requests of the people served. Input is received through focus groups and participant committees and is an essential component in fulfilling the mandate of a community health centre.

CUPS seeks through compassionate health care and social and educational services to nurture and promote healing to those who have rejected or have been rejected or neglected by society.

The programs and services available include:

- Health clinic that provides a variety of services such as a hepatitis C clinic, a perinatal program, a shared care mental health program as well as general health care by a multidisciplinary team
- An outreach team that focuses on basic needs such as housing, transportation, crisis counselling, etc. Team members spend considerable time in the community.
- Volunteers who provide basic services such as referrals, clothing, showers, laundry, and food. Bus tickets are provided to many people who are searching for employment or need transportation to other appointments.
- Many people of various First Nations use the services of CUPS; cultural sensitivity is achieved by using Aboriginal staff and volunteers. An Elder is available at CUPS to provide wisdom in issues of significance for Aboriginal people.
- The Family Resource Centre program offers support for basic needs, an opportunity to connect with other families, and some counselling to almost 1700 families annually, many of them homeless. Educational and support programs help low-income parents with many of the day-to-day challenges they face.
- The goal of the One World Development Centre educational program for children and parents is to reverse the cycle of poverty and assist children to enter school with similar opportunities as other children.
- Calgary *Street Talk* is a monthly paper that provides a medium for presenting information on poverty and other social justice issues and serves as a community voice. It employs about 30 people who learn a variety of skills such as writing and sales.

For more information: www.cupshealthcentre.com

BOX 5-2. DEFINITIONS OF TERMS

- *Equity:* fairness in the distribution of resources, particularly for those in need
- *Rights:* equality of rights established and promoted for all people
- *Access:* fair access for all people to economic resources, services, and rights essential to their quality of life
- *Participation:* opportunity for all people to genuinely participate in the community and be consulted on decisions which affect their lives

---

negotiating on "a sure footing of respect rather than charity" (Novak, 2000). However, community facilitators should never use their skills and knowledge to empower "racists, sexists, fascists, militarists, or religious bigots, for to do so would be to contribute to violation of the very premise of human fulfillment" (Laue & Cormick, 1978, p. 222, as cited in Novak, 2000). Empowerment is the guarantor of equity and justice, and freedom is the result—freedom to fully participate in public decisions.

Participation

Engaging people in determining how a society guides its actions, makes decisions on public policy, and delivers programs and services is called public participation, or citizen engagement. The desired outcome of participation in decision-making is greater social cohesion as evidenced by the creation of shared values, the reduction of health and wealth disparities, and the building of community spirit and capacity for action.

Formal community agencies (e.g., health and social services departments) are increasingly seeking means to help people to become aware of opportunities to take part in decision-making processes such as needs assessments, service planning, and program evaluation. Because a range of approaches and strategies can facilitate and support informed and meaningful public participation, a public involvement strategy must be designed and planned in collaboration with stakeholders, taking into account:

◆ What is the nature and scope of the issue?
◆ Who is interested in and most affected by possible decisions?
◆ Why is public involvement in the decision-making process important?
◆ What are the expected outcomes of the process?

Public consultation is part of, but not the same as, public involvement. Public *consultation* involves collecting comments and input as part of a larger decision-making process. Consultation should *not* take place if there is an urgent need for action, if the issue is technical, trivial, or routine, or if there is no chance that the public can influence the decision. Consultation may not be possible with matters that involve secrecy or confidentiality.

The many terms associated with public participation are defined in Table 5-2. Health Canada (2000) describes five levels of public involvement (Fig. 5-1). Box 5-3 lists the criteria for selecting a level. It is worth noting, however, that "hybrid" strategies that bridge levels may be needed depending on:

◆ Goal and phase of decision-making
◆ Nature and complexity of the issues
◆ Level of influence and involvement participants expect to have on the outcomes
◆ Mix of participants, whom they represent, and their prior experiences with participation
◆ Staff expertise, stakeholder support, and agency commitment to the process
◆ Timelines and costs
◆ Degree of public concern and media attention

TABLE 5-2 ◆ DEFINITIONS OF COMMONLY USED TERMS IN PUBLIC PARTICIPATION

Public	The general public, consumers, and communities of interest (e.g., consumer groups, industry, scientific and professional associations)
Involvement	A range of activities and relationships, including two-way communications, public education, stakeholder consultation, citizen engagement, advisory bodies, partnerships, and joint decision-making. Involvement implies a continuing dialogue where all participants are mutually open to influencing decisions.
Stakeholder	An individual, group or organization with a stake in an issue, its outcome, and/or the overall public involvement process
Community of interest	A stakeholder group assembled around a common issue, viewpoint, or concern, as opposed to geography, discipline, or occupational background, often for a self-limiting period of time
Partner	An individual, group, or organization that may participate in or be responsible for implementing various aspects of a public involvement plan, or the policy or program decisions related to the plan
Citizen engagement	The process of informed dialogue and deliberation among individual citizens, usually involving the exchange of ideas and values, opportunities to learn from each other, decisions on best ways to move toward action, and formation of partnerships to act on solutions agreed on
Consultation	Canvassing of views of stakeholders and clients in the process of developing sound public policy, often through forums, roundtables, and advisory bodies.

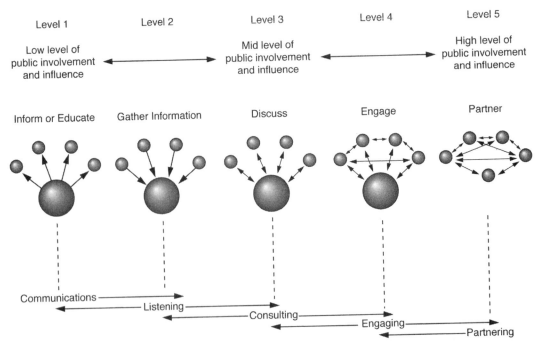

Figure 5-1 ◆ Health Canada's public involvement continuum. (From *Health Canada policy toolkit for public involvement in decision-making*. Ottawa: Health Canada, p. 12.)

Who should be involved are those who will be affected by the issue (or potentially affected in the future) and those who can contribute to a solution. Some groups (e.g., consumer groups, advocacy agencies) will insist on being present and cannot be left out. Other agencies, politicians, and segments of the community might also be included (e.g., academics, marginalized populations, industry representatives) as appropriate to the issue. Neither sceptics nor vested interests should be excluded from participation. Although they may cause some disruption and seek undue attention, a good facilitator will balance their views with those of the other groups in attendance. "Community leaders" may or may not represent their constituencies well, so planners should seek to ensure that there is good communication and feedback to the community at large.

A checklist for the public participation planning process is shown in Figure 5-2. Done well, public involvement in decisions that affect people's health or quality of life addresses the ethical principles of justice and autonomy and ensures that decisions taken will be beneficial and not cause harm. Further, community capacity can be enhanced as people become empowered for social action, resulting ultimately in equity, access, social justice, and the prevention of human rights abuses.

BOX 5-3. LEVELS OF PUBLIC INVOLVEMENT

Level 1— Inform/Educate When:
- Factual information is needed to describe a policy, program or process
- A decision has already been made (no decision is required)
- The public needs to know the results of a process
- There is no opportunity to influence the final outcome
- There is need for acceptance of a proposal or decision before a decision may be made
- An emergency or crisis requires immediate action
- Information is necessary to abate concerns or prepare for involvement
- The issue is relatively simple

Level 2—Gather Information/Views When:
- The purpose is primarily to listen and gather information
- Policy decisions are still being shaped and discretion is required
- There may not be a firm commitment to do anything with the views collected (we advise participants from the outset of this intention to manage expectations)

Level 3—Discuss or Involve When:
- We need two-way information exchange
- Individuals and groups have an interest in the issue and will likely be affected by the outcome
- There is an opportunity to influence the final outcome
- We wish to encourage discussion among and with stakeholders
- Input may shape policy directions/program delivery

Level 4—Engage When:
- We need citizens to talk to each other regarding complex, value-laden issues
- There is a capacity for citizens to shape policies and decisions that affect them
- There is opportunity for shared agenda setting and open time frames for deliberation on issues
- Options generated together will be respected

Level 5—Partner When:
- We want to empower citizens and groups to manage the process
- Citizens and groups have accepted the challenge of developing solutions themselves
- We are ready to assume the role of enabler
- There is an agreement to implement solutions generated by citizens and groups

Health Canada. (2000). *Policy toolkit for public involvement in decision making.* Ottawa: Author.

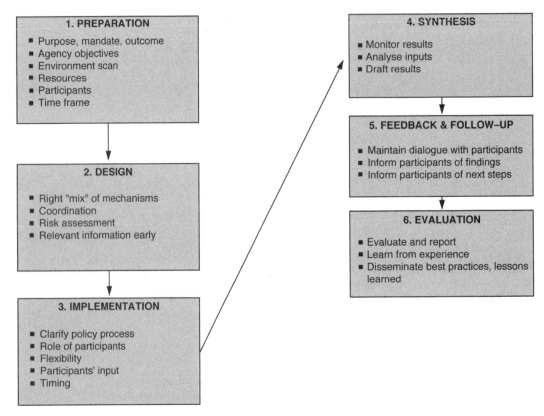

Figure 5-2 ◆ Planning checklist.

Empowerment

Is empowerment an end result or a process? Kreisberg (1992) defines it as a process of developing knowledge and skills that increase one's mastery over decisions that affect one's life. To gain mastery, people must be able to predict, control, and participate in their environment (Rappaport [1984] as cited by Helvie, 1998, p. 328). At the community or population level, empowerment is an outcome that has been described as *community competence* (Eng & Parker, 1994) and exhibits the following dimensions:

◆ Participation
◆ Commitment
◆ Self-other definition and clarity of a situational definition
◆ Articulateness

◆ Conflict containment and accommodation
◆ Management of relations with the wider society
◆ Machinery for facilitating participant interaction and decision-making
◆ Social support

Empowerment, therefore, can be either a process (an ongoing action process, often facilitated by community-professional collaboration that is enabling and transformative) or an end result (an outcome of the action process that transforms people or communities from passive recipients to involved participants in community life).

Barriers

Israel and colleagues (1994) describe several obstacles to the implementation of effective community empowerment strategies:

◆ Past experiences with community interventions that lead people to think they are not influential
◆ Differences in social status, race, or ethnicity between community members and community workers hindering trust, communication, and collaboration
◆ Community members and workers experiencing role-related tensions and differences related to values and interests, resources, skills, politics, control, rewards, and costs
◆ Challenges to measuring progress or change
◆ Resistance to change on the parts of community members, agencies, or the community workers
◆ Short-time-frame expectations versus long-term commitments of financial and personal resources needed
◆ Perceived inaction during the data collection and analysis phases
◆ Perception that a community focus is not adequate in the global world in which we live now

Obstacles and barriers can be overcome by close attention to process and effective communication among all parties. Bracht (1990) identifies the following factors for success:

◆ People involved are concerned about their community
◆ People involved have leadership experience in the community
◆ Confidence that competent people can be recruited to support the project

◆ Resources available
◆ Good faith among sponsors
◆ Clearly defined citizen authority roles
◆ Ability to create, sustain, and control a community organization
◆ Knowledge of community history
◆ Early identification and discussion of barriers to change
◆ Clearly stated volunteer roles and time commitments
◆ Project staff who are committed to community ownership/partnership
◆ Recognition and rewards to reinforce participation
◆ Timely use of conflict resolution when required

Summary

Philosophical and ethical perspectives provide the foundation for community practice. If access, equity, and social justice are important outcomes of community intervention, then practices related to advocacy and public participation are necessary processes by which those societal objectives can be achieved. As facilitators of community empowerment, community workers must avoid taking an expert approach, but instead work *with* others as partners in determining the destiny of the community. To direct, to judge, to preach, or to do *to* or *for* flies in the face of the foundation on which community practice is based.

References

Advocacy Institute. (2001). What is 'advocacy'? Downloaded from website http://www.advocacy.org/definition.htm.

Bracht, N. (Ed.). (1990). *Health promotion at the community level* (pp. 99–108). Newbury Park, CA: Sage.

Clark, M. J. (2000). *Nursing in the community* (3rd ed., pp. 303–316). Norwalk, CT: Appleton & Lange.

Coughlin S. S., Soskolne, C. L., & Goodman, K. W. (1997). *Case studies in public health ethics.* Washington, DC: American Public Health Association.

Eng, E., & Parker, E. (1994). Measuring community competence in the Mississippi Delta: The interface between program evaluation and empowerment. *Health Education Quarterly, 21,* 199–220.

Health Canada. (2000). *Policy toolkit for public involvement in decision making.* Ottawa: Author. www.hc-sc.ca

Helvie, C. O. (1998). *Advanced practice nursing in the community* (pp. 327–374). Thousand Oaks, CA: Sage.

Israel, B. A., Checkoway, B., Schultz, A., & Zimmerman, M. (1994). Health education and community empowerment: Conceptualizing and measuring perceptions of individuals, organizations and community control. *Health Education Quarterly, 21,* 149–170.

Kreisberg, S. (1992). *Transforming power: Domination, empowerment and education.* New York: SUNY Press.

Laue, J., & Cormick, G. (1978). The ethics of intervention in community disputes. In G. Bermant, H. Kelman, & D. Warwick (Eds), *The ethics of social intervention* (pp. 205–232). Washington, DC: Halstead Press.

Novak, M. (2000). Defining social justice. *First Things: A Journal of Religious and Public Life, 108*(12), 11–13.

Oberle, K., & Tenove, S. (2000). Ethical issues in public health nursing. *Nursing Ethics, 7*(5), 425–437.

Pojman, L. P. (1992). *Life and death: Grappling with the moral dilemmas of our times.* Boston: Jones & Bartlett.

Rappaport, J. (1984). Studies in empowerment: Introduction to the issue. *Prevention in Human Services, 3,* 1–7.

Schroeder, C., & Gallow, S. (2000). An advocacy approach to ethics and community health. In E. T. Anderson & J. McFarlane (Eds.), *Community as partner: Theory and practice in nursing* (3rd ed., pp. 78–91). Philadelphia: Lippincott Williams & Wilkins.

6

Public Participation for Healthy Communities and Public Policy

WILFREDA E. THURSTON
CATHERINE M. SCOTT
ARDENE ROBINSON VOLLMAN

CHAPTER OUTLINE

OBJECTIVES

After studying this chapter, you should be able to:

◆ Describe the policy-making processes
◆ Discuss the role of public participation in policy development
◆ Acknowledge the need for critical social analysis throughout the policy cycle
◆ Outline the community development process
◆ Understand the roles of partnerships in population health promotion

Introduction

Healthy public policies are those that influence the health of populations; they are described as "ecological in perspective, multisectoral in scope and participatory in strategy" (Milio, cited in Pederson et al., 1988, p. iii). This chapter provides the relevant theory behind the practice of community professionals and informs the process of community development. Fundamental to community development is public participation, intersectoral and multidisciplinary partnerships and collaboration, and the creation of public policy that supports the health of Canadians. In this chapter we present a framework for understanding the development of public policy. We discuss how the public can participate in development of such policy and we argue that the processes of policy development and participation must be analyzed critically if reduction of health inequities is an intended outcome of public policies.

What Is Public Policy?

Public policy as defined by Pal (2001) is "a course of action or inaction chosen by public authorities to address a given problem or interrelated set of problems" (p. 2). Once a problem or issue has been given public attention, inaction or failure to formulate a response is a deliberate policy decision. "We have no position" is a policy statement. Public policies deal with public problems, not with the operations and structures through which the policies (or lack of policy) will be implemented. Public policies act as a set of guidelines or as a framework for action. Once a problem has been identified, governments have three general categories of policy instruments: do nothing; act indirectly (e.g., educate, provide funds); or act directly through state agencies, corporations or in partnership with private or nonprofit organizations (Pal, 2001).

Public policy in a democracy is made by elected officials (Pal, 2001). Thus it is distinguished from the organizational policies made by administrators, managers, or front-line staff within public organizations. Public policy is also separate from corporate policy or policies made by nongovernmental organizations. That does not mean that there is no interaction among these various locations of policy.

How Does Public Policy Get Developed?

Howlett and Ramesh (1995) present five aspects of a policy cycle:

◆ Agenda setting
◆ Policy formulation

◆ Decision-making
◆ Policy implementation
◆ Policy evaluation

Figure 6-1 is a representation of how the processes work together. These processes are not considered to be linear because there may be several iterations for each before a public policy is stated. This should be contrasted with what Pal (2001) identified as the more commonly promoted rational decision-making model that assumes that a linear process where problems and the solutions are broken into discrete parts would result in a more efficient and predictable government. According to Pal (2001), those models have "deep roots in an impulse to centralize, categorize, and control" (p. 20). We argue that linear models are incompatible with public participation in policy processes because such participation inevitably reveals the complexity and nonlinear nature of most problems and their solutions (Miller et al., 1998). Healthy Cities (HC) projects as described

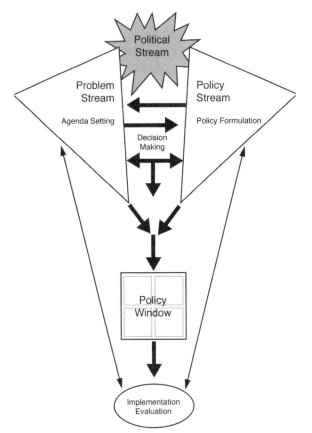

Figure 6-1 ◆ A non-linear, non-rational policy process.

by the World Health Organization (WHO) are examples of ecological, multisectoral, and participatory healthy public policy initiatives. HC initiatives focus on the setting where people live and work (e.g., home, school, work, community) to support the development of policies that address broad determinants of health (e.g., income and social status, social support networks, education, working conditions, social environments, physical environments, gender, culture; WHO, 2003). Knowledge of public policy processes and theory provides a foundation for such population health initiatives.

Agenda Setting

Agenda setting is the process through which problems come to the attention of elected officials or policymakers. This is the problem recognition stage. The *problem stream* is the process whereby a problem or lack of an ideal state becomes perceived as a problem that public bodies should address. Decision-makers receive feedback from both external and internal sources. (Howlett et al., 1995). The strength of the policy network (to be discussed later) clearly affects this feedback process. Pal (2001) emphasizes the difference between problem recognition and problem definition. The way a problem is defined shapes the options available.

Policy Formulation

The *policy stream* is the process whereby experts and analysts pose solutions to the problem and is consistent with the stage of *policy formulation*. When solutions become joined to problems, argued Kingdon (cited in Howlett et al., 1995), and a favourable political stream exists, a policy window opens. The *political stream* refers to social and political context. The *policy window* refers to a favourable opening for a public policy. Even if the work of the problem and policy streams goes well, if the political stream is not favourable, for instance, if any public policy is going to attract vociferous opposition, then the policy window may never open. For example, when the issue of domestic violence was first raised in the House of Commons in 1982 some members made jokes and laughed. In general, the public was outraged by the response of some of their elected officials. Public pressure widely reported in the media prompted the House of Commons report on domestic violence (Standing Committee on Health, 1982).

The latter example also highlights the influential role of the media (Phillips & Orsini, 2002) in both reflecting and shaping the political stream. Pal (2001) writes about "ideas in good currency," ideas that "sound right to most people"

(p. 121). Similarly, Engberg-Pedersen and Webster (2002) talk about a political space for the poor where public policies can be generated. An important aspect of political space is the range of ideas that are circulating in the political stream.

Decision-Making

In the *decision-making stage*, policymakers select from among policy options developed in the formulation stage. Even at this stage the policy-making process may cease. Alternatively, politicians may float a policy idea to gauge public reaction. Sufficient negative reaction may mean that the policy never sees implementation.

Policy Implementation and Evaluation

Policy implementation is the process by which governments put solutions or policies into effect. *Policy evaluation* includes processes by which results of policies are monitored. Evaluation can lead back to a fuller understanding of either the problem or potential solutions.

Public Participation

Participation is a major tenet of health promotion and is encapsulated in its Ottawa Charter definition: "health promotion is the process of enabling people to increase control over and to improve their health" (WHO, 1986b). Fostering public participation is one of three strategies for health promotion encouraged in early policy documents from the Canadian government (Epp, 1986). Partnerships between organizations is one form of participation that has been posed as a solution to many health problems (Feldberg & Carlsson, 1999; Giachello, 1995; Jadad, 1999; Zaini, 1998). Participatory action-research (Smith, Pyrch, & Lizardi, 1993), participatory research (Plaut, Landis, & Trevor, 1992), and participatory development (Kelly & Vlaenderen, 1995) are just some of the activities thought to improve the chances of success in health promotion. In the 1950s, community development, which encompasses some of the work of health promotion (Bhatti & Siler-Wells, 1987), was synonymous with participation (Abbott, 1995) (Box 6-1).

One of the recent trends in public policy is the desire of people to have input into the processes (Pal, 2001). Participation has become a key part of the discourse in the health sector in the last few years. Participation was central to the

---

BOX 6-1. PARTICIPATORY ACTION RESEARCH

Participatory action research (PAR) is a philosophical approach to research
that recognizes the need for persons being studied to participate in the design
and conduct of all phases (e.g., design, execution, and dissemination) of any
research that affects them. Its purpose is to foster empowerment, community
capacity development, social change, democracy, participation, access, and
social justice.

---

concept of primary health care introduced in the 1970s (Fournier & Potvin,
1995), but has moved beyond that to a broader inclusion in health policy documents. One regional health authority in Alberta recently developed a Public
Participation Framework intended to guide practice throughout the health
authority (Maloff, Bilan, & Thurston, 2000). Recognition that the broad determinants of health (Evans, Barer, & Marmor, 1994) and that other sectors influence the health of populations, has also increased the demand for intersectoral
action (Draper, 1995). The social service and nonprofit sectors include many
organizations that advocate for specific groups of people and some of these are
participating in health policy development through consultation and partnerships.

Despite the widespread support of participation, there is little consensus
about what it means in practice and the literature on participation is fraught
with inconsistency (Cleaver, 2001; Fournier & Potvin, 1995; Hailey, 2001).
Similarly, the term partnership is used to denote many different relationships
and understandings such as coalitions, networks, coordinating committees,
and work groups. The partner relationships, therefore, range from instances
where organizations or individuals are consulted on a topic to involvement in
decision-making, to delegated authority over a program (e.g., in a formal collaboration or partnership). The health authority Public Participation
Framework mentioned earlier (Maloff et al., 2000) acknowledges a range of participation from information exchange to delegation of authority (Fig. 6-2).

One of the debates around participation is whether it is a means to some
other end or an end in and of itself. Cleaver (2001) characterizes this as a distinction between "efficiency arguments" and "equity or empowerment arguments" (p. 37). A focus on efficiency involves maximizing project outcomes
(e.g., attendance at mammography clinics), whereas empowerment is focused
on enhancing capacity. Cleaver (2001) concluded that empowerment of marginalized people in development work has become "depoliticized" (p. 37), with a

Two assumptions are relevant to the level provided below:
a) the publics are informed about the issue and process at each level
b) regardless of the level selected, the RHA is accountable for the decisions and outcomes

Level	Objective
Information Publics ◄─────── RHA	Publics are informed about the issue and process; misconceptions are clarified; communication of decisions made.
Input Publics ───────► RHA	Publics' perceptions, opinions and advice are sought and may be used in decision making. Decision making is retained by the RHA.
Consultation Publics ◄──────► RHA	Publics' informed perceptions, opinions and advice are sought and may be used in decision making regarding the issue. Consultation is an interactive exchange. Decision making is retained by the RHA.
Partnership Publics ◄──────► RHA	Publics participate in a partnership process. Decision making is joint between the RHA and the public.
Delegation RHA ───────►Publics	Decision making is delegated to the publics.

Figure 6-2 ◆ Levels of public participation with a regional health authority.

focus on individuals and little attention to changing social structures. Cowen (2001) points out that because people use the same terminology (e.g., empowerment, partnerships), this does not mean that they share common meanings and values. Poland (1992) challenges health professionals to "walk the talk."

One of the challenges for the student of participation is a failure on the part of practitioners and researchers to clarify the underlying assumptions and associated values of public participation initiatives (Fournier & Potvin, 1995; Hailey, 2001). As Weiss (1995) indicates, this is a general failure around comprehensive community initiatives. Fournier and Potvin (1995) identify three goals of public participation with different underlying values: maximizing the outcomes of a program (a utilitarian view), helping people take control of their lives (conscientization), and acting as a democratic tool to extend and protect the power of marginalized peoples. These are not mutually exclusive goals. However, if the underlying value of participation is linked to the utilitarian view, then increasing enrolment in a program can be achieved without concern about the philosophy of the partner organization. If the underlying value of participation is linked to the democratic view, then involving women who advocate for a return of women to the home can be argued to be appropriate. These women might, for instance, be very successful in having other women, even some marginalized women, participate in a child health initiative. If the underlying value, however, is an enhanced civil society that strives for equity for all women, poor women, women of colour, lesbians, women with disabilities, or immigrant women then the philosophy of the partner organization must be feminist (Elliott & Mandell, 1998, cited in Crow & Gotell, 2000).

Policy Communities, Networks, and Coalitions

People who are concerned about a particular policy issue are considered by Howlett and Ramesh (1995) to form a *policy community* (Fig. 6-3). These people may include members of the general public, representatives of organizations, government employees, and elected or appointed officials. They further distinguish the actors in the policy cycle. "Policies are made by *policy subsystems* consisting of actors dealing with a public problem. ... Policy subsystems are forums where actors discuss policy issues and persuade and bargain in pursuit of their interests" (Howlett & Ramesh, 1995, p. 51). Some members of the policy community interact on a regular basis and these form a *policy network*. *Advocacy coalitions* form yet another subset of the policy community and comprise "actors from a variety of public and private institutions at all levels of government who share a basic set of beliefs (policy goals plus causal and other perceptions) and who seek to manipulate the rules, budgets and personnel of governmental institutions in order to achieve these goals over time" (Howlett &

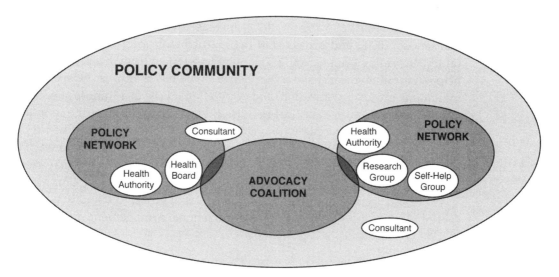

Figure 6-3 ◆ Policy subsystems: policy communities, networks; and advocacy coalitions.

Ramesh, 1995, p. 126). Doern and Phidd (1992) suggest "Bureaucracy is also a system of delegation that immediately creates an impetus for 'bottom-up' policy initiatives emanating from departments that possess their own agendas reinforced and challenged by their policy communities" (p. 154). Actors in the policy subsystem vary in knowledge and expertise and in ultimate goals. The arrows in Figure 6-1 point to the importance of a varied membership in a policy network and the role of advocacy coalitions and the broader policy community. The problem and policy streams rely on experts and analysts examining problems and proposing solutions, but these people need accurate information to do their jobs well.

Howlett and Ramesh (1995) suggest that dense policy networks, where both the government and society are strong and close partnerships between the two are possible, result in more "cohesive and long-term policies" (p. 65). Networks where the government and society are both weak will produce "ineffective and short-sighted policies" (p. 65). Doern and Phidd (1992) go further in saying that the absence of a network* "may make coherent policy impossible" (p. 77). This would suggest that strengthening policy networks might be necessary in some instances. Further, it is important to keep in mind that other advocacy coalitions can create competition for the time and attention of the policymakers.

A number of goals of participation are discussed in the literature. These range from informing individuals to increasing community cohesion, understanding community needs (Cooke & Kothari, 2001), mobilizing opposition to organizational change (Carnall, 1986), or encouraging organizational learning (Detert, Schroeder, & Mauriel, 2000). Some unintended outcomes include burnout (Huxham & Vangen, 2000), increased competition among agencies (Alexander, 2000), and project staff in a participatory project being viewed as underperforming (Mosse, 2001). The point to be taken from this is that any participation initiative can have a number of outcomes that must be specified at individual, group, organization, and population levels. In addition, attention to unintended outcomes is critical because these may undermine the long-term goals. A number of people with a stake in the initiative might influence outcomes and the potential for conflicting goals should not be ignored. This process of articulating underlying assumptions or program theory may be difficult, but it can be a learning experience in and of itself (Weiss, 1995).

We would argue that discussion and analysis of power and equity must be a central focus of the purpose of interorganizational arrangements, or participa-

---

*They actually speak of the policy community and do not make the distinction between communities and networks.

tion is more likely to be about social control than social change (Cooke & Kothari, 2001). It is the critical analysis that distinguishes social justice participation from social control participation. One of the unintended consequences of ignoring power and equity is that participation of social elites can be strengthened at the expense of redistribution of power (Hildyard et al., 2001). The interactions among citizens, social movements, the political representation system, and government apparatus create opportunities for participation (Briskin, 1999). In the next two sections, we briefly outline strategies and frameworks for citizen participation in public policy.

Participation in Healthy Public Policy Formation

Healthy public policy strengthens communities, and a policy process built on participation strengthens the ability of communities to develop the ways and means to address its issues, to nurture the talent and leadership that enhance the quality of community life, to tackle problems that threaten the community, and to take advantage of opportunities that can help create conditions for people to mutually support and care for each other. In this section we review how individual citizens and communities develop this capacity and what it contributes to health and quality of life.

Community Development

Community development is the building of collective commitment, resources, and skills that can be deployed for purposive community change to build on community strengths and address community problems. It means developing the capacity and competencies of the members of a community in such a way that they are better able to identify and help meet their needs and to participate more fully in society. Community development is therefore concerned with providing opportunities for people to learn through experience and involving people in collective effort so that they gain confidence in their own abilities and their ability to influence decisions that affect them. Thus individual involvement and collective activity go hand in hand; the aim is to encourage people in a community to join together with others so as to provide through collective effort what the community needs, but in such a way that those taking part also develop their own potential as members of society (Box 6-2).

BOX 6-2. DEVELOPING COMMUNITIES:
WHERE DO WE START?

"Start where people are, because it reflects a respect for the rights of individuals and communities to affirm their own values and ways of living. Secondly, one should recognize and build on community strengths instead of only assessing the community needs. Thirdly, while we need to work closely with communities, to respect their capacities and rights to self-determination, we must at the same time strive to live up to our own ethical standards and those of our profession in not letting blind faith in the community prevent us from seeing and acting on the paramount need for social justice. Fourth, high level community participation must be fostered. Fifth, commitment is that one should not forget sense of humour in their work. Sixth, the role of political analysis and activism in health education must be recognised. Health problems and their solutions need to be re-framed in terms of their political, economic and social contexts. Think globally, act locally, foster individual and community empowerment and finally work for social justice." (Minkler, 1994)

Building Community Capacity

What does it mean to develop community capacity? It means making a positive difference to the capacity and skills of the members of a community in question because they participate with other members of that community in activities directed toward meeting their needs in some way. Sometimes this process is described as "empowerment." In more specific terms, this is likely to involve:

- ◆ Equipping people with skills and competencies that they would not otherwise have
- ◆ Realizing existing skills and developing potential
- ◆ Promoting people's increased self-confidence
- ◆ Promoting people's ability to take responsibility for identifying and meeting their own, and other people's, needs
- ◆ Encouraging people to become involved in their community and wider society in a fuller way

Not every activity that benefits a community can be seen as promoting community capacity building in the sense described above. Kretzmann and McKnight (1993) describe community development as "building community from the inside out." They suggest that people external to the community of interest (e.g., urban planners, professionals from public, private, and non-profit organizations) traditionally view communities as entities with deficits or problems to be addressed, usually through the provision of services. Thus, community residents begin to view themselves as victims that need the services of outside agencies to survive. The pervasive nature of this deficiency model has a devastating effect on a community and its residents. Residents become demoralized and dis-empowered, mutual support and community problem-solving abilities weaken, and hope for improvement disappears as funding for services is ever dependent on problems being worse than last year or more intractable than the problems of other communities, or funding will disappear. A cycle of dependence is the result, community leadership is undermined, and incentive to change the social construction of their lives is lost.

An alternative is to focus not on problems associated with a deficiency model, but to take a capacity-oriented approach. Evidence indicates that when local community members are committed to investing in citizens and their community, they can successfully develop and mobilize their assets, capacities, and abilities to construct a new social reality—one that is based on opportunity, competence, and empowerment. This community development approach focuses on community assets, not deficiencies.

Asset-Based Community Development

Asset-based community development (ABCD) is based on four key factors:

◆ Assets: what is present in the community; the capacities of all residents (even those who are traditionally marginalized—the young, old, mentally ill); the associational and institutional base of the area
◆ Internal focus: the focus is on the agenda-building and problem-solving capacity of local residents, associations, and organizations to stress the importance of local definition, investment, creativity, hope, and control
◆ Relationship driven: developing, maintaining, and sustaining connections and affiliations among residents, local businesses and associations, public institutions (e.g., schools, libraries, health centres, police), and faith communities
◆ Action orientation: stakeholders are actively involved in creating conditions for action, fostering relationships and opportunities for action, and rely more on "doing" things than "talking" about them

Methods of Community Development

Although there are no prescribed methods to community development because each community will have unique challenges and assets, several social and environmental conditions can facilitate the process:

◆ Trust and the presence of community bonds
◆ Effective and inclusive communication methods
◆ Presence of responsive organizations and community facilities
◆ Adequate and appropriate levels and mix of skills across the community
◆ Preparedness to engage with government and external stakeholders
◆ Shared commitment and entrepreneurial spirit
◆ Resilience and flexibility to deal with conflict and change
◆ The ability to sustain its commitments, networks, and outcomes

External champions in the form of local politicians or professional service providers (e.g., community workers) are helpful to the community development process, but such supporters must take care to allow community control over directions, agendas, and processes, and not highjack the process for their professional purposes.

The Community Development Process

Often there is an external catalyst that brings people together against a common "foe." In some instances, it has been reactions against crime (e.g., gangs, prostitution, violence); in others it has been a result of externally imposed decisions (e.g., urban renewal, school closings, hospital relocations) or a common issue facing many residents (e.g., poverty, AIDS, homelessness). Whatever the impetus, people come together to take action. It is in these initial gatherings that community development begins, gains momentum, creates leaders, focuses efforts, and campaigns for solutions (Table 6-1). There are several steps in the process of developing community:

◆ Defining the issue—articulate the issue, what is known about it, and who is affected.
◆ Initiating the process—research the veracity of the issue and perspectives, identify the full range of stakeholders, gather people together to create commitment for action.

TABLE 6-1 ◆ CHECKLIST FOR ISSUE DEFINITION	
Who says there is an issue?	Is it a person or group with expertise in the area?
	Are they representing others or speaking for themselves?
	On what basis do they say there is a problem?
	How much information do they have?
	Who and how many people are affected, either primarily or secondarily?
How real is the problem?	Are there any indicators or measures of the extent of the problem?
	What is the problem trend?
	Is it increasing or decreasing?
	Is the nature of the problem changing, if not increasing in occurrence?
	Is the problem linear, discontinuous, or cyclical?
	Is it a "new" problem?
	Is there knowledge about it?
	What are the underlying causes?
What do people believe about the issue?	What are the values of the stakeholders?
	What are the government's values?
	Is there a way of ranking the various values involved?
What can be done about the issue?	By government?
	By other groups (e.g., business, nongovernment organizations)?
	Through coordinated effort?

◆ Planning community conversations—invite all stakeholders to participate; develop both informal and formal processes of consultation that allow all viewpoints to be properly aired.

◆ Talking, discovering, and connecting—prepare handouts that outline the issue, why you are gathering information and mobilizing the community, connect with key people and community members, share information and garner support.

◆ Creating an asset map—develop lists as you talk to people and initiate relationships, communicate regularly and widely, attract resources.

◆ Mobilizing the community—bring people together in central locations to discuss options, share experiences, create a common vision, and plan activities.

◆ Taking action—involve and educate community members, help shape opinion, and galvanize commitment.

◆ Planning and implementing community-driven initiatives—have a vision in mind of what must change to improve the situation, organize people and work, and sustain efforts.

The community development process involves commitment, resources, and skills. Each community has its unique starting point. For instance, some communities know exactly what they want but either do not know how to get there or need leadership. Other communities rarely get decisions made because of deep-rooted conflicts or historical divisions among groups of people who stubbornly refuse to cooperate. Some communities have experienced too much change too quickly, and old-timers and newcomers have not yet formed a common bond. Other communities have given up trying to do anything because too many people have moved away and the energy of those remaining has been sapped and there is general apathy. Whatever the starting point, and no matter what the community is facing, certain time-tested principles must be kept in mind:

♦ Have patience: community development takes time.
♦ Be flexible: there will be ups and downs.
♦ Be resilient: adversity builds character.
♦ Encourage others: many hands make light work.
♦ Be organized: you will be ready when opportunity knocks.
♦ Embrace challenge: opportunities are often found in threats.
♦ Build networks: champions are sometimes located in strange places.
♦ Communicate, communicate, and communicate!

There are many positive consequences of community development, among them:

♦ Greater citizen participation—an ever-increasing number and diversity of people take part in all types of activities and decisions.
♦ Expanded leadership base—the opportunity to engage in leadership activities is important to the development of individual and collective capacity.
♦ Strengthened individual skills—as people develop new skills and expertise the level of volunteer service is raised.
♦ Wide sharing of values and vision—the more widely a vision is shared, the stronger will be the motivation of the community to achieve it, and there will be less conflict.
♦ A strategic community agenda—helps to understand, embrace, and manage change proactively.
♦ Consistent, tangible progress toward goals—celebrating achievements turns plans into results, sets milestones, creates momentum, and creates a bias for action.
♦ More effective community organizations and institutions—when civic clubs and local institutions are effective, the community is strengthened.
♦ Improved utilization of community resources—duplication is minimized, gaps are filled, and self-reliance is balanced with the use of outside resources.

Measuring Success
in Community Development

America Speaks [http://www.americaspeaks.org] (1996) developed the following criteria for determining if citizen engagement is sustainable over the long term:

◆ Political, civic, and corporate leadership have vision and understand the importance of listening to all voices in the community.
◆ Community activists have vision, are self-initiating, and focus on the common good.
◆ Institutional and grassroots leaders recognize that the changes necessary are systemic and both individuals and institutions carry responsibility for making the necessary changes.
◆ Media outlets, print, television, radio, and the Internet, have embraced civic/public journalism values and commit resources to building community.
◆ Sufficient technology infrastructure is in place to support community-wide and region-wide dialogue and deliberation processes.
◆ Community projects flow across political jurisdictions and reflect a natural ecological and economic region.
◆ There is an existing infrastructure of citizen involvement so that people who participate in the project have opportunity to stay involved for the long term.
◆ Resources are committed to capacity building for people at all economic levels in the community, reflecting the skill sets needed for leadership in the next century.
◆ There is an established and expressed public trust, respect, and compassion among the people engaged in the civic life of the community.

Partnerships

Addressing complex societal issues requires that stakeholders work together to explore disparate perspectives. Widespread recognition of the need for partnerships is necessary to ensure the effective development and delivery of health services and supports that contribute to health (Baier, 1995; DiStefano, 1990; Gillies, 1998; Gordon, Plamping, & Pratt, 1999; Hennekens & Buring, 1987; Hornby, 1993; Jadad, 1999; Kemm & Close, 1995; MacKean & Thurston, 1996; Vancouver/Richmond Health Board, 2000; WHO, 1986a). Interdependence among sectors that influence the health of populations has made this critical. In Canada, emphasis has been placed on the need for intersectoral action to effectively address the broad determinants of health (Draper, 1995; Evans et al., 1994; Federal/Provincial/Territorial Advisory Committee on Population Health, 1991). Strengthening the impact of intersectoral policy requires detailed knowledge of collaborative planning and evaluation strategies. In this section we present an overview of collaboration literature and describe a partnership framework and process model that has been used effectively for planning and evaluation (Scott, 2000; Scott & Thurston, 1997, 1998).

Collaboration and Partnerships

Collaboration and partnerships are terms that are frequently used synonymously. Although they are closely linked, they have distinct meanings.

Collaboration is a strategy for building relationships and doing work (Winer & Ray, 1997). Gray (1989) and Winer and Ray (1997) make clear distinctions between collaboration, coordination, and cooperation. Gray (1989) suggests that cooperation and coordination "often occur as part of the process of collaboration" (p. 15). They are informal interactions that lay the foundation for the development of more formal relationships. Similarly, Winer and Ray (1997) suggest that all three of these concepts exist along a continuum of increasing intensity with cooperation at one end, coordination in the middle, and collaboration representing the more intense end of the relationship scale (Box 6-3).

Partnerships are a type of collaboration. *Partnerships* occur when the purpose of collaboration is to advance a shared vision of a need and the expected outcome is to develop a joint agreement to address the problem and bring the vision into reality. As a result, referent organizations (i.e., managing bodies

---

BOX 6-3. DEFINITIONS OF COLLABORATIVE PROCESSES

Barbara Gray defines collaboration as "a process in which those parties with a stake in the problem actively seek a mutually determined solution" (Gray, 1989, p. xviii). Collaboration may be motivated by a desire to advance a shared vision or a need to resolve conflict. The expected outcome of collaboration may be the exchange of information or the development of a joint agreement (Gray, 1996). Participating organizations form a new structure to address the mission. Such relationships involve detailed planning and communication as well as the pooling of resources.

BOX 6-4. WHAT IS A REFERENT ORGANIZATION?

A referent organization is formed as a result of a collaborative effort. The functions of this organization include regulation of relationships and activities, appreciation of emergent trends and issues, and infrastructure support (Gray, 1989; Trist, 1983)

---

such as committees) are usually created to address agreements (Scott-Taplin, 1993) (Box 6-4).

Some commonly identified characteristics of partnerships include:

◆ Shared authority, responsibility and management
◆ Joint investment of resources (time, work, funding, material, expertise, information) and reputation
◆ The development of a new structure
◆ Comprehensive planning
◆ Detailed communication strategies
◆ The distribution of power, which may be unequal
◆ Shared liability, risk-taking, accountability, and rewards

(Health Canada, 1996; Winer & Ray, 1997)

Over the past 10 years, there has been an explosion of literature on the topic of partnerships. Partnership theory derives from many different theoretical perspectives and practice situations; correspondingly, a number of collaboration and partnership frameworks and models have developed (Box 6-5). By their very nature, frameworks and models leave out much of the detail

---

BOX 6-5. DEFINITIONS: FRAMEWORK AND MODEL

Framework—"Descriptive categories are placed within a broad structure of both explicit and assumed propositions...its propositions summarize and propose explanations for vast amount of data. It is not a theory, however, because the propositions are not systematically derived in a deductive fashion" (Denzin, 1970).
Models—Symbolic representation of the concepts that make up a theory, may draw on a number of theories or empirical findings to further understanding of a problem in a specific context (Polit & Hungler, 1995).

---

of the propositions or theories they represent and frequently do not make explicit links to theories from which they are derived. Application of such tools therefore involves acknowledging their contextual (ir)relevance and applying them with a measure of flexibility that accounts for contextual realities. A recent study (Scott, 2001) reviewed several frameworks and models of partnership that were developed in the following contexts: government-funded partnerships, public health, health care, community agencies, vulnerable groups, campus/community initiatives, nongovernmental agencies, and business.

When analyzed thematically, partnership and collaborative models clearly share characteristics. This brief overview that we provide below highlights common themes that are repeated many times in the literature (Agger, 1994; Beynon et al., 1999; Courtney et al., 1996; Dayton, Anetzberger, & Matthey, 1997; Fawcett et al., 2000; Gillies, 1997; Harris et al., 1995; Health Canada, 2000; Hulme, 1998; Joint Working Group on the Voluntary Sector, 1999; Kuhn, Doucet, & Edwards, 1999; Lasker, 2000; Parker et al., 1998; Quigley, 1999; Scott & Thurston, 1997, 1998). The factors that influence partnerships include environment or context or external factors, common interest or domain, characteristics of the partnership (principles, common purpose, vision, culture, structures, processes, representation, reputation, resources, outcomes), characteristics of the members or partners (culture, structures, resources, representation, reputation), and communication (open, frequent, formal and informal, shared language, respectful). The processes were generally described as flexible and iterative. Partnership development usually commences with a few potential partners exploring issues of common interest and articulating a common vision and a preliminary strategy before approaching other potential partners. Before commitment to proceed is achieved, many relationship-building activities are required (e.g., developing clear roles and guidelines, accepting accountability, discussing and resolving issues of power, identifying resources, developing and implementing a plan of action, and agreeing on communication strategies). Many process descriptions emphasized the importance of evaluation strategies throughout (Beynon et al., 1999; Gillies, 1997; Harris et al., 1995; Joint Working Group on the Voluntary Sector, 1999; Kuhn et al., 1999; Lasker, 2000;). Resources that were frequently discussed in relation to the process were people, time, and commitment. In the following sections we describe a partnership framework and models that reflect these themes. The tools that we describe were originally developed based on a qualitative study conduced in 1993, which focused on the development of partnerships among community agencies working with vulnerable groups (Scott-Taplin, 1993).

The Partnership Framework

The partnership framework (Table 6-2) comprise six categories: extra-local relations, domain, partner characteristics, partnership characteristics, communication, and operations. Each of these categories is defined below.

Table 6-2 ◆ PARTNERSHIP FRAMEWORK

Categories	Partnerships		
	Properties	Dimensions	
Extra-local factors	Administrative	Organizational	
	Service provision	Individual	
		Community	
Domain	Recognition	Funders	
	Support	Community	
		Vulnerable group	
		Partners	
		Personnel	
Partnership characteristics	Groundwork	Research	Activities
	Organizational structure	Administrative	
		Operational	
	Resources	Funding	Space
		Personnel	Time
		Material	
	Representation	Areas	Characteristics
	Reputation	Positive	Negative
Partner characteristics	Organizational structure	Administrative	
		Operational	
	Resources	Commitment	Funding
		Knowledge	Time
		Skills	
	Representation	Areas	Characteristics
	Reputation	Partners	
		Personnel	
		Vulnerable group	
Communication	Type	Formal	Informal
	Area	Service recipient	
		Personnel	
		Partnership	
		Partner	
		Community	
Operations	Type	Administrative	
		Service provision	
	Area	Service recipient	
		Personnel	
		Partnership	
		Partner	
		Community	

Adapted from Scott-Taplin, C. M. (1993). *The development of partnerships among community agencies working with vulnerable groups* (p. 107). Calgary: University of Calgary.

Extra-Local Relations

Extra-local relations are described as the external influences on the partnership, including the social context and the political and economic systems within which the partnership is based. All programs are situated within social contexts. Although extra-local relations may not play a predominant role in a partnership, they must always be considered. Extra-local relations that may influence the partnership are distinguished by whether they exert influence at the administrative level or at the service provision level. Organizations, individuals, and communities external to the partnership are potential sources of external influence.

Domain

The *domain* is the sphere of interest at the partnership level. Partners may come to a partnership representing interests in several different domains. However, at the partnership level, these disparate interests are focused in an attempt to address one particular domain. If the existence of the domain is recognized and supported by all players (i.e., funders, the community, potential partners, and program personnel), partnership initiatives are more likely to succeed.

Partner Characteristics

Partner characteristics are those factors that distinguish the partners. Each partner will bring distinctive characteristics to the partnership that will directly and indirectly influence its development. These characteristics include:

◆ The organizational structure of the partner agency
◆ The resources that the partner and the partner representative are able to contribute to the partnership initiative
◆ Representation of the target group in the partner agency
◆ The reputation of the partner, of the personnel working for the partner, and of the group(s) served by the partner agency

The importance of formal representation of the target group in the partner agency is something that needs to be discussed by all informants. The characteristics of this representation will vary from partnership to partnership. For example, some agencies might involve the target group at the board/management committee level, whereas other agencies might seek such feedback through questionnaires or informal meetings.

Partnership Characteristics

Each partnership initiative is unique. This uniqueness is a function of the way in which a partnership is established and the individuals and organizations that participate in its development. The characteristics that distinguish a partnership include:

◆ The groundwork completed before the initiation of the partnership initiative
◆ The organizational structure of the partnership
◆ The resources available to the initiative
◆ The representation of the target group within the partnership
◆ The reputation of the partnership

Partnerships that are effective are those that develop partnership characteristics to break down professional territorial barriers. These characteristics include the implementation of communication strategies and professional development opportunities that encourage collaboration (Scott-Taplin, 1993).

COMMUNICATION

Communication affects all of the categories previously discussed. Recognition of formal and informal types of communication is vital to the success of a partnership. The type of communication that occurs between partners will directly or indirectly affect the partnership. There is a need for both formal and informal communication strategies. It is suggested that ongoing evaluation of communication strategies will facilitate the determination of strategies that are appropriate for the partnership at a given time (Scott-Taplin, 1993).

OPERATIONS

Operations are the administrative and service provision activities performed on behalf of the partnership. The operations clearly influence the success of the partnership. The type of operations that are carried out in all areas that are associated with the partnership may directly or indirectly affect the extra-local relations, the domain, partner characteristics, partnership characteristics, and communication. Care must be exercised to ensure that the type of activities that are performed and the manner in which they are performed will advance the vision of the partnership. The types of activities performed by the partnership are influenced by the time frame for completion, the available resources, and knowledge of similar programs.

Partnership Configuration

The configuration of categories, properties, and dimensions must be unique to the specific requirements of the partnership. It is recommended that all six categories and their associated properties and dimensions be appraised and adapted to meet the specific needs of individual partnership initiatives.

Although properties and dimensions reinforce the distinctiveness of each of the categories, these categories must never be considered in isolation. Each of these categories interacts with each of the other categories. Changes in one area may directly, or indirectly, influence changes in all other categories. Just as the cogs within a toy must all work together to propel the toy, within this framework, all of the categories and their properties and dimensions must be considered and configured to advance the partnership toward a common vision.

The configuration will vary from partnership to partnership with some categories taking precedence in some partnerships and other categories taking precedence in other partnerships. Failure to assess each of the elements in the framework to determine its appropriateness for a specific partnership model may result in some essential elements being neglected (Fig. 6-4), some nonessential elements being implemented (Fig. 6-5), or some essential elements being implemented improperly (Fig. 6-6). In any of these situations, the result may be that increased work will be required to ensure the success of the partnership or the partnership may fail to achieve the vision.

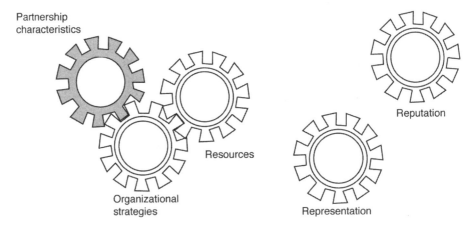

Figure 6-4 ◆ Failure to include essential elements in the partnership. In this example, the partnership has failed to address the issue of representation of the partners. As a result, the partnership is not as successful as it otherwise would have been. (Redrawn from Scott-Taplin, C. M. [1993]. *The development of partnerships among community agencies working with vulnerable groups.* Unpublished Master's thesis. Calgary, AB: University of Calgary.)

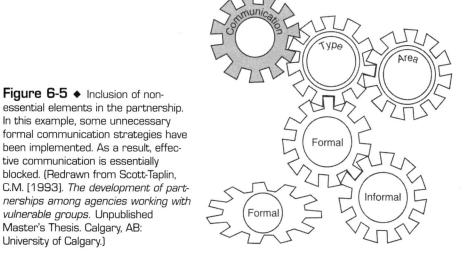

Figure 6-5 ◆ Inclusion of non-essential elements in the partnership. In this example, some unnecessary formal communication strategies have been implemented. As a result, effective communication is essentially blocked. (Redrawn from Scott-Taplin, C.M. [1993]. *The development of partnerships among agencies working with vulnerable groups.* Unpublished Master's Thesis. Calgary, AB: University of Calgary.)

Partnership Organization

The model of partnership organization (Fig. 6-7) extends the description of partnership configuration. This model portrays the categories of the partnership framework enmeshed in the partnership culture. All of the categories are displayed in a relationship of mutual dependency. The linkages (direct and indirect) between each of the categories within the model will vary from partnership to partnership.

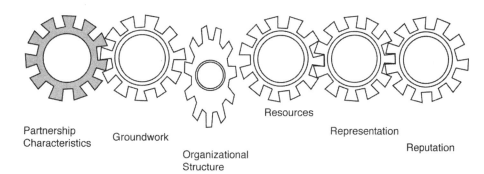

Figure 6-6 ◆ Improper configuration of elements in the partnership model. In this example, the organizational structure that has been selected does not meet the needs of all of the partners. As a result, more work is required to advance the vision of the partnership. (Redrawn from Scott-Taplin, C. M. [1993]. *The development of partnerships among community agencies working with vulnerable groups.* Unpublished Master's thesis. Calgary, AB: University of Calgary.)

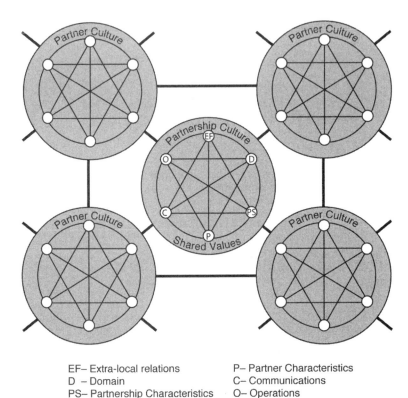

EF– Extra-local relations   P– Partner Characteristics
D – Domain   C– Communications
PS– Partnership Characteristics   O– Operations

Figure 6-7 ◆ A model of partnership organization.

It is important to note that although the characteristics of the partners are part of the partnership culture, the organizational culture of individual partners may overlap with, or be distinct from, the partnership culture. The similarity between the partnership culture and the culture of the individual partners should be carefully considered when forming a partnership. If the partnership and partners' cultures are in conflict, decisions will have to be made about whether the partnership is appropriate for some partners or whether the inclusion of those partners is important enough to warrant extra resources being devoted to support their participation. For example, some additional strategies may be required to make successful a partnership between a government organization that is based on hierarchical structures and a nonprofit organization based on feminist principles of equity and consensus building. It is also important to recognize that partners may develop relationships with one another that are external to the partnership. Consideration should be given to how such external relationships may influence the partnership.

A Process Model
of Partnership Development

It is one thing to recognize that specific elements in the partnership framework are essential or nonessential for the development of a partnership; it is quite another to determine when to implement each of these elements. The process model describes some phases of partnership development (Fig. 6-8).

The development of a partnership is an iterative process. The elements of the process are arranged around a circle. However, after the partnership has been initiated, the order in which these activities occur will vary from one partnership initiative to the next. As the partnership evolves, some elements of the process may need to be revisited.

The process begins with the awareness of a need. It is important to discuss the formation of the partnership with potential partners early in the process.

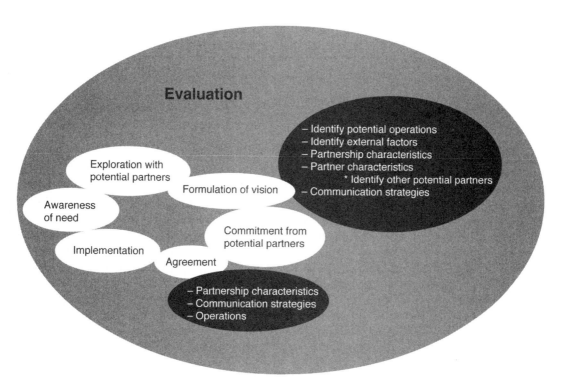

Figure 6-8 ◆ A process model for partnership development.

This informal group will formulate a vision for the collaborative initiative. When the vision has been formulated, this group will be able to:

◆ Identify potential actions/operations that will advance the vision
◆ Identify extra-local relations which may affect the partnership
◆ Identify essential partnership characteristics
◆ Identify the characteristics of other potential partners
◆ Contact the partners that are so identified
◆ Identify communication strategies

The next stage of the process involves going to the identified partner agencies to discuss their potential commitment to the project. Before proceeding, it is recommended that potential partners achieve agreement on issues relating to partnership characteristics, communication strategies, and operations. Once these factors have been established, the partnership initiative can be implemented. Evaluation procedures are an integral part of the entire development process.

Application of the Tools—Key Considerations

Complex interactions within and among categories imply that there is no single right way to develop and structure a partnership initiative (Scott & Thurston, 1997). The proposed framework and models must only be used to guide such initiatives. This being said, the framework suggests some actions that may encourage the success of these ventures.

Prior to developing a relationship of the intensity and formality of a partnership, some coordinating activities are necessary. The completion of groundwork prior to the establishment of a partnership and the implementation of ongoing program evaluation may facilitate the identification of the elements of the framework that are required for a specific partnership. Issues relating to extra-local relations, domain, partnership characteristics, partner characteristics, communication strategies, and potential operations should be discussed early in the development of a partnership initiative.

Failure to complete these activities may result in some essential elements of the framework not being identified or being improperly implemented. When all elements of the partnership framework have been reviewed and appropriately implemented, the partnership is more likely to succeed.

An evaluative component should permeate every aspect of the partnership. An overall commitment to evaluation may ensure that the partnership is responsive to the external environment and that it meets the changing needs of the people that it serves.

Partner Identification

Partners may be identified based on their ability to contribute to the goals of the project. Before entering into partnership agreements, it is necessary to identify preliminary criteria to guide the identification of potential partners.

Each potential partner will seek specific benefits from participation in the partnership. These reasons for participation should be acknowledged through open discussion. If it is not possible for the partnership to meet these individual needs, partners should be given the opportunity to withdraw from the initiative.

It is particularly important that the people who are approached to act as partner representatives be committed to the issue that will be addressed by the partnership. It is essential to develop strategies to maintain a high level of commitment as experienced partner representatives leave and as new partner representatives join the partnership.

In the current economic climate there is increasing pressure on partnership initiatives to achieve the objectives that they identify. In this environment, it will be necessary that partner representatives possess the skills and knowledge required to advance the partnership toward the shared vision. Care should be taken to select partner representatives who will provide different skills required for advancing the partnership. An additional factor to consider in the identification of potential partners is the implications of differences between the organizational culture of the partnership and the organizational culture of potential partners.

Partnership Characteristics, Communication Strategies, and Operations

It is not possible to overemphasize the importance of clearly describing the reason for the partnership. It is essential to develop agreement on definitions regarding the vision, goals, and objectives of the partnership. All of the partner representatives must be talking the same language when they come to the partnership table. Agreement on these and other partnership characteristics, communication strategies, and partnership operations should be in place before a partnership is formally established. Some more successful partnerships have implemented a formal time for discussing partnership issues during each partnership meeting.

Guiding Principles

The results of research regarding the development of partnerships have emphasized the need for partners to agree on the basic guiding principles for the partnership. Although specific principles that are adopted by a partnership will vary, the following general principles have been identified as being valuable for creating sustainable partnerships:

◆ Membership is not assumed. Partners will agree to the mission, goals, objectives, activities, and guiding principles that have been established for the partnership.
◆ All partners and partner representatives are recognized for their unique and essential contributions to the partnership.
◆ All partners agree to share the risks, responsibilities, and rewards associated with the partnership.
◆ All partners agree to the distribution of power within the partnership. Power is shared but may not be equally distributed among the partners.
◆ All partners recognize the need for the partnership to enhance the capacity of individual partners while working to achieve a common purpose.
◆ The structure of the partnership will remain flexible to accommodate changing needs.
◆ Administration of partnership contracts will be assigned to members as appropriate.
◆ All communication (formal and informal) on behalf of the partnership or relating to the partnership will embody the principles of health promotion.
◆ All activities performed on behalf of the partnership will embody the vision and values of health promotion.
(Himmelman, 1996; Labonte, 1993; Thurston & Scott, 1996; Winer & Ray, 1997)

Summary

"Public policy is a highly complex matter, consisting of a series of decisions, involving a large number of actors operating within the confines of an amorphous, yet inescapable, institutional set-up, and employing a variety of instruments. Its complexity poses grave difficulties for those seeking a comprehensive understanding of the subject" (Howlett & Ramesh, 1995, p. 198).

In this chapter we provide a brief introduction to the literature on public policy with the intent of emphasizing the complexities of policy processes. Policy that is designed to effectively address population health must do so with a critical social lens to scrutinize all elements of the policy cycle from construction of the problem to evaluation of solution. We have also linked the purposes, processes, and outcomes of developing strong communities and strengthening social action to the policy development process. The positive effects of healthy communities become evident as citizens participate in making choices and decisions that affect the quality of community life.

References

Abbott, J. (1995). Community participation and its relationship to community development. *Community Development Journal, 30,*158–168.

Agger, N. (1994). *Defining collaboration in the context of inter-agency relationships: An overview and an attempt at re-definition.* Calgary: United Way of Calgary.

Alexander, J. (2000). Adaptive strategies of non-profit human service organizations in an era of devolution and new public management. *Nonprofit Management and Leadership, 10,* 287–303.

Baier, A. C. (1995). A note on justice, care, and immigration policy. *Hypatia, 10,* 150–152.

Beynon, C., Abbott, M., Cashmore, A., Leffley, A., Mai, V., Sussex, B., Boratto, L., Broomfield, E., Feniak, M., & Shular, S. (1999). *Mapping the journey for a successful partnership. Our partnership model.* London, ON: Middlesex-London Health Unit.

Bhatti, T., & Siler-Wells, G. (1987). Strengthening community health means strengthening communities. *CPHA Health Digest, 11,* 2–7.

Briskin, L. (1999). Mapping women's organizing in Sweden and Canada: Some thematic considerations. In L. Briskin & M. Eliasson (Eds.), *Women's organizing and public policy in Canada and Sweden* (pp. 3–47). Montreal: McGill-Queen's University Press.

Carnall, C. A. (1986). Toward a theory for the evaluation of organizational change. *Human Relations, 39,* 745–766.

Cleaver, F. (2001). Institutions, agency and the limitations of participatory approaches to development. In B. Cooke & U. Kothari (Eds.), *Participation: The new tyranny?* (pp. 36–55). London, England: Zed Books.

Cooke, B., & Kothari, U. (2001). The case for participation as tyranny. In B. Cooke & U. Kothari (Eds.), *Participation: The new tyranny?* (pp. 1–15). London, England: Zed Books.

Courtney, R., Ballard, E., Fauver, S., Gariota, M., & Holland, L. (1996). The partnership model: Working with individuals, families, and communities toward a new vision of health. *Public Health Nursing, 13,* 177–186.

Cowen, E. L. (2001). Ethics in community mental health care: The use and misuse of some positively valenced community concepts. *Community Mental Health Journal, 37,* 3–13.

Crow, B., & Gotell, L. (2000). Introduction: What is women's studies? In B. A. Crow & L. Gotell (Eds.), *Open boundaries: A Canadian studies reader* (pp. xii–xviii). Toronto: Prentice-Hall Canada.

Dayton, C., Anetzberger, G. J., & Matthey, D. (1997). A model for service coordination between mental health and adult protective services. *Journal of Mental Health and Aging, 3,* 295–307.

Denzin, N. K. (1970). *The research act: A theoretical introduction to sociological methods.* Chicago: Aldine Publishing.

Detert, J. R., Schroeder, R. G., & Mauriel, J. J. (2000). A framework for linking culture and improvement initiatives in organizations. *Academy of Management Review, 25*, 850–863.

DiStefano, C. (1990). Dilemmas of difference: Feminism, modernity, and postmodernism. In L. J. Nicholson (Ed.), *Feminism/postmodernism* (pp. 63–82). New York: Routledge.

Doern, G. B., & Phidd, R. W. (1992). *Canadian public policy: Ideas, structure, process* (2nd ed.). Toronto: Nelson.

Draper, R. (1995). *Perspectives in health promotion: A discussion paper.* Ottawa: Canadian Public Health Association.

Engberg-Pedersen, L., & Webster, N. (2002). Introduction to political space. In N. Webster & L. Engberg-Pedersen (Eds.), *In the name of the poor: Contesting political space for poverty reduction* (pp. 1–29). London, England: Zed Books.

Epp, J. (1986). *Achieving health for all: A framework for health promotion.* Ottawa: Minister of Supply and Services.

Evans, R. G., Barer, M. L., & Marmor, T. R. (1994). *Why are some people healthy and others not? The determinants of health populations.* Hawthorne, NY: Aldine de Gruyter.

Fawcett, S. B., Francisco, V. T., Paine-Andrews, A., & Schultz, J. A. (2000). A model memorandum of collaboration: a proposal. *Public Health Reports, 115*, 174–190.

Federal/Provincial/Territorial Advisory Committee on Population Health. (1991). *Strategies for population health: Investing in the health of Canadians.* Ottawa: Health Canada.

Feldberg, G., & Carlsson, M. (1999). Organized for health: Women's activism in Canada and Sweden. In L. Briskin & M. Eliasson (Eds.), *Women's organizing and public policy in Canada and Sweden* (pp. 347–374). Montreal: McGill University Press.

Fournier, P., & Potvin, L. (1995). Participation communautaires et programmes de sante: Les fondements du dogme. *Sciences Sociales et Sante, 13*, 39–59.

Giachello, A. L. (1995). Cultural diversity and institutional inequality. In D.L. Adams (Ed.), *Health issues for women of color: A cultural diversity perspective* (pp. 5–26). Thousand Oaks, CA: Sage.

Gillies, P. (1997). *The effectiveness of alliances or partnerships for health promotion. A global review of progress and potential consideration of the relationship to building social capital for health (Conference Working Paper).* Jakarta, Indonesia: Fourth International Conference on Health Promotion.

Gillies, P. (1998). Effectiveness of alliances and partnerhsips for health promotion. *Health Promotion International, 13*, 99–120.

Gordon, P., Plamping, D., & Pratt, J. (1999). Partnership: fit for purpose? In S. Schruijer (Ed.), *Multi-organizational partnerships and cooperative strategy* (pp. 149–153). Tilburg, The Netherlands: Dutch University Press.

Gray, B. (1989). *Collaborating—Finding common ground for mulitparty problems.* San Francisco: Jossey-Bass.

Gray, B. (1996). Cross-sectoral partners: Collaborative alliances among business, government and communities. In C. Huxham (Ed.), *Creating collaborative advantage* (pp. 57–79). Thousand Oaks, CA: Sage.

Hailey, J. (2001). Beyond the formulaic: Process and practice in South Asian NGOs. In B. Cooke & U. Kothari (Eds.), *Participation: The new tyranny?* (pp. 88–101). London, England: Zed Books.

Harris, E., Wise, M., Hawe, P., Finlay, P., & Nutbeam, D. (1995). *Working together: Intersectoral action for health.* Canberra, Australia: Commonwealth of Australia.

Health Canada. (1996). *Health partners: a report on Health Canada community health initiatives in Alberta.* Edmonton: Health Canada, Health Promotion Programs Branch, Alberta, Northwest Territories Region.

Health Canada. (2000). *Intersectoral action toolkit: The cloverleaf model for success.* Edmonton: Health Canada.

Hennekens, C. H. & Buring, J. E. (1987). *Epidemiology in medicine.* Toronto: Little, Brown.

Hildyard, N., Hegde, P. H., Wolvekamp, P., & Reddy, S. R. (2001). Pluralism, participation and power: Joint forest management in India. In B. Cooke & U. Kothari (Eds.), *Participation: The new tyranny?* (pp. 56–71). London, England: Zed Books.

Himmelman, A. T. (1996). On the theory and practice of transformational collaboration: From social service to social justice. In C. Huxham (Ed.), *Creating collaborative advantage* (pp. 19(–43). Thousand Oaks, CA: Sage.

Hornby, S. (1993). *Collaborative care: Interprofessional, interagency and interpersonal.* London, England: Oxford/Blackwell Scientific Publications.

Howlett, M., & Ramesh, M. (1995). *Studying public policy: Policy cycles and policy subsystems.* Toronto: Oxford University Press.

Hulme, A. (1998). *An analysis of collaboration in the municipal public health plan process in a number of Victorain municipalities.* Unpublished master's thesis. Melbourne, Australia: Deakin University.

Huxham, C., & Vangen, S. (2000). Leadership in the shaping and implementation of collaboration agendas: How things happen in a (not quite) joined-up world. *Academy of Management Journal, 43,* 1159–1175.

Jadad, A. R. (1999). Promoting partnerships: Challenges for the Internet age. *British Medical Journal, 319,* 761–764.

Joint Working Group on the Voluntary Sector. (1999). *Building the relationship between national voluntary organizations working in health and Health Canada.* Ottawa: Health Canada.

Kelly, K., & Vlaenderen, V. (1995). Evaluating participation processes in community development. *Evaluation and Program Planning, 18,* 371–383.

Kemm, J., & Close, A. (1995). *Health promotion: theory and practice.* London, England: Macmillan Press.

Kretzmann, P., & McKnight, J. (1993). *Building communities from the inside out: A path toward finding and mobilizing a community's assets.* Evanston, IL: Institute for Policy Research.

Kuhn, M., Doucet, C., & Edwards, N. (1999). *Effectiveness of coalitions in heart health promotion, tobacco use reduction, and injury prevention: a systematic review of the literature 1990–1998.* Ottawa: Community Health Research Unit.

Labonte, R. (1993). Community development and partnerships. *Canadian Journal of Public Health, 84,* 237–240.

Lasker, R. D. (2000). *Promoting collaborations that improve health.* San Francisco: Community-Campus Partnerships for Health.

MacKean, G., & Thurston W. E. (1996). A Canadian model of public participation in health care planning and decision making. In M. Stingl & D. Wilson (Eds.), *Efficiency versus equality: Health reform in Canada* (pp. 55–69). Halifax: Fernwood Publishing.

Maloff, B., Bilan, D., & Thurston, W. E. (2000). Enhancing public input into decision making: Development of the Calgary Regional Health Authority Public Participation. *Family and Community Health, 23,* 66–78.

Miller, W. L., Crabtree, B. F., McDaniel, R., & Stange, K. C. (1998). Understanding change in primary care practice using complexity theory. *Journal of Family Practice, 46,* 369–376.

Minkler, M. (1994). Challenges for health promotion in the 1990s: Social inequities, empowerment, negative consequences, and the common good. *American Journal of Health Promotion, 8*(6), 403–413.

Mosse, D. (2001). "People's knowledge," participation and patronage: Operations and representations in rural development. In B. Cooke & U. Kothari (Eds.), *Participation: The new tyranny?* (pp. 16–35). London, England: Zed Books.

Pal, L. A. (2001). *Beyond policy analysis: Public issue management in turbulent times.* (2nd ed.) Scarborough, ON: Nelson Thomson Learning.

Parker, E. A., Eng, E., Laraia, B., Ammerman, A., Dodds, J., Margolis, L., & Cross, A. (1998). Coalition building for prevention. *Journal of Public Health Management Practice, 4,* 25–36.

Pederson, A. P., Edwards, R. K., Marshall, V. W., Allison, K. R., & Kelner, M. (1988). *Coordinating healthy public policy: An analytic literature review and bibliography.* Ottawa: Minister of National Health and Welfare.

Phillips, S. D. & Orsini, M. (2002). *Mapping the links: Citizen involvement in policy processes* (Rep. No. CPRN Discussion Paper No. F/21). Ottawa: Canadian Policy Research Networks.

Plaut, T., Landis, S., & Trevor, J. (1992). Enhancing participatory research with the community oriented primary care model: A case study in community mobilization. *The American Sociologist, 23,* 56–70.

Poland, B. D. (1992). Learning to 'walk our talk': The implications of sociological theory for research methodologies in health promotion. *Canadian Journal of Public Health, 83,* S31–S46.

Polit, D. F., & Hungler, B. P. (1995). *Nursing research, principles and methods.* (5th ed.) Philadelphia: Lippincott.

Quigley, M. A. (1999). *Strategic alliances in health care: The way of the future.* Capital Health Authority: 4th annual designing health conference. New partnerships for a new millennium. Edmonton: Capital Health Authority.

Scott, C. M. (2000). http://www.apha.ab.ca/ptnr-m.html.

Scott, C. M. (2001). *Partnership theory for Canadian health systems: An analysis of research and practice.* Unpublished doctoral dissertation. Calgary: University of Calgary.

Scott, C. M., & Thurston W. E. (1997). A framework for the development of community health agency partnerships. *The Canadian Journal of Public Health, 88,* 416–420.

Scott, C. M., & Thurston, W. E. (1998). Community development and partnerships in health promotion research: An evaluation model. In W. E. Thurston, J. D. Sieppert, & V. J. Wiebe (Eds.), *Doing health promotion research: The science of action.* Calgary: Health Promotion Research Group.

Scott-Taplin, C. M. (1993). *The development of partnerships among community agencies working with vulnerable groups.* Calgary: University of Calgary.

Smith, S. E., Pyrch, T., & Lizardi, A. O. (1993). Participatory action-research for health. *World Health Forum, 14,* 319–324.

Standing Committee on Health, Welfare and Social Affairs. (1982). *Report on violence in the family: Wife battering.* Ottawa: Queen's Printer for Canada.

Thurston, W. E., & Scott, C.M. (1996). *Lessons learned from health promotion initiatives in Alberta. A report prepared for the Health Promotion Research Group.* Calgary: University of Calgary.

Trist, E. L. (1983). Referent organizations and the development of inter-organizational domains. *Human Relations 36,* 269–284.

Vancouver/Richmond Health Board. (2000). *Women's health planning project: Final report.* Vancouver: Author.

Weiss, C. H. (1995). Nothing as practical as good theory: Exploring theory-based evaluation for comprehensive community initiatives for children and families. In J. P. Connell, A. C. Kubisch, L. B. Schorr, & C. H. Weiss (Eds.), *New approaches to evaluating community initiatives: Concepts, methods, and contexts* (pp. 65–92). Washington DC: Aspen Institute.

Winer, M., & Ray, K. (1997). *Collaboration handbook: Creating, sustaining, and enjoying the journey.* Saint Paul, MN: Amherst H. Wilder Foundation.

World Health Organization. (1986). *Intersectoral action for health.* Geneva, Switzerland: Author.

World Health Organization. (1986). *Ottawa charter for health promotion.* Geneva, Switzerland: Author.

World Health Organization. (2003). *Healthy cities.* Available: http://www.who.int/hpr/archive/cities (accessed on April 1, 2003).

Zaini, J. (1998). Women: Consumers as activists. *Community Development Journal, 23,* 235–242.

7

Cultural Competence in Partnerships With Communities

ADAPTED FROM THE ORIGINAL CHAPTER BY JUDITH C. DREW

Being the other is feeling different; it is an awareness of being distinct; it is consciousness of being dissimilar. Otherness results in feeling excluded, closed out, precluded, even disdained and scorned. ... On the one hand being the other frequently means being invisible ... Or inevitably seen stereotypically. For the majority, otherness is permanently sealed by physical appearance. For the rest, otherness is betrayed by ways of being, speaking, or of doing. (Madrid, 1988, pp 10–11, 16)

Arturo Madrid tells his story of being different, its significance, and its consequences. His poignant expressions of "otherness" are wakeup calls for us. Our sensitivities may be sharpened if we consider that, in any place, at any time, we might just be an "other."

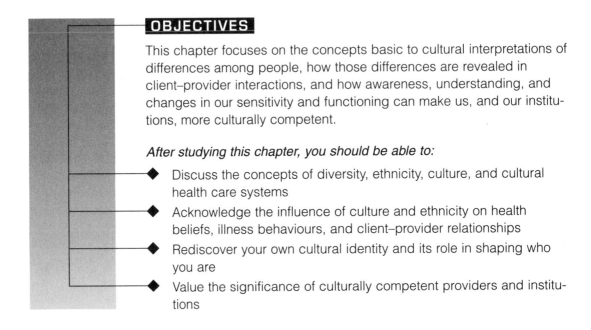

OBJECTIVES

This chapter focuses on the concepts basic to cultural interpretations of differences among people, how those differences are revealed in client–provider interactions, and how awareness, understanding, and changes in our sensitivity and functioning can make us, and our institutions, more culturally competent.

After studying this chapter, you should be able to:

◆   Discuss the concepts of diversity, ethnicity, culture, and cultural health care systems

◆   Acknowledge the influence of culture and ethnicity on health beliefs, illness behaviours, and client–provider relationships

◆   Rediscover your own cultural identity and its role in shaping who you are

◆   Value the significance of culturally competent providers and institutions

Introduction

This chapter presents concepts that will assist you in building cultural competence, beginning with an enlightened awareness of diversity, ethnicity, and culture, and illustrating their influence on individuals' and communities' health and illness beliefs and practices. Self-assessment and an analysis of client–provider interactions are presented as learning experiences with implications for practice. After all, successful health promotion intervention strategies and outcomes depend on our abilities to competently reach and work with the diverse communities we serve.

Diversity, Ethnicity, and Culture

Derived from the Latin *divertere*, diversity implies the condition of being different or having differences. There is no attempt made here to imply a ranking, ordering, or prioritizing of differences; they simply exist. How we look at and deal with differences in human attributes can either build bridges or construct barriers with individuals in and across groups and communities. Rather than thinking of differences as sources of conflict, we should view them as part of a whole process of social and individual identity. A celebration of differences can become commonplace when we understand that the principal strengths on which our country is built suggest a tolerance for individual uniqueness and a collective creativity (Drew, 2000). Recognizing that each of us differs in what we think is functional in our lives, we must understand that those who act differently from the mainstream are not deficit in something or "disadvantaged"; they are rich in a different culture and are "other-advantaged" (Dervin, 1989; Lyons, 1972).

Ethnicity and race are overlapping concepts (Centers for Disease Control and Prevention, 1993); *race* usually refers to a group of people who share common biologic features and ethnicity is a classification based on some commonality or affiliation. *Ethnicity* includes a shared culture rather than shared biologic characteristics. *Culture* is the learned and shared behaviour and understanding that acts as a behavioural map and perceptual filter. Culture, ethnicity, and race are often used interchangeably, creating confusion about their respective meanings (Strasser, 1995).

In daily practice, community workers provide services to individuals, families, and communities from around the globe. Yet we know little about the basic cultures, beliefs, and values that shape our clients' health and well-being, healing beliefs, and behaviours. Asking clients to teach us about themselves will extend to others our sensitivities about being different and will empower others to share their own awareness and may allow providers to administer better care. Taking the time to value both the differences and commonalities across ethnic and cultural groups will provide us with valuable insights into the human experience and enable us to build bridges between providers and the growing numbers of diverse individuals (Drew, 2000).

Historical Context

> As a society built around existing Aboriginal peoples, based on two founding European cultures, and expanded through successive waves of immigration, Canada has ... been at the forefront of debates about the recognition of cultural diversity. Not only are some of the leading scholars in the field Canadians, but Canada is also to a certain extent a laboratory in terms of policy development in response to such challenges. (Jenson & Papillon, 2000)

Since 1971, the Government of Canada has promoted its official policy of multiculturalism that is often termed a "cultural mosaic" in contrast to the United States' assimilation model or "melting pot." To the extent that cultural rights exist, they are intended to enhance individuals' freedom to choose to live according to their own cultural heritage (Jenson & Papillon, 2000).

Multiculturalism policy promotes tolerance through antiracist programs and programs that enhance access (e.g., to education, health, employment, language training, etc.) to minority groups.

Canada recognizes national minorities in facing the challenges of a diverse population (Jenson & Papillon, 2000). Traditionally this discourse has involved the place, rights, responsibilities, cohesion, and attachment to the nation of French- and English-speaking Canadians in the various provinces. Quebec views itself as a "distinct society" and has achieved independence from the federal government in a number of portfolios, including immigration. More recently, Aboriginal people have sought recognition of certain privileges and rights not available to other Canadians on the basis of their status as First Nations that allows them to exercise a limited sovereignty over the lands granted to them under treaties with the Crown and the people residing on those lands (Jenson & Papillon, 2000).

There have been many waves of immigration to Canada; from 1860 to 1998 nearly 15 million people have immigrated. Prior to the outbreak of the Civil War in the United States in 1861, 30,000 slaves came to Canada. In the 1870s, Canada averaged 33,000 immigrants annually; in 1871 (Canada's first official census) two thirds of the people of Ontario identified themselves as Irish. Many Irish had come to Upper Canada to work on the construction of the Rideau Canal with Colonel By in the wake of potato famines in their home country. In the 1880s, many Chinese were brought to Canada to help with building the Canadian Pacific Railway; however, in 1885 an act was passed to restrict Chinese immigration once the railroad was completed. In the 1890s, an advertising campaign attracted many Europeans to Canada as homesteaders to populate the prairies and, by the end of the first decade at the turn of the century, 28% of Canada's population were immigrants. In fact, the largest number of immigrants to Canada was in 1913 when 400,810 people arrived.

There are some dark moments in Canada's immigration history with evidence of anti-Semitism, racism (particularly against people of African ancestry), intolerance (e.g., the internment of "foreign aliens" in times of war), and outright discrimination against certain groups of people. In 1914, Indian nationals aboard the *Komagata Maru* were denied access (Box 7-1); until 1925 orphaned British "home children" were sent to Canadian farms as apprentices. From 1920 to 1929, 138,000 Jews immigrated to Canada, many of them refugees fleeing organized massacres in Czarist Russia and Eastern Europe; in several subsequent years no Jews were admitted. In the 1930s, immigration was restricted because of the Great Depression; only American and British citizens were allowed entry. After World War II, immigration levels again climbed and in 1947 the first Immigration Act was proclaimed, followed by the formation of the Department of Citizenship and Immigration. The next two decades saw

---

BOX 7-1.   IMMIGRATION OF INDIANS

In 1914, the ship called *Komagatu Maru* arrived in Vancouver, having sailed from China with 376 Indian nationals aboard, who were refused admittance to Canada. After 2 months in the harbour, and following an unsuccessful appeal to the BC Supreme Court, the boat sailed back to China. Between 1914 and 1920 only one Indian was admitted to Canada as an immigrant.

---

many refugees accepted from the 1957 Hungarian uprising and the 1967 Prague spring. In the 1970s, immigration was closely related to economic activity, and in 1978 Parliament enacted a policy to reunite close family members. The United States was the largest source country of immigration in 1971–1972, in part because of the large numbers (an estimated 40,000) of "draft dodgers" unwilling to fight in Vietnam who found refuge in Canada. Although a recession was responsible for halving immigration numbers in the early 1980s, Canada received the 1986 Nansen Medal for its support of the Southeast Asian "boat people." Immigration targets are currently set at approximately 200,000 annually; the largest numbers were entering from Eastern Asia (252,340), Southeast Asia (118,265), and Southern Asia (140,055) in the 5 years between 1991 and 1996 (Statistics Canada, 2002).

Cultural Barriers to Health Care

Despite Canada's policy of equal access to health care, significant barriers exist due to language, culture, and ethnicity. Most programs in Canada rely on the ability to communicate in English (except in Quebec where the official language is French), are oriented toward people in the middle income bracket, and are based on Western values and concepts of socialization, child development, and family structure (Centre for Addiction and Mental Health, 1999). Consequently, people from ethnocultural communities may not make use of existing services. They may feel that care does not respond to their needs; their need for help is a shameful reflection on them; they have not yet exhausted the family or folk remedies for their condition; they fear stigma; they perceive distance and cost to be barriers; they may not be aware of services available; they cannot speak the language of the new country and there are no human service providers that speak their language; they lack trust in the system; they fear discrimination and racism; and they have less opportunity than Canadian-born workers to take time off from work to attend appointments. Community workers may have difficulty working in ethnic communities because of communication problems, literacy issues, misunderstanding about experiences (e.g., torture, poverty), inadequate translation, and stereotyping.

Beyond awareness and understanding, health care providers must develop skills to work with culturally diverse individuals, their families, and communities. Many believe that these skills are learned rather than innate and that they require commitment and nurturing. Such an imperative also suggests that programs and services be designed so that they are available, acceptable, and appropriate to the cultures they seek to serve (Adams, 1990). This "cultural competence" demands that practitioners and delivery systems understand a client's, family's, and even a community's perception of their health needs (Campinha-Bacote, 1995; Cross, 1987), including their health status and acceptable sources of help during vulnerability and illness (Box 7-2).

According to Sockalingam (2002), several elements contribute to becoming culturally competent: valuing diversity, conducting cultural self-assessment, understanding the dynamics of cultural differences, institutionalizing cultural knowledge, and adapting to diversity. Cultural competence is built on a strengths model, not a deficit model. Traditionally the human service community has dealt with minority populations on the basis of deficits, that is, that they are somehow lacking or insufficient in some way, compared to the rest of the population

Culture, for the purposes of this chapter, is a concept that includes not only ethnic groups but also (to name but a few) women, people of different age groups and sexual orientation, people with disabilities, people living in poverty, people with mental illness, overweight people, smokers, alcohol or drug abusers, street people, and religious minorities. Such groups often have their needs and perspectives ignored or demeaned by mainstream health providers. Refugees, for instance, may require specialized services to adjust to the new community.

As we partner with communities to improve the health of Canadians, it is important that we examine issues of white privilege, social identity, and domi-

---

BOX 7-2. CULTURAL COMPETENCE

Cultural competence is a set of congruent behaviours, practices, attitudes, and policies that come together in a system or agency or among professionals, enabling effective work to be done in cross-cultural situations (Cross et al., 1989).

nation in Canadian society as we endeavour to determine priorities, solutions, and strategies. Many collaborations between mainstream service organizations and minority communities fail because agencies use strategies that are based on mainstream values and beliefs, forgetting to recognize that aspects of collaboration (such as building trust, determining positions and interests, having effective communication, building consensus, and resolving conflicts) are also culturally bound (Sockalingam, 2002).

Valuing Diversity

Wirth (1945, p. 347) has suggested that a minority is "a group of people who, because of their physical or cultural characteristics, are singled out from others in the society in which they live, for differential and unequal treatment, and who therefore regard themselves as objects of collective discrimination." Health care providers need to appreciate the special histories of ethnic minority groups, how their identities are preserved, their variant subcultures, and their unique coping structures—all of which have been challenged by change, exploitation, and prejudice (Moore, 1971). We still have a long way to go to improve the health status of groups who are at great risk. To do this, we must understand that there may be differences in health and healing beliefs between care providers and care recipients. Those differences are rooted in heritage, ethnicity, and culture, but they represent potential barriers to healing relationships.

Whether ethnicity is associated with minority or majority populations, ethnic groups are composed of persons who share a unique cultural background and social heritage that is passed from one generation to another. Ethnicity should be understood as a social differentiation that engenders in us a sense of self-awareness and exclusivity, a sense of belonging. Our ethnicity gives us a membership in a distinct social group and differentiates us from those in other groups. Our distinction is often based on such cultural criteria as a common ancestry, shared history, a common place of origin, language, dress, food preferences, and participation in rituals, networks, clubs, or activities (Holzberg, 1982). The passing of these beliefs, values, knowledge, and practices occurs through the rituals of sharing and participating in cultural events and celebrations.

It may be helpful to think of your own ethnic culture. What group(s) do you identify with and why? What are your common bonds? What cultural rituals do you celebrate and with whom? What are the purposes and meanings of your gatherings and celebrations? What types of things are shared and learned when people get together? What types of foods are prepared for the event? Are there dances, special rites, or ceremonies? Each of us can probably identify several shared beliefs, values, and practices that make us members of unique collectives, and many of us strive to preserve our rich cultures and histories by passing them on to each successive generation. Foods, languages, and other bonds of common ancestry are the cultural aspects of ethnicity that offer consistency and structure to life and provide individuals with abilities to interpret life events as significant and meaningful (Royce, 1982).

In health and illness, an ethnic group's shared beliefs, symbols, and customs serve as common reference points that members use to judge the appropriateness of their decisions and actions (Kleinman, 1986). However, attention must be given to the variations within and between generations that are sometimes attributed to acculturation, socioeconomic status, and education (Congress & Lyons, 1992). Caution should be taken by all health care providers not to generalize beliefs and practices to every member of an ethnic group or culture (Campinha-Bacote, 1995). Although ethnicity captures the larger cultural component of human experiences, we must not permit our awareness of a culture to erode its members' individual identities and dignity.

Gender Discrimination

Discrimination does not affect women and men the same way; minority women often face multiple forms of discrimination (Box 7-3). The Office of the High Commissioner for Human Rights (OHCHR) at the United Nations (2001) reports that women suffer the following forms of discrimination:

◆ Gender-based violence—Women tend to face higher rates of violence because gender discrimination renders them among the most powerless members of society. Because racial discrimination often results in violence,

---

BOX 7-3. WHAT IS DISCRIMINATION?

Discrimination means to treat someone differently or unfairly because of a personal characteristic. The Supreme Court of Canada describes discrimination as a "distinction which, whether intentional or not but based on grounds relating to personal characteristics of the individual or group, has an effect which imposes disadvantages not imposed upon others or which withholds or limits access to other members of society" *Andrews v. Law Society of BC* (1989) 1 S.C.R.p.1144).

Canadian Human Rights Commission (2001)

women who face both race and gender discrimination are doubly at risk from violence.

◆ Poverty—The majority of the global population living in poverty are women. With lack of access to education and training programs, women have limited employment options.

◆ Education—Worldwide the literacy rate for men is 84% and 71% for women. In developing countries, 60% of men are literate compared with 40% of women. Two thirds of illiterate adults are women.

◆ Labour market—Exploitative labour practices disproportionately affect women of disadvantaged communities; women are subjected to poor working environments, minimal or no social protection, low wages, and abusive conditions.

◆ Trafficking in humans—Limited avenues for legal migration make women vulnerable to trafficking, forced labour, or slavery-like practices. Women are lured into underground networks with promises of jobs in the West only to suffer humiliation, prostitution, and threats from crime rings. When apprehended, they suffer at the hands of law enforcement officials, are criminalized, and deported back to the country of origin without recourse.

◆ Health—Racial discrimination is among the factors that can prevent women from receiving adequate health care. Many lack power over their bodies and sexual lives, may be stigmatized by HIV or other infections, may also be forcibly sterilized, or subjected to coercive measures (e.g., female circumcision), while showing low rates of preventive screening (e.g., Pap smears, mammography) and high rates of maternal mortality.

◆ Armed conflict—Violence against women is often part of a war strategy to undermine the morale of a community. Violence, rape, genital mutilation, forced pregnancy or abortion, and sexual slavery are used as a means of ethnic cleansing. After the conflict, women who have experienced these atrocities are shunned or ostracized from their communities, experience guilt and stigma, and suffer from mental health consequences that often go untreated.

◆ Politics and decision-making—In no country of the world are women represented in the same numbers as men in positions of power and authority. Few women are legislators, heads of corporation, or in senior justice positions, thus further marginalizing minority women and creating an inequitable society (OHCHR, 2001) (Box 7-4).

Not only are people treated differently on the basis of their sex, but for other reasons also. Age, religion, and ethnic affiliation are also causes for discrimination. Youth and seniors are often treated unfairly because of their age and lack of power, and history is rife with examples of religious prejudice. It is beyond the scope of this text to deal with all situations that cause inequity and injus-

---

BOX 7-4. FAMOUS FIVE

In 1927, Emily Murphy and four other prominent Canadian women—Nellie McClung, Irene Parlby, Louise McKinney and Henrietta Muir Edwards—asked the Supreme Court of Canada to answer the question, "Does the word 'person' in Section 24 of the BNA Act include female persons?" After 5 weeks of debate and argument the Supreme Court of Canada decided that the word "person" did *not* include women.

The five women, nicknamed "The Famous Five," were shocked by the Supreme Court decision but did not give up the fight. Instead they refused to accept the decision and took the Persons Case to the Privy Council in England, which in those days was Canada's highest court.

On October 18, 1929, Lord Sankey, Lord Chancellor of the Privy council, announced the decision of the five Lords. The decision stated "that the exclusion of women from all public offices is a relic of days more barbarous than ours. And to those who would ask why the word 'person' should include females, the obvious answer is, why should it not?"

The Famous Five achieved not only the right for women to serve in the Senate, but they and their many contributions paved the way for women to participate in other aspects of public life and the assertion of women's rights is now honoured by the Governor General's Awards in Commemoration of the Persons Case.

Status of Women Canada, 2000.

---

tice, but the principles of dealing with one form of "ism" are transferable to others. In the next section, change the term "ethnocultural" to seniors, youth groups (gangs), disabled people, or "Hamiltonians, Manitobans, mainlanders" and you will see how the principles apply.

Racism and Prejudice

Ethnocultural communities are not homogeneous; many smaller groups may be contained within the larger community. For instance, recent immigrants will have needs different from those people who have been in Canada for a generation or more; they may need second language training to prepare for prospective employment and education. Some people within a community will be wealthy and others will be disadvantaged in several ways (e.g., poverty, illiteracy, age, and gender). Community workers cannot assume that just because a translator is available to make communication possible that all aspects of culture can be interpreted and that all questions will be answered fully and truth-fully. Language interpreters are not necessarily cultural interpreters; issues of "class, power, disparate beliefs, lack of linguistic equivalence, or the disparate use of language" (Kaufert & Putsch [1997] as cited in Oelke, 2002) are much more difficult to address.

To create an environment that promotes health, community workers must act to strengthen community action and increase social support, mutual aid, and coping skills. In other words, community development is the key to social action.

Culture, Health, and Illness

Ethnic culture is the medium through which an individual's beliefs, standards, and norms for health and illness behaviours are structured, learned, shared, practised, and judged. Cultural beliefs give meaning to health and illness experiences by providing the individual with culturally acceptable causes for illness, rules for symptom expression, interactional norms, help-seeking strategies, and determining desired outcomes (Harwood, 1981; Kleinman, 1980). For example, when you awake before school with dryness in your throat and cramps in your stomach, several beliefs about what could be wrong and how you should act in response to what is wrong are set into action. What is causing this to happen to me? What can I do about it? Should I stay home from school? Who should I call for help? What will people think if I stay home today? The answers to these questions and the actions you take are learned and are influenced by the experiences you have had with your family and the larger ethnic aggregate. In some cultures, a special home remedy tea can be taken for specific complaints of dry throat and cramps and going to work or school is an expectation. Other cultural groups may expect you to be visited by a healer, stay home from work or school, and tell no one else about your problem (Drew, 2000).

Noted psychiatrist and anthropologist Arthur Kleinman studied members of many diverse ethnic groups to gain an understanding of the links between cultural beliefs and health and illness behaviours and actions (Kleinman, 1980). The findings of his studies are especially helpful in guiding community practitioners who interact with clients in their homes and various types of community institutions. He found, like other researchers, that cultural beliefs based in shared meanings, values, and norms are the basic guidelines people use for recognizing that something is wrong, interpreting what it might be, and organizing a plan of appropriate actions (Kleinman, 1986). For example, before action is taken in response to a problem, individuals and family members must first agree that the symptoms represent a problem. Next, there is an examination of all possible and probable causes, which may range from behaviours and foods to violations of cultural norms. Once a cause is identified, a plan of action is made and appropriate treatment is determined. In addition, how we act when we are "ill" is determined by our ethnic culture. Some cultures have specific norms for sick role behaviour, whereas other cultures suggest that you continue to carry out your everyday role to the best of your abilities. In this overall illness recognition and management process, cultural beliefs influence the reasons the client formulates to explain the illness, the language and terms used for communicating the health problem, the choice of whom one talks to about the problem, the range of acceptable healing alternatives, how choices are made, and expectations for treatment outcomes (Helman, 1984; Kleinman, 1980; Mechanic, 1986). In Box 7-5, an example of community workers attempting to deal with a feral cat problem is presented to illustrate the process of solving a community health problem in a culturally appropriate manner.

For those of us in the helping professions, culturally sensitive health care continues to be a central focus of a holistic and humanistic philosophy that guides our practice (Aamodt, 1978; Leininger, 1991; Munet-Vilaro, 1988). The role of cultural beliefs in guiding a client's (whether individual, family, or community) health practices and responses is an important concern to community health workers (Whall, 1987).

The healing goals of culturally sensitive care can only be achieved through conscious efforts at gaining knowledge of different groups' ways of explaining, understanding, and treating health problems. Certainly gaining this knowledge and putting it to use will take some time, but it is important for practitioners to learn the strategies presented in this chapter for eliciting cultural models for health, illness, help seeking, and healing.

Strasser (1995) identifies the following key concepts as central to understanding cultural communities:

◆ Time and space. The Western view of time is linear, divided into parts with a beginning and an end. A circular view of time is a perception that time is a never-ending unity, part of a continuous whole. A linear view sees time as a commodity to be used and controlled; in a circular view time is perceived as a gift to be enjoyed.

   Different cultures structure space in different ways; space is linked with territoriality, or the creation of physical boundaries. Some cultures are accustomed to very little distance in personal space; others are more comfortable with larger distances. When space is invaded, people may become angry or intimidated. Land and personal property are seen by various cultures as communal or as individual; shared spaces as informal or formal.

BOX 7-5. SOLVING A HEALTH ISSUE IN AN ETHNIC COMMUNITY: CONTROL OF FERAL CATS

The control of feral cats in ethnic communities requires special care because cultural attitudes towards cats vary. This includes:

- Attitudes about allowing them inside a human dwelling
- Whether neutering is permissible according to religious observances
- Whether other forms of contraception are permissible
- Whether euthanasia is permitted

Practical Problems Facing Cat Workers

The most obvious problem facing cat workers in some Asian communities is that many of the older residents do not speak good English. Some, particularly the middle-aged and older women, do not speak any English at all. Some households may be very traditional and the women may live in total seclusion (purdah); they are fully robed (in chadors) when outside and will not speak to strangers. However, the children are usually bilingual and act as translators; they are also interested in the cats and are often eager to help the cats.

Posters and information leaflets therefore have to be translated, or even better, presented in bilingual form, and it is appreciated when cat workers learn some basic language skills—again, the children are most eager to help.

The community is very important and there is likely to be a gathering place (often as part of, or close to, a place of worship) and in traditional communities, elders are greatly respected. If cat workers are invited into a mosque, they are advised to observe dress rules: for women this means modest dress with shoulders and arms covered, though head-covering is not mandatory in all areas. A donation to the mosque collection is a welcome gesture of respect. Though Westerners may consider some religious observances "sexist," these views must be put aside to gain respect and be able to carry out cat work. In very strict households a woman may not give instructions to a man, and cat worker recommendations (which might be relayed through a junior male member of the household) must be phrased tactfully so that they do not appear to be orders.

Out of respect for the teachings of the Koran on the subject of birth control, cat welfare projects are best not promoted as neutering schemes unless the community has already expressed willingness in this matter. The emphasis should therefore be placed on improving the quality of life and welfare of the cats; the subject of neutering should be approached with considerable tact and diplomacy. Abortion is anathema to Muslims; therefore, the spaying of obviously pregnant cats is distressing to the community.

Neutering will reduce the amount of caterwauling. Hindus consider caterwauling to be an omen of a death in the vicinity (much like a wailing banshee). Cats are believed to be very paranormal animals, able to see the spirits or messengers who come to collect the souls of the dead. When they see such a spirit they wail, and this is a sign that someone in the area is about to die.

(continued)

BOX 7-5. SOLVING A HEALTH ISSUE IN AN ETHNIC COMMUNITY: CONTROL OF FERAL CATS (*Continued*)

Among Muslims who own cats, the attitude toward neutering will depend on whether they are traditional or moderate in their interpretation of the Koran and whether the individual feels himself to be doing God's work in preventing suffering rather than infringing on God's work. Because tomcats spray smelly urine, neutering may be seen as a cleanliness issue and some may consider neutered cats "cleaner." Each person's beliefs must be dealt with individually, being aware that people who agree to neutering may face hostility from their community.

An alternative to surgical neutering is contraceptive implants for female cats—the cat continues to cycle but cannot conceive.

Although euthanasia is strictly against the teachings of the Koran, many Muslims accept that on occasion euthanasia will be necessary to relieve or prevent suffering. Some, however, will insist that nature take its course in which case pain-relieving treatment must be tactfully recommended.

A community centre may make a suitable base to hold a regular clinic for residents who want general advice on cat care or who would like help with veterinary treatment, neutering, or the re-homing of kittens. It should be possible to find volunteers from within the community who will assist with practical aspects of a cat welfare project and who will later monitor feeding sites and shelters. Local volunteers can also help with cat care education programs working with neighbours and with children so that future generations grow up with an awareness and understanding of feline welfare.

Excerpted and adapted from Hartwell (2000, 2001)

These values determine how space is used and the degree to which certain areas are "off limits" to others.

◆ Rites and rituals. A *rite* is an event that marks a change in status from a lower to a higher level; a *ritual* is a prescribed manner or process related to a culture's ideology (Strasser, 1995). Some rites happen at certain ages (e.g., birth), certain life events (e.g., marriage), and at certain festivals (e.g., religious holidays). Events of separation (e.g., divorce), intensification (e.g., renewal of wedding vows on one's 25th anniversary), incorporation (e.g., admission to school or club, making a sports team), or passage (e.g., graduation, confirmation, bar mitzvah) contain rituals that celebrate, through food, social gatherings, and emotion, some achievement.

◆ Culture and health. Religion and spirituality are increasingly recognized as influencers of cultural identity, moral belief systems, and ethical codes of conduct. Dietary practices, health practices and behaviours, decision-making, and the cultural context of seeking professional help create situations where community health workers must assess the availability, accessibility, acceptability, and appropriateness of services provided to different population groups.

Family and kinship are the foundation of many cultures; definitions may differ between legal interpretations and practical applications. In communal living situations, family may be determined through consensual processes rather than by marriage or blood relationships. Children may be raised intergenerationally (i.e., by grandparents) or in different households on different days. Community workers may experience complications related to formal consent procedures and other legal issues as a consequence.

◆ Social roles. Gender roles are culturally constructed; boys/men and girls/women have different expectations and are treated differently in different societies. Sexual orientation and reproductive health practices are controversial topics in many cultures and can be very emotionally charged. How cultural groups deal with sexuality determines the social rules and restrictions placed on people and events. Community health workers need to be aware of the implications of cultural values and beliefs to understand the various taboos and restrictions placed on men and women in different situations.

◆ Language and communication patterns. Language may be a barrier to understanding a culture; if one cannot communicate, it is difficult to gain the critical awareness or acquire the information required to become culturally competent. Sometimes translators are needed. A translator simply puts the words used into the language of the health care worker; an interpreter provides cultural context for the language as well as translation. Family members may be asked to translate, but issues of personal privacy may arise, or lay translators may not know health terminology or idioms of speech to translate accurately. Community members may not be acceptable as translators because of status, age, sex, and privacy. Written resources may not be appropriate because community members may not be literate in either their home or new languages. Creativity and sensitivity are required to overcome barriers created by language.

Strasser (1995) offers a tool for cultural assessment that includes: definition of self, definition of others, definitions of health and illness, beliefs about health and illness, life ways and meanings, time, space, physical objects, food customs, religions, clubs, work, education, play, power, environment, in- and out-migrants and migration, deviance, change, sick role, death ways and meanings, sexuality and gender roles, childbearing, child rearing, growth and development across the life span, reciprocity and exchange, customs and laws, and health care providers (pp. 150-152).

Cultural Health Care Systems

Basic to successful interactions between clients and providers is the understanding that we are all different from one another, with different ethnic and cultural backgrounds, and, therefore, different health and illness beliefs and practices. There's that word again: "different." But despite our differences, we come together at a mutually agreed on place to achieve a common goal: to maintain or regain health. The dilemma presented here is that health means different things to each of us; we recognize it and measure changes in it differently, act in diverse ways when faced with these changes, and seek different methods for achieving healing outcomes (Drew, 2000). The settings where we meet and interact with each other may take on different veneers and titles, but they are all what Kleinman calls "cultural health care systems" (Kleinman, 1980). The simple fact that culture influences health and illness beliefs and behaviours serves as a constant reminder to us that wherever clients and providers interact, there is a system, and it is influenced by the beliefs, values, norms, and standards that each of us brings to it. Cultural health care systems are made up of individuals experiencing and treating illness and the social institutions where interactions between clients and providers occur (Kleinman, 1980, 1986). Each cultural health care system can have several recognized sectors. The three sectors Kleinman's model addresses are referred to as popular, folk, and professional. Typically, the popular sector is composed of ordinary people, families, groups, social networks, and communities. Lay practitioners and healers comprise the folk sector, whereas the professional sector is composed of the licensed health professionals (Kleinman, 1980). Let us look at these sectors in some detail.

Popular

The popular sector of cultural health care systems is made up of informal healing relationships that occur within one's own social network. Although the family is at the nucleus of this sector, health care can take place between people linked by kinship, friendship, residence, occupation, or religion (Helman, 1984). In Canada, there are as many versions of the popular sector as there are ethnic cultures. In neighbourhoods where many ethnic groups have settled, popular sectors of health care systems are found to have several different ways of managing health, illness, and healing.

In the popular sector, the process of defining oneself as ill begins with a self-diagnosis confirmed by significant others based on the implicit standards of what it means to be well (Angel & Thiots, 1987; Eisenberg, 1980; Helman, 1984). Consequently, a person is defined as ill when there is agreement between self-perceptions of impairment and the perceptions of those around him or her (Helman, 1984; Weiss, 1988). The social, ethnic, and cultural values on which the illness judgment is based focus on the experience of discomfort, failure to function as expected, and a change in physical appearance. Whether a symptom is recognized as significant or normal is also influenced by the occurrence, persistence, and prevalence of the symptoms among group members (Angel & Thiots, 1987; Helman, 1984). For instance, in rural Canada people consider themselves healthy as long as they can work, do chores, and carry out daily activities (Weinert & Long, 1991). Professionals (such as social workers, nurses, physicians, police, and teachers) are often recruited from outside the community and are not consulted until other remedies, carried out in collaboration with local family and social networks, have been exhausted. To use a rural example once again, graffiti on town buildings may be dealt with according to local custom (such as clean-up day after high school graduation celebrations) rather than by calling in law enforcement. Bereavement and grief experiences are met by local action such as neighbourhood "pot luck" suppers, hampers, and other help rather than intervention by professionals. What is done for an occasion is usually based on beliefs, standards, and norms passed down from previous generations or elders. Within the popular sector, both the care recipient and the network counsellors share similar assumptions about the issue and recommended healing strategies. Therefore, misunderstandings are rare, and the healer's credentials are based on experience rather than professional education and licensure (Chrisman, 1977; Kleinman, 1980).

Folk

The folk sector of cultural health care systems includes the interaction between an individual and sacred and secular healers. Most healers share the same basic cultural values and beliefs as their constituents. In many cases, family members and others in the social network work alongside the client and the healer to discover and treat the problem. Sources of holistic health problems are believed to include relationships the client has with other people, with the natural environment, and with supernatural forces (Helman, 1984).

Treatment rituals and strategies are prescribed to correct disequilibrium and to promote healing. Healers have little formal training, although some have served an apprenticeship with another, more accomplished healer. Most are believed to receive healing powers through family position, inheritance, signs, revelations, or gifts (Lewis, 1988).

Within the folk sector, illnesses are defined as syndromes from which members of a group suffer and for which their culture provides a cause, a diagnosis, preventive measures, and regimens of healing (Rubel, 1977). It is very important that beliefs about causes of illnesses be compatible with selected treatments. In some cases, family and folk healers may be the only persons who can effectively recommend or perform healing rituals. For example, some Hispanics believe that *susto* (fright) results from a traumatic experience or that sickness is a punishment from God. Some Latin peoples recognize it as an illness that includes the loss of one's spirit from the body. Symptoms include crying, loss of appetite, listlessness, insomnia, nightmares, and withdrawal. *Susto* requires treatment by a *curandero* whose healing rituals attempt to get the individual's spirit back into the body. Sometimes complementary and supportive treatment from a psychiatrist is sought (Rivera & Wanderer, 1986; Ruiz, 1985). Working with clients and families to learn acceptable forms of healing for these problems is imperative. Community issues, such as petty crime or vandalism, might be addressed through healing circles in some Aboriginal or rural towns.

Professional

The professional sector of cultural health care systems is made up of organized health professionals who are formally educated and legally sanctioned (Kleinman, 1980). Unlike the popular and folk sectors, the clients and the providers in the professional sector typically differ in their social and cultural values, beliefs, and assumptions. Based on these differences, as well as the unfamiliar surroundings and rules of the institutions where care is given in the professional sector, the client–provider relationship may be one of mistrust, suspicion, and conflict.

Although many collaborative, complementary, and alternative models of healing are gaining popularity, practices in the professional sector remain dominated by a Western orientation. A Western orientation suggests that problems have a direct cause, solutions can be prescribed, and as long as people comply with the "rules," the problem will be solved. This view is exclusive of and counter to the popular, holistic view of meaningful experiences perceived and constructed in sociocultural context (Allan & Hall, 1988; Angel & Thiots, 1987).

Oelke (2002) learned, in a Canadian study of urban Sikh women about cervical screening for cancer, that the following strategies were recommended for outreach:

◆ Media—various ethnic-specific media (e.g., television, radio, newspapers and magazines, particularly magazines that are available free of charge) with programming in Punjabi
◆ Small group education—"education camps" held at the *gurdawara* (temple) or other community facilities, accompanied by simultaneous screening clinics. With transportation and time being an issue, these clinics would provide women an opportunity for same-day screening.
◆ One-to-one education—use of the existing informal network of friends and family is a way to get information to women in the Sikh community. Women will generally seek information from a friend first; information from family members will then follow depending on the relationship among them; and in some cases a friend may also be a close confidante.
◆ Bilingual resource materials—Punjabi and English materials placed in physicians' offices, the *gurdawara*, beauty salons and Indian stores

Before launching a campaign through ethnic media, however, several things should be considered:

◆ **Identify** your target group and be specific, not only about ethnicity, but also about age group, location or neighbourhood. Are you targeting newly arrived immigrants or established newcomers?
◆ **Examine** the capacity within your program for working with the specified target group. If you are going to offer a particular service, begin with those groups for which you already have established contacts, relationships, resources, and skilled staff to handle cultural issues. Start out slowly by seeking small successes and build on these to expand services to other populations.
◆ **Demonstrate** to ethnic media the value and need for the service or program you provide. Share neighbourhood or ethnic-specific data and explain why the issue is a concern to their public.
◆ **Be creative** in your outreach to media; perhaps editors would appreciate a column in which you discuss issues related to the health of the community.
◆ **Be sensitive** to cultural practices, such as obtaining permission, seeking approval from elders or those who hold informal or formal positions of leadership (New York City Public Health Partnership, 2002).

Cultural Sensitivity

Ethnocentrism is the tendency to believe one's ways are best and to act superior in relation to other ways as a result. Bennett (1986, as cited in Helvie, 1998) suggests the process of moving along a continuum from ethnocentrism to cultural competence involves several steps:

◆ Denial—cultural blindness and ethnocentrism; no recognition of cultural differences and different behaviour is viewed as deviant
◆ Defence—cultural differences are recognized, but one's own beliefs are defended as correct or superior
◆ Minimization—cultural differences are recognized, but differences are minimized
◆ Acceptance—different cultural beliefs and practices are recognized and valued
◆ Adaptation—rare; adaptation to another culture results, and stereotypes are minimized
◆ Integration—very rare; comfortable movement between cultures occurs and differences are accepted (pp. 137–138)

Leininger's (Leininger & McFarland, 2002) theory of transcultural nursing and the Sunrise Model (Leininger, 1991) provide a framework for understanding the cultural foundations of a community and for developing cultural knowledge to guide practice. The Sunrise Model is a cognitive map of components that influence care patterns and well-being of individuals, families, and communities (Fig. 7-1). Three types of care decisions guide practice:

◆ Cultural care preservation and/or maintenance—actions that support, assist, or enable clients of any culture to preserve or maintain health, recover from illness or injury, or face death
◆ Cultural care accommodation and/or negotiation—actions that assist the client to negotiate a beneficial health status
◆ Cultural care repatterning or restructuring—actions that assist clients to change traditional life ways for new or different patterns that are culturally meaningful and satisfying and support beneficial and healthy life choices (Leininger, 1991)

A rural community health team investigating the high incidence of hypertension in a Hutterite colony found that residents consumed a traditional diet of meat and vegetables prepared in a communal kitchen. However, the food was prepared in a manner that made it high in fat, salt, and carbohydrates.

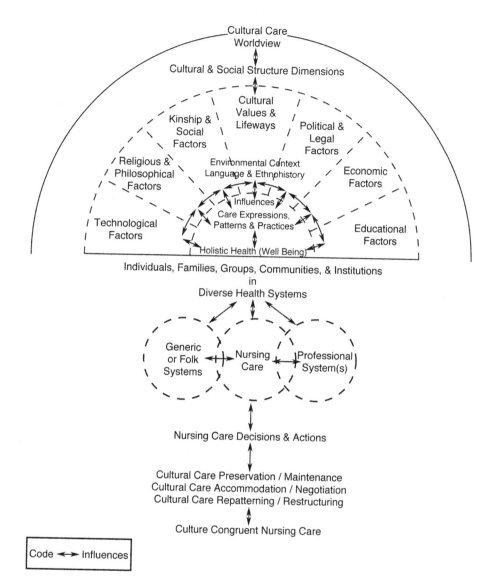

Figure 7-1 ◆ Leininger's Sunrise Model to depict theory of cultural care diversity and universality. (Redrawn from Leininger, M. M. [1991. The theory of culture care diversity and universality. In M. M. Leininger [Ed.], *Culture care diversity and universality: A theory of nursing.* New York, NY: National League for Nursing Press.)

Adults, as a group, had an average body mass index higher than recommended, several had high-normal blood glucose levels, and on average, blood lipid levels were elevated. There was no shortage of food, but supplies were closely monitored. Once the community was informed of the results of the research, a delegation came to the community health centre to find out what could be done to prevent more people from becoming hypertensive and what those with high blood pressure could do to prevent complications. Because no individual had control over his or her diet, the head cook and other influential elder women had to be convinced to adapt their recipes and food preparation methods to low-salt, low-fat versions. The Head Man had to approve the purchase of blood pressure monitoring equipment and the training of people to take measurements. A blood glucose monitor was also purchased with his permission.

The public health nurse visited the colony weekly to monitor those residents who had been identified as at risk. The nurse also taught those who had received prescriptions for medication about its administration and the need to take their pills at regular times of the day. In their communal living context, it was not uncommon for medications to be "shared"—if it worked for one person, it could work for another; the nurse explained the dangers of this practice. The social worker on the team provided information and counselling on stress relief and relaxation. The public health inspector collected water samples and tested for mineral content that may affect blood pressure. The teacher created appropriate written/graphic information resources.

The most difficult challenge was to initiate a "healthy activity" program; as farmers, they felt they were active enough, but the men spent much time on tractors and in trucks and the women were busy in the kitchen and in the sewing rooms and gardens. However, as they examined their patterns of activity, they began to see room for more planned exercise. A walking program was proposed by the active living and health promotion team from the nearby health centre; they would come to the colony at a set time in the middle of the afternoon three times a week to lead the women on a "power walk." Soon, the men asked for a program (separate from the women, and done on their own); the team provided a plan to follow each day that included a morning warm-up, aerobic exercise, and flexibility activities.

After a year of experimentation with menus, the cooks provided the community health team with recipes that were printed and made available to other colonies; average weights and blood pressure levels had declined, and colony residents expressed satisfaction with their adapted patterns of eating and activity. As residents migrated to establish new colonies, the adapted patterns of eating and activity were disseminated more widely. At a recent community "Walk for the Cure" event in support of breast cancer, several women from the colony walked the route with their daughters.

Recently, one of the women had been diagnosed with breast cancer, and the health centre had been able to convince the Head Man to encourage the women to attend a screening clinic for the first time, receive instruction on monthly breast self examination, and undergo a mammogram. He also agreed that the public health nurse could teach cancer prevention methods to the older girls in school.

Decision-Making

People who become ill or who want to remain healthy make choices about who to consult in the popular, professional, or folk sectors of the cultural health care system. Those choices are influenced by the subjective definition of health and illness by individuals, the family, and community; what health and illness means to them; and the expected course of events across the life cycle. Attitudes toward different types of providers, and decisions about who to consult for assistance, vary according to how the symptom or issue is interpreted and what it means as a significant life event to the people involved. Typically, people make their help-seeking choices based on prior learning, symptom significance, compatibility between the philosophies of the sectors, and evaluation of the treatment outcome (Blumhagen, 1982; Chrisman, 1977; Kleinman, 1980; Young, 1982). It seems logical that clients, in the process of seeking help, may involve a network of potential consultants ranging from informal structures in the nuclear family to select laypeople and professionals (Friedson, 1961; Roberts, 1988).

Specific knowledge about a culture is necessary for a community partnership to be structured within a helping framework. Bringing down barriers and facilitating the negotiation of plans for community action will support positive health outcomes for all clients. The ultimate goal in planning collaborative approaches to community practice is to preserve the dignity of the client (individual, family, aggregate) and to foster health promotion and healing programs that are likely to meet with adherence because they support rather than offend the people who use the services (Drew, 2000).

Drew (2000) suggests the following questions community workers may ask to understand a situation or issue:

◆ What do you call your problem?
◆ What worries you most about having this problem?
◆ How did you come to know that you were having a problem?
◆ What do you think caused this problem?
◆ Why do you think it started when it did?
◆ How long do you think it will last?
◆ What has been done about the problem?

◆ With whom have you discussed the problem?
◆ What kind of help and from whom would you like to receive help for the problem?
◆ How will you know when your problem is getting better?

Answers to these questions may take time and will take a conscious effort to collect and use. However, the process is well worth the time and commitment as we gain a greater understanding and respect for all clients' health beliefs and practices. This understanding can lead to both improved client–provider relationships and intervention outcomes. An analysis of the answers to these questions and much introspection will enable community workers to understand the complexities of cross-cultural interactions (Drew, 2000) (Table 7-1).

Conflict Among Sectors

Given our diverse cultural backgrounds, we should not be surprised to find that research across many health-related disciplines provides evidence that barriers, conflicts, and misunderstandings among the system's sectors are, in part, related to the differences in cultural beliefs about illness causation and management (Chavez, 1984; Roberson, 1987).

Although we may never have viewed conflicts through Kleinman's (1980) perspective before, we have all encountered conflicts between providers and clients. Even after students in undergraduate and graduate programs acquire a greater knowledge of ethnicity and culture, conflicts in beliefs and practices between sectors and resultant barriers to effective health care remain unresolved. The lack of progress in reducing barriers can be linked to professional providers' relative inattention to the popular sector of cultural health care systems. Drew (2000) asks: Have you ever heard a professional provider say, "This client is difficult" or "This client is noncompliant with his medicines and he won't follow his diet"? Perhaps you have made such comments yourself without thinking that what has been prescribed or recommended may not be compatible with the client's beliefs about treatment and healing. The problem could be more basic than a mere treatment conflict; perhaps the client and provider have incongruent beliefs about what is wrong and what caused the symptom of illness. In the popular or folk sector, illness is sometimes thought to be a physical manifestation (*somatization*) of a client's uneasiness with a stressful relationship, the natural environment, or supernatural forces. Because belief systems in the popular and folk sectors have often been termed as "unorthodox," "lay," "subjective," or "nonscientific" (Roberson, 1987) and have been associated with non-Western societies, a client's preference for such healing practices has been dismissed by some professional community workers.

TABLE 7-1 ◆ COMMUNITY CULTURAL ASSESSMENT: AN APPLICATION

The community centre administrator was approached by a prominent member of a community of recent immigrants about how to deal with an issue that had arisen at the school. Teachers were concerned about the number of early teen pregnancies (age 14) among this group and had contacted the community health centre to provide contraception education and counselling to the girls. The health centre administrator asked the following questions, and actively listened to the responses, to assess the situation and determine a course of action:

Question	Response
What is the problem?	Unacceptable teachings for girls at school
What worries you most about having this problem?	Our young women will be shunned if they use unnatural methods to prevent having children. Women will not keep their place in the home if they are too educated.
How did you come to know that you were having a problem?	The nurse came to homes in our community and told us it was not right that so many girls were pregnant at school. So, we kept them home from school. Now we are told they have to go to school until they are 16. We don't understand.
What do you think caused this problem?	Teachers and nurses don't understand that girls are betrothed at the time of their first bleed (menstruation) and are married 2 years later. It is expected that they will bear children when they are young, even though they remain at their paternal home until the husband is ready to support them. The men must be educated first, and the girls' fathers must have time to prepare the dowry.
Why do you think it started when it did?	When we came to this country, our children were young. Now they are growing up and we must do the right thing according to our culture. This year four girls were betrothed and two became married and pregnant. They stayed in school and the teachers told the nurse about it. They want the girls to go to the doctor, go to special birth classes, and take pills (prenatal vitamins).
How long do you think it will last?	I don't know. We have many young children now that we are in this country—and they are all healthy. Soon more will be betrothed.
What has been done about the problem?	I talked to the parents; we went to the midwife; we prayed at the temple. Now the police tell us we have to send the girls to school.
With whom have you discussed the problem?	You are the first person outside the community we have come to. Fathers are worried their daughters will be disgraced and their husbands won't take them away.
What kind of help and from whom would you like to receive help for the problem?	Can you tell the schools that the girls are not a problem? Fathers are still in charge of the daughters so the school should listen to them. It is good they are pregnant—they will learn to care for children and a home from their mothers.
How will you know when your problem is getting better?	Fathers will not be so upset; daughters will stay in school but will not have to go to classes or take pills; husbands will not shun their wives.

This is problematic because if recommended treatments do not fit the perceived cause, then the client may not follow suggested protocols. Appropriate advocacy must be based on the ability to understand the popular sector's realities and to translate and negotiate between the system's sectors with the goal of reducing barriers to culturally sensitive care (Chrisman, 1977). Without a doubt, differences are sources of conflict and misunderstanding in client–provider relationships (Angel & Thiots, 1987; Blumhagen, 1982). A detailed understanding of cultural health care systems will provide us with many reasons for the existence and resolution of real and potential barriers between providers and lay people in the care-giving process. Beyond a basic understanding of the ingredients for conflict, this paradigm of differences should be used by providers, partners, and communities as a guide for becoming culturally competent (Drew, 2000).

The Culturally Competent Provider

Cultural competence implies an awareness of, sensitivity to, and knowledge of the meaning of culture and its role in shaping human behaviour (McManus, 1988). If culture, broadly defined, is socially transmitted beliefs, values, ways of knowing, and patterns of behaviour characteristic of a designated population group (Kleinman, 1980; Wood, 1989), then cultural competence is the ability to express an awareness of one's own culture, to recognize the differences between oneself and others, and to adapt behaviours to appreciate and accommodate those differences (Dillard et al., 1992). Cultural competence depends on the development of an attitude among community workers that begins with one's willingness to learn about cultural issues, proceeds with the commitment to incorporate at all levels of care the importance of culture, and is operationalized by making adaptations in services to meet culturally unique needs. Although some practitioners may have specific knowledge of the languages, values, and customs of other cultures, the most challenging tasks are understanding the dynamics of difference in the helping process and adapting practice skills to fit a community's cultural context (Drew, 2000).

Developing an awareness and acceptance of cultural differences is required as a first step in the process of becoming a culturally competent individual (Cross et al., 1989; McManus, 1988). Differences must be explored and understood so barriers to seeking health care can be reduced. Understanding differences begins with an awareness that they exist and continues with a willingness to accept them (Drew, 2000). In the next section, there is a suggested exercise to enhance your awareness of your own culture.

A Cultural Awareness Exercise

A major component of cultural competence is an acknowledgement and awareness of one's own culture and a willingness to explore one's own feelings and biases. Each person is responsible for building an awareness of how culture influences his or her own ways of thinking and making decisions. Included in this awareness must be an acknowledgement of how day-to-day behaviours reflect cultural norms and values perpetuated by our families and larger social networks.

One strategy used in teaching diversity awareness to students in the helping professions is a cultural assessment project that serves as a purposeful self-examination and an exercise in appreciating differences. The exercise asks you to begin by identifying your own cultural beliefs and values about health and illness, education and vocation, foods, religion, and role expectations. (You can do this now as you read this section.) Once identified, think through your responses and make notations about how you remember being taught about some of those values, practices, expectations, habits, and traditions.

◆ Where and how was knowledge about your heritage passed on to you?
◆ Who are the persons in your social network responsible for influencing and shaping the lives of the young people?

Proceed with this exercise by seeking out someone known to you but who has a background, heritage, or ethnicity different from your own.

◆ Ask that person's permission for an interview and ask them the same things you asked yourself in establishing your basic cultural richness.
◆ When you have the data you gathered to compare with information about yourself, sit down and analyze what sociocultural similarities and differences the two of you have.

This exercise is particularly beneficial to the beginner who has not ventured into self-awareness projects from a perspective of cultural beliefs and values. Having analyzed similarities and differences, proceed with your analysis and focus on predicting potential areas of conflict between the two views as well as the positive, congruent strengths. These may be as simple as food preferences and celebrated holidays or as complex as preferred vocations, generational hierarchies, and healing rituals. You may complete the practice exercise by asking the following question:

◆ What potential strengths in similarities between us should I build on to begin interactions with this person?

As the preceding cultural exercise points out, all interacting parties bring with them unique histories, communication styles, and learned expectations. Together, these contribute to potential misunderstandings and misinterpretations that manifest the dynamics of difference. Therefore, strategies of relating with community partners must include eliciting information about their health and illness practices, as well as basic ethnic and cultural norms (Drew, 2000).

Summary

Community-based educators and human service providers must remember that ethnicity provides a sense of belonging to people in a pluralistic society; a celebration of differences in identity, strength, and survival. An understanding of ethnic, religious, age, and gender cultures is functional for coping with and appreciating differences. Research supports the roles of heritage and identity in influencing people's behaviours and attitudes and the perpetuation of culture throughout generations. Cooperation with and respect for others with different heritages rather than eradication of differences, stimulation of conflict, and goals for sameness must be the focus of practice and research. Cultural competence is an imperative for health promotion and successful outcomes of life experiences. Many of the skills needed by providers are in place and available for enrichment through awareness, specialty and continuing education, and careful listening to what our communities teach us (Drew, 2000).

References

Aamodt, A. (1978). The care component in a health and healing system. In E. Bauwens (Ed.), *The anthropology of health*. St. Louis, MO: Mosby.

Adams, E. V. (1990). *Policy planning for culturally comprehensive special health services*. Rockville, MD: United States Department of Health and Human Services, Maternal and Child Health Bureau.

Allan, J. D., & Hall, B. A. (1988). Challenging the focus on technology: A critique of the medical model in a changing health care system. *Advances in Nursing Science, 10*(3), 22–34.

Angel, R., & Thiots, P. (1987). The impact of culture on the cognitive structure of illness. *Culture, Medicine, and Psychiatry, 2,* 465–494.

Blumhagen, D. (1982). The meaning of hypertension. In N. J. Chrisman & T. W. Maretzki (Eds.), *Clinical applied anthropology: Anthropologists in health science settings*. Boston: Reidel.

Campinha-Bacote, J. (1995). The quest for cultural competence in nursing care. *Nursing Forum, 30*(4), 19–25.

Canadian Human Rights Commission. (2001). *Race, colour, national or ethnic origin: Antidiscrimination casebook*. Ottawa: Minister of Public Works and Government Services Catalogue No. HR21-56-2001.

Centers for Disease Control and Prevention. (1993). *Morbidity and Mortality Weekly Report, 42*(RR10), 15.

Centre for Addictions and Mental Health. (1999). Q & A: Common questions about ethnocultural diversity. *Journal of Addiction and Mental Health, 2*(4).

Chavez, L. R. (1984). Doctors, curanderos, and brujas: Health care delivery and Mexican immigrants in San Diego. *Medical Anthropology Quarterly, 15*(2), 31–37.

Chrisman, N. (1977). The health seeking process: An approach to the natural history of illness. *Culture, Medicine, & Psychiatry, 1,* 351–377.

Congress, E. P. & Lyons, B.P. (1992). Cultural differences in health beliefs: Implications for social work practice in health care settings. *Social Work in Health Care, 17*(3), 81–96.

Cross, R. L. (1987). Cultural competence continuum. *Focal Point: The Bulletin of the Research and Training Center to Improve Services for Seriously Emotionally Handicapped Children and Their Families, 3*(1), 5.

Cross, T. L., Bazron, B. J., Dennis, K. W., & Issacs, M. R. (1989). *Towards a culturally com-

petent system of care (Vol. I). Washington, DC: Georgetown University Child Development Center, CASSP Technical Assistance Center.

Dervin, B. (1989). Audience as listener and learner, teacher, and confidante: The sense-making approach. In R. E. Rice & C. K. Atkin (Eds.), *Public communication campaigns*. Newbury Park, CA: Sage.

Devore, W., & Schlesinger, E. (1991). *Ethnic-sensitive social work practice*. New York: Macmillan.

Dillard, M., Andonian, L., Flores, O., Lai, L., MacRae, A., & Shakir, M. (1992). Culturally competent occupational therapy in a diversely populated mental health setting. *American Journal of Occupational Therapy, 46*(8), 721–726.

Drew, J. C. (2000). Cultural competence in partnerships with communities. In Anderson, E. T. & McFarlane, J. *Community as partner* (3rd ed., pp. 116–135). Philadelphia: Lippincott, Williams & Wilkins.

Eisenberg, L. (1980). What makes persons patients and patients well? *American Journal of Medicine, 69*(2), 277–286.

Friedson, E. (1961). *Patient's view of medical practice*. New York: Russell Sage.

Hartwell, S. (2000, 2001). Cat welfare and feral cat control in ethnic communities. Retrieved from the Internet: http://messybeast.com/ethnic-cat.htm.

Harwood, A. (1981). *Ethnicity and medical care*. Cambridge, MA: Harvard University Press.

Helman, C. (1984). *Culture, health, and illness: An introduction for health professionals*. Boston: Wright.

Helvie, C. O. (1998). *Advanced practice nursing in the community*. Thousand Oaks, CA: Sage.

Holzberg, C. S. (1982). Ethnicity and aging: Anthropological perspectives on more than just the minority elderly. *The Gerontologist, 22*(3), 249–257.

Jenson, J. & Papillon, M. (2000). Citizenship and the recognition of cultural diversity: The Canadian experience. Backgrounder for *A structured dialogue on diversity: The values and political structures that support it*. May 12, 2000. Ottawa, Canada.

Kleinman, A. (1980). *Patients and healers in the context of culture*. Berkeley, CA: University of California Press.

Kleinman, A. (1986). Concepts and a model for the comparison of medical systems as cultural systems. In C. Currer & M. Stacy (Eds.), *Concepts of health, illness, & disease: A comparative perspective*. New York: Berg.

Leininger, M. M. (1991). The theory of culture care diversity and universality. In M. M. Leininger (Ed.), *Culture diversity and universality: A theory of nursing*. New York: National League for Nursing Press.

Leininger, M., & McFarland, M. R. (2002). *Transcultural nursing concepts, theories, research and practice* (3rd ed.). New York: McGraw-Hill.

Lewis, M. C. (1988). Attribution and illness. *Journal of Psychosocial Nursing, 26*(4), 14–21.

Lyons, J. (1972). Methods of successful communication with the disadvantaged. In *Communication for change with the rural disadvantaged*. Washington, DC: National Academy of Sciences.

Madrid, A. (1988). Diversity and its discontents. *Black Issues in Higher Education, 5*(4), 10–18.

McManus, M. (1988). Services to minority populations: What does it mean to be a culturally competent professional? *Focal Point: The Bulletin of the Research and Training Center to Improve Services for Seriously Emotionally Handicapped Children and Their Families, 2*(4), 1–17.

Mechanic, D. (1986). The concept of illness behavior: Culture, situation, and personal predisposition. *Psychological Medicine, 16*(1), 1–7.

Moore, J. (1971). Situational factors affecting minority aging. *The Gerontologist, 11*, 88–93.

Munet-Vilaro, F. (1988). The challenge of cross-cultural nursing research. *Western Journal of Nursing Research, 10*(1), 112–115.

New York City Public Health Partnership. (2002). Reaching out through ethnic media. In *Working together to create healthy communities.* NYCPHP Bulletin no. 9; June-July 2002.

Oelke, N. D. (2002). An exploration of cervical cancer screening among women in an urban Sikh community. Unpublished master's thesis, Faculty of Nursing, University of Calgary, November 29, 2002.

Office of the High Commissioner for Human Rights. (2001). *Gender dimensions of racial discrimination.* Geneva, Switzerland: United Nations.

Rivera, G., & Wanderer, J. (1986). Curanderismo and childhood illnesses. *Social Science Journal, 23*(3), 361–372.

Roberson, M. (1987). Folk health beliefs of health professionals. *Western Journal of Nursing Research, 9*(2), 257–263.

Roberts, S. J. (1988). Social support and help seeking: Review of the literature. *Advances in Nursing Science, 10*(2), 1–11.

Royce, A.P. (1982). *Ethnic identity: Strategies of diversity.* Bloomington, IN: Indiana University.

Rubel, A. J. (1977). The epidemiology of a folk illness: Susto in Hispanic America. In D. Landy (Ed.), *Culture, disease, and healing: Studies in medical anthropology* (pp. 119–128). New York: Macmillan.

Ruiz, P. (1985). Cultural barriers to effective medical care among Hispanic-American patients. *Annual Review of Medicine, 36,* 63–71.

Sockalingam, S. (2002). Cultural competence in developing health promotion and intervention strategies: Rhetoric or reality. Retrieved from: http//depts.Washington.edu /obesity/DocReview/Suganya/basedoc.html

Statistics Canada. (2002). *1996 Census nations tables.* From: www.statcan.ca

Status of Women Canada. (2000). *The "Famous Five" and the Persons case.* Ottawa: Author.

Strasser, J. (1995). The cultural context for community health nursing. In Smith, C. M., & Maurer, F. A. (Eds.), *Community health nursing theory and practice* (pp. 141–151). Toronto: Saunders.

Weinert, C., & Long, K.A. (1991). Theory and research base for rural nursing practice. In Bushy, A. (Ed.), *Rural nursing* (Vol. 1, pp. 21–38). Thousand Oaks, CA: Sage.

Weiss, M. G. (1988). Cultural models of diarrheal illness: Conceptual framework and review. *Social Science & Medicine, 27*(1), 5–16.

Whall, A. (1987). Commentary. *Western Journal of Nursing Research, 9*(2), 237–239.

Wirth, L. (1945). The problem of minority groups. In R. Linton (Ed.), *The science of man in the world crisis* (p. 347). New York: Columbia University Press.

Wood, J.B. (1989). Communicating with older adults in health care settings: Cultural and ethnic considerations. *Educational Gerontology, 15,* 351–362.

Young, A. (1982). The anthropology of illness and sickness. *Annual Review of Anthropology, 11,* 257–285.

Internet Resources

BC Teacher's Federation: **www.bctf.bc.ca/Social**

Canadian Council for Multiculturalism and Intercultural Education: **www.ccmie.come/siteinternet**

Canadian Human Rights Commission: **www.chrc-ccdp.ca**

Canadian Race Relations Foundation: **www.crr.ca**

Centre for Intercultural and International Education: **www.cam.org/~ceici/index.html**

Equal Opportunity Education: **www.equalopp.web.net**

First Nations on SchoolNet: **www.schoolnet.ca/aboriginal/menu-e.html**

United Nations Office of Human Rights: **www.unhchr.ch/**

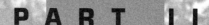

PART II

The Process of Community as Partner

8

A Model to Guide Practice

OBJECTIVES

Models that serve as guides for practice, education, and research have become important tools for community health workers. This chapter, in which we begin our examination of the process as applied to the community as partner, focuses on the use of one model to guide practice.

After studying this chapter, you should be able to:

◆ Define model
◆ Describe the purposes of a model
◆ Begin to use a model in practice

Introduction

Health disciplines have developed models for practice that provide the boundaries needed to define areas of concern for each professional group and a conceptual map that is a necessary guide for action. This is particularly true when practice focuses on the entire community. The community-as-partner model provides us with both the map and the boundaries and will be used throughout this chapter.

Models

A conceptual model is the synthesis of a set of concepts and the statements that integrate those concepts into a whole. A community process model can be defined as a frame of reference, a way of looking at a community, or an image of what working in and with a community encompasses. A model is a representation of practice, not a reality. Other types of models that are used to represent realities are model airplanes, blueprints, chemical equations, and anatomic models.

A model with which health workers identified for many years was the medical model, that is, a disease-oriented, illness- and organ-focused approach to patients, with an emphasis on pathology. This model has served us well in our quest to eliminate childhood communicable diseases and common preventable illness. However, reliance on the medical model that focuses on individuals excludes health promotion and the holistic focus that is central to population wellness and community health. Additionally, important aspects of care, such as psychological, sociocultural, and spiritual areas, are not explicitly included in the medical model. Thus, a community-as-partner model should encompass all aspects of health and incorporate long-range goals and planning.

As a representation of reality, a model can take numerous forms. Because they describe professional practice, all models are narrative; that is, words are the symbols that are used by workers (e.g., nurses, social workers, nutritionists, etc.) to define how they view their practice. And although all models are described in words, many are clarified further through the use of diagrams or illustrations. Diagrams are an efficient and effective way of depicting models; the use of such images allows the model builder to show relationships and linkages among the concepts in the model. The diagram is often thought of as the model itself, with the accompanying text then seen as the elaboration or explanation of the model.

The method chosen to depict a model reflects the model builder's own philosophy and preference; no one method is accepted as the best. There are, however, certain components that must be included in any health-related model. Table 8-1 presents these essential elements. There is general agreement that four concepts are central to health disciplines: person, environment, health, and the body of knowledge relating to the specific health discipline (e.g., nursing, social work, medicine, nutrition). *Concepts* are defined as general notions or ideas and are considered the building blocks of models. How each of the four concepts is defined will both dictate the organization of the model and be illustrated in that model. For example, health may be defined on a continuum with wellness at one end and death at the other, as a dichotomy wherein one is seen as well or ill, as the outcome of numerous biopsychosocial and spiritual forces, or as the interaction of these same forces. In the medical model, health has been

TABLE 8-1 ◆ ESSENTIAL UNITS OF A NURSING MODEL

Essential Unit	Description of Unit
A goal of action	The mission or ideal goal of the profession expressed as the end product desired (a state, condition, or situation)
A descriptive term for the patient population	That concept that best isolates who or what is acted on to achieve a goal; that is, those aspects of the person (as patient) or the organization or those aspects of their functioning toward which attention is to be directed; the target of action
The actor's role	A descriptive label that indicates the nature of the nurse's (the actor's) actions on patients
Source of difficulty	The origin of deviations from the desired state or condition
Intervention focus	The kind of problems found when deviations from the desired state occur; the kinds of disturbances in patients that are to be prevented or treated. Mode is the major means of preventing or treating such problems (the kinds of levers that can be used to change the course of events toward the desired end).
Consequences intended	Outcomes of action that are desired, stated in more abstract or broader terms than the mission, or including significant corollaries of the intended outcomes. Unintended outcomes may follow and may or may not be desirable.

Data from Riehl, J. P. & Roy, C. (1980). *Conceptual models for nursing practice* (2nd ed.), p. 2. New York: Appleton-Century-Crofts; from unpublished lecture notes of D. Johnson, UCLA, Fall 1975.

defined traditionally as the absence of disease. Figure 8-1 depicts four ways to view health and illustrates these definitions. Notice that the diagrams vary widely, reflecting the fundamental differences among these views of health.

What, then, are the purposes of a model of practice? Think for a moment of what a model is to you and how a model might be useful in your practice. Although you may not have formulated your own model of practice, you have been influenced greatly in your education by the model or models on which your professional curriculum is based. Does your faculty subscribe to one particular model? Just as the choice of a model creates a basis for curriculum planning and decisions, a model can also provide a basis for practice.

What does professional practice mean to you? If you can express an answer to that question, you have begun to describe your model of practice. A model serves the following purposes:

◆ Provides a map for the problem-solving process
  ◆ Gives direction for assessment
  ◆ Guides analysis
  ◆ Dictates community health diagnoses
  ◆ Assists in planning
  ◆ Facilitates evaluation
◆ Provides a curriculum outline for education
◆ Represents a framework for research
◆ Provides a basis for development of theory

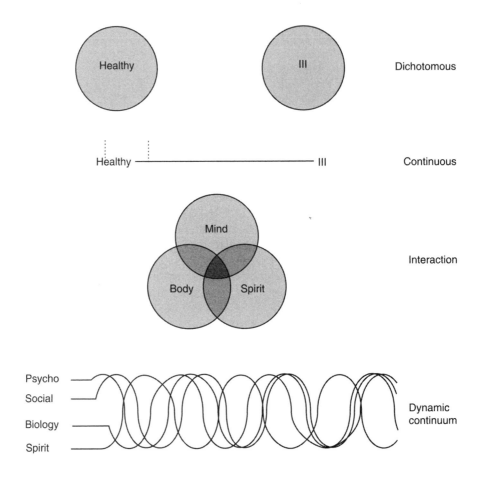

Figure 8-1 ◆ Four models of health.

A model is nothing more or less than an explication of practice. A model not only describes what is but also provides a framework for making decisions about what could be.

Community-as-Partner Model

Based on Neuman's 1972 Systems Model of a total-person approach to viewing client problems, the community-as-client model was developed by Anderson and McFarlane in 1986 to illustrate the definition of community health nursing as the synthesis of public health and nursing. The model has been renamed the community-as-partner model to emphasize the underlying philosophy of multidisciplinary primary health care and the evolving respect for public participation in health decision-making. Beddome (1995) expanded the utility of the model to aggregates within the community as well as to the geopolitical community itself.

The phenomena of interest are the community system and its related environment. The environment can be internal, external, or created. It is based on a social ecological foundation. The objective of the care provider (community health worker) is to prevent fragmentation of care to the community. The care provider's goal is to intervene to either (1) decrease the potential of the community system to encounter stressors, or (2) limit the impact or effects of stressors on the community through prevention interventions.

Consider the community-as-partner model (Fig. 8-2). There are two central factors in this model: a focus on the community as partner (represented by the community assessment wheel at the top, which incorporates the community's people as the core) and the use of the problem-solving process. The model is described in some detail to assist you in understanding its parts so you may use it as a guide to your practice in the community. Refer now to Figure 8-3 for the following discussion.

The *core* of the assessment wheel represents the people who make up the community. Included in data to describe the community's core are the population's social demographics (e.g., age, sex and ethnic distribution, culture, education and employment levels, socioeconomic status) and the community values, beliefs, and history. This core must be maintained to ensure the survival of the community. When the core does not survive, for instance when a mine shuts down and the economic base of the town is gone, people move away and what remains is referred to as a "ghost town."

As residents of the community, people are affected by and, in turn, influence the eight *subsystems* of the community. These subsystems, representing the broad determinants of health, are physical environment, education, safety and transportation, politics and government, health and social services, communication, economics, and recreation. The eight subsystems are divided by broken lines to remind us that they are not discrete and separate but influence (and are influenced by) one another. (Remember that one of the principles of ecology is that everything is connected to everything else. This also applies to the community as a whole.) The eight divisions both define the major subsystems of a community and provide the community health worker with a framework for assessment.

The solid line surrounding the community core and its subsystems represents its *normal line of defence* (NLD), or the level of health the community has

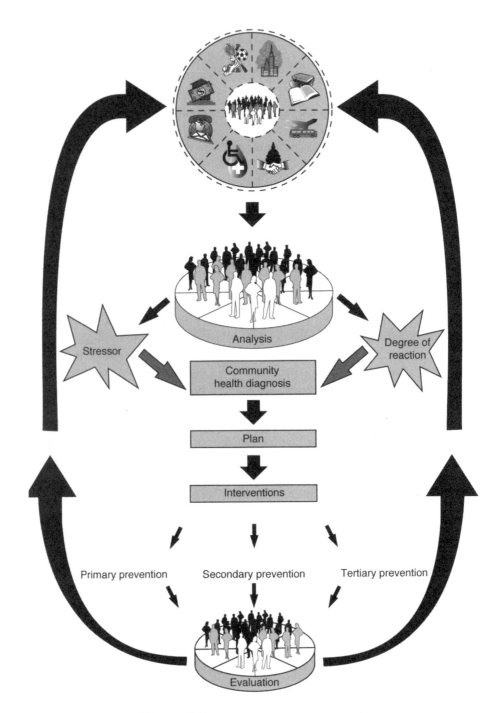

Figure 8-2 ◆ Community-as-partner model.

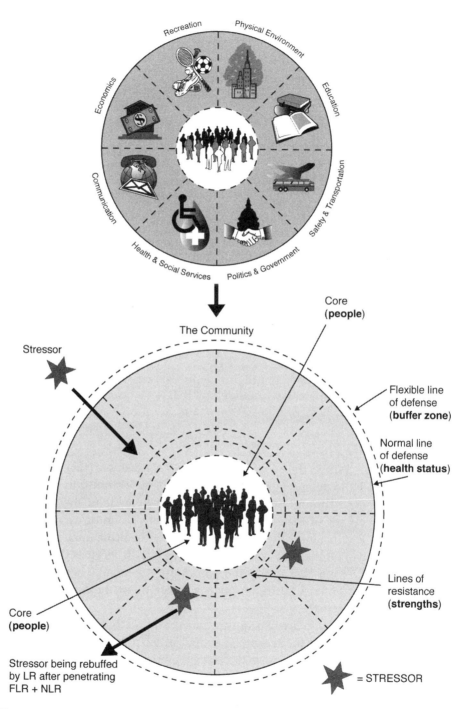

Figure 8-3 ◆ The community assessment wheel, featuring lines of resistance and defense within the community structure.

reached over time. The NLD may include epidemiologic and health status measurements such as birth, mortality, and morbidity rates; incidence and prevalence of disease and injury; presence and prevalence of risk factors; community capacity; social capital; and other health-related statistics. The NLD also includes usual patterns of coping and problem-solving capabilities; it represents the health of the community.

The *flexible line of defence* (FLD), shown as a broken line around the community and its NLD, is a buffer zone representing a dynamic level of health resulting from a temporary response to stressors. It prevents stressors from penetrating through the NLD. An example of a temporary response may be that, in the time of an economic crisis, inner-city churches will provide temporary shelter and the food bank will offer food to a wider clientele when the weather suddenly turns cold. Temporary responses are used until more permanent solutions are found (e.g., the economy recovers and people find jobs and housing, or the weather improves).

✎ TAKE NOTE

Take a moment to examine the selection of subsystems that have been identified. Can you think of any that have been omitted? Think of the community where you live. What examples of each subsystem can you identify?

Within the community are *lines of resistance* (LR), internal mechanisms that act to defend against penetration of the community core by stressors. The LR exist throughout each of the subsystems, and their strength influences the degree of reaction to a stressor that a community or aggregate experiences. For instance, the availability of teen health clinics near public transit routes can offer sexual and reproductive health services that prevent teen pregnancy from disrupting the community system. These services, as well as the community attitudes that support them, represent community assets and capacity.

Stressors are tension-producing stimuli that have the potential of causing disruption in the system. They may arise from the internal environment, the external environment, or the created environment. Stressors, then, may be intrasystem (originating within the geopolitical community, population or aggregate), extrasystem (originating outside of the community and its people), or intersystem (originating from interactions among the subsystems).

Let's use the issue of hypertension on a Hutterite colony to illustrate the model concepts (Table 8-2). A stressor (hypertension) has penetrated the flexi-

TABLE 8-2 ◆ APPLICATION OF COMMUNITY-AS-PARTNER MODEL CONCEPTS TO A HEALTH PROBLEM IN A POPULATION GROUP

Model Concept	Community Response
Stressor	Several people diagnosed with high blood pressure
Degree of reaction	Two older residents experienced symptoms needing medication; some midlife adults are too fatigued to work a full day and need to rest in the afternoon; kitchen requested to prepare special diets for those affected.
Core	Mature community with three generations living on it. Head Man and Cook have been leaders for many years. Hutterites live communally on a farm with ready access to meat, vegetables, fruit, and milk. Everyone contributes to the life of the colony. Children go to school on the colony until age 16.
Normal line of defence	Increased incidence of hypertension, moderately high mean blood sugar levels among midlife women and men. Cultural practice of sharing prescriptions
Flexible line of defence	Multidisciplinary health team mobilizes to provide education, screening, and support.
Lines of resistance	Nearby community health centre; on-site school; communal living increases social support; cooks willing to try new recipes. Head Man approves the purchase of blood pressure monitors and training in their use.

ble and normal lines of defence, resulting in disruption of the community. The *degree of reaction* is the amount of disruption that results from stressors impinging on the community's lines of defence. The degree of reaction may be reflected in changes to mortality and morbidity rates (impact on the community core), unemployment (effect on the economic subsystem), or crime statistics (effect on the safety subsystem), for instance. In the case of the Hutterite colony, the *stressor* has caused several individuals to experience symptoms and require medication. The community has also been affected because these individuals need to rest during the day and have special diets; because food is prepared and served communally, accommodations need to be made by the cooks and other colony members. The affected individuals need to be treated differently to regain and maintain their health, which counters the prevailing cultural values of colony life.

Stressors and degree of reaction become part of the *community health diagnosis*. To continue the analysis of the exemplar, the problem is the community adaptation to members of the colony needing special care (a degree of reaction by the community core) related to hypertension (a stressor) caused by a combination of genetic endowment, diet, and physical inactivity. Data that illustrate the health problem may be increased physician visits for hypertension, costs of medications and equipment (*health services subsystem*), and changes to the communal cooking practices and dietary menus (*physical environment subsystem*). When the regular service provided by the community health nurse (*line of resistance*) is supplemented by a monthly blood pressure clinic and wellness activities (healthy weight and healthy activity programs) in response to the alteration in the *normal line of defense* (health status of the community), this service is considered to be a *flexible line of defense*, temporarily put in place in response to the colony's need.

TAKE NOTE

The outcome of a stressor impinging on a community is not always negative. Often it is positive. For example, in the face of a crisis, people may band together and develop a community group to deal with the crisis. This group may continue to function after the crisis is over, strengthening the community and continuing to contribute to its health. (Advocacy for gun control laws and the implementation of antibullying programs in schools after a shooting at a school are examples of positive outcomes following a stressor.)

Assessment

The community's core and subsystems comprise assessment parameters for the community worker. A variety of methods are used to complete a community assessment (described in Chap. 9), and the data are organized in ways to allow the interdisciplinary community health team to understand the community core (people), its lines of defence and resistance, any stressors, and the community or aggregate response (degree of reaction) to any stressors present or threatening. Because community work is founded on the principles of primary health care, public participation is a critical component of all steps in the community action process. A team that assesses from a distance will not gain the insider knowledge important to making accurate and appropriate interpretations of the collected data.

Diagnosis and Planning

The community health diagnosis (see Chap. 10) gives direction to both the community health team's goals and intervention planning. The goals are derived from the impact of stressors (degree of reaction caused) and are aimed to reduce community encounters with the stressor or to limit the effects of a stressor through prevention activities that strengthen the community's lines of defence. To be relevant, acceptable, and successful, the processes of analysis and planning must include representatives of the target population, just as the assessment process included community participants. Planning processes are detailed in Chapter 11.

> ✎ **TAKE NOTE**
>
> The term community health diagnosis is preferred over community nursing diagnosis for three reasons: it is holistic and does not imply that only a nurse can address the identified problem; it underscores that work in the community is by nature inter- and intradisciplinary (not only confined to health professions but incorporating many others); and it places the emphasis once again on the community, which is the focus of our practice. For the purposes of planning nursing interventions, however, do use a community nursing diagnosis; for social workers, use a community social work diagnosis, and so on.

Intervention

In this model, all community interventions are considered to be preventive in nature. There are three levels of prevention at which interventions are aimed. The process of implementing community interventions is detailed in Chapter 12.

Primary prevention focuses on risk factors and health promotion. Health education and awareness programs that foster social justice, reduce inequities, and encourage healthy lifestyles are examples of primary prevention interventions. These programs assist the community in strengthening its ability to respond to stressors by expanding its FLD. Primary prevention strategies help the community retain its system stability. Consider the previous exemplar of hypertension in a Hutterite colony: Primary prevention could be education about healthy eating and regular exercise for the colony youth at school; an activity program instituted at school; annual screening of adults for blood pressure and blood glucose levels; and changes in colony food preparation.

Secondary prevention is used after a stressor has penetrated the community subsystems. The focus is on treating responses to stressors and focuses on early case finding, symptom management, and correction of maladaptive responses. Such interventions strengthen the lines of resistance by building on the capacities and assets of the community so that it can attain system stability. An example of secondary prevention would be the monitoring of blood pressure and glucose for those with high blood pressure, education about safe and appropriate medication administration, and supportive diet, exercise, and stress reduction programs for those affected.

Tertiary prevention activities focus on residual consequences of stressor impact by strengthening and re-expanding the flexible line of defence to the previous level (or a new level) in an effort to maintain system stability. For instance, weight loss maintenance and healthy activity programs to maintain healthy blood pressure and blood sugar levels of colony residents, development of a cookbook so novice cooks will learn healthy ways of food preparation, and a resulting change in the prevailing diet and activity norms of the colony would be examples of tertiary prevention. Tertiary prevention interventions are aimed at re-establishing equilibrium in the community.

✎ TAKE NOTE

Many single interventions address more than one level of prevention. In the Hutterite community example, tertiary prevention is illustrated, but actions that build trust will have primary preventive qualities as well. The community's capacity to act in concert with the health care providers will be enhanced by improved communication networks and mutual trust should future events occur.

Evaluation

Feedback from the people in the community provides the basis for evaluation of community health interventions (see Chap. 13) just as involvement of community people in all steps of assessment and planning processes ensures relevance to the community. The community health diagnosis sets the parameters for evaluation (as described in Chap. 10). The target population for the intervention is identified by the reaction of the population to the stressors. The goals and objectives of the intervention are related to the stressor that caused the reaction, and indicators for success are established by the manifestations of the reaction (see Chap. 11). Such is the process of working with the community as partner. Interconnections, overlap, and interdisciplinary considerations are the rule rather than the exception.

Summary

Consider the community-as-partner model (see Fig. 8-1) once more. The goal represented by the model is system equilibrium, a healthy community, and includes the preservation and promotion of community health.

> ✎ **TAKE NOTE**
>
> Health may not be a primary goal of the community (although it may be that of the community health worker). It is, however, an important resource for the community to meet its goals. Realizing that we do not always share the same goals is important for anyone working in the community and must at least be considered (if not reconciled) as we plan, implement, and evaluate programs aimed at improving health.

The model's target is the total community, the population and its aggregates, and, as such, includes individuals and families. The community worker's role is to assist the community to attain, regain, maintain, and promote health, that is, to act as a facilitator, catalyst, and advocate for health so the community is empowered to regulate and control its responses to stressors that are the source of difficulty. The intervention focus is the actual or potential disruption experienced by the community or an inability of the community to function. The intervention mode comprises the three levels of prevention: primary, secondary, and tertiary. The consequences intended in this model include a strengthened normal line of defence, increased resistance to stressors, and a diminished degree of reaction to stressors by the community. Congruent with the principles of primary health care, it is the community's competence to deal with its own problems, strengthen its own lines of defence, and resist stressors that dictates the interventions and measure their success. Let us now begin the process.

References

Anderson, E. T. & McFarlane, J. (2000). *Community as partner* (3rd ed., pp. 153–164). Philadelphia: Lippincott Williams & Wilkins.

Beddome, G. (1995). Community-as-client assessment. In B. N. Neuman, (Ed.), *The Neuman systems model* (3rd ed., pp. 567–580). Norwalk, CT: Appleton & Lange.

Neuman, B. N. (Ed.). (1995). *The Neuman systems model* (3rd ed). Norwalk, CT: Appleton & Lange.

Suggested Readings—Model Examples

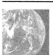

Clark, M. J. (1996). *Nursing in the community* (2nd ed., pp. 895–900). Norwalk, CT: Appleton & Lange.

Ervin, N. E. (2002). Exploring frameworks for guiding a community assessment. In N. E. Ervin (Ed.), *Advanced community health nursing practice* (pp. 8–10, 83–108). Upper Saddle River, NJ: Prentice Hall.

Lancaster, D. R. (1996). Neuman's systems model. In J. J. Fitzpatrick & A. L. Wahll (Eds.), *Conceptual models of nursing: Analysis and application* (3rd ed., pp. 199–224). Norwalk, CT: Appleton & Lange.

Mill, J. E. (1997). The Neuman systems model: Application in a Canadian HIV setting. *British Journal of Nursing, 6*(3), 163–166.

9

Community Assessment

OBJECTIVES

Preceding chapters have focused on the foundational concepts for community practice. A model was introduced in Chapter 8 to guide the process of working with communities and populations. This chapter and those that follow in this section focus on the application of the community-as-partner process in the community. Consequently, the objectives will be primarily practice oriented.

After studying this chapter, you should be able to:

◆ Complete a community assessment using the community-as-partner model

◆ Discuss the challenges of working with communities and populations

◆ Detail the processes that are helpful in overcoming barriers and resistance

◆ Describe the various methods of data collection and their strengths and weaknesses

◆ Begin organizing data for analysis

Introduction

Community assessment is a systematic process; it is the act of becoming acquainted with a community. The people in the community are your partners and contribute throughout the process; the assessment phase is their point of entry into the processes of inquiry, planning, implementing programs, and evaluating their success. The purpose for assessing a community is to identify factors (both positive and negative) that impinge on the health of the people to develop strategies for health promotion. As Hancock and Minkler (1997, p.140) point out, "For health professionals concerned with ... community building for health, there are two reasons for [conducting] community health assessments: information is needed for change, and it is needed for empowerment." Haglund, Weisbrod, and Bracht (1990) suggest several additional purposes for community assessment: preintervention planning, developing health risk profiles, evaluating needs for health promotion actions, assessing community readiness and leadership capacity for planned interventions, preparing funding proposals, and setting the stage for ongoing monitoring of processes and progress toward health goals.

In this chapter, we first discuss how to enter into the community assessment process and then we move into sources and types of data and methods that can be used to collect information. We will use the community assessment wheel (Fig. 9-1) as a framework for the assessment itself and the preparation of the data for the next stage in the process—analysis. (For a specific assessment guide for industry, see Appendix A. Appendix B includes the completed assessment of one industry.)

Rarely does an individual professional conduct a community assessment alone; rather, it is a team effort that brings together different disciplines, perspectives, agendas, and approaches. It is also critical to have community members on the team to facilitate the processes of the assessment, analysis, planning, implementation, and evaluation. Remember, we work *with* the community.

The outcome of a community assessment is a realistic profile of the community, its people, and its subsystems that allows a meaningful determination of strengths and capacities as well as an identification of risks to population aggregates and the environment. Assessment goes beyond documenting types of needs, it also helps to examine why the needs are occurring, the prevalence and urgency of concerns, and the capacity of communities to address the issues it faces, and may point to some possible solutions.

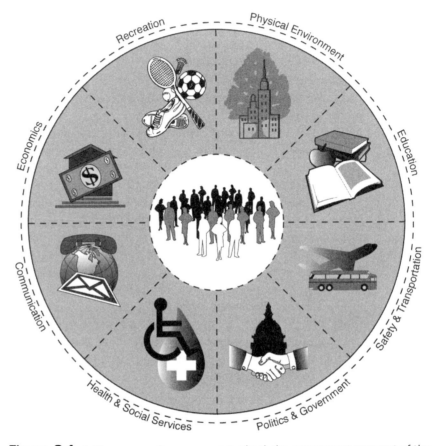

Figure 9-1 ◆ The community assessment wheel, the assessment segment of the community-as-partner model.

Getting to Know the Community

One of the enduring challenges facing the team is the entry into the community and access to people with information. In many cases team members will be outsiders—they will not live in the community of interest or they may not be of the population of interest. It is necessary to get to know the people, how the community is organized formally and informally, and to build rapport and trust. Sometimes being an agent of an organization is helpful in entering the community; other times it may be an impediment. For instance, the school nurse may be a valued outsider with a history of positive engagement in the community who will be accepted more readily than a probation officer who may be perceived as a punitive force and a person to be avoided. Building trust and rapport takes time; often teams do not allow enough time for this important process. How can this process be facilitated?

1. Select a spokesperson or lead agency that already has a relationship with the community.
2. Make contact with the formal community leaders.
3. Be physically present, available, and visible in the community.
4. Engage with people in nonthreatening ways; be open and honest in your actions.
5. Communicate—keep the people involved in decisions and processes.

In particular, sites and moments for informal dialogue can be created through informal, unstructured personal contacts (e.g., at coffee breaks). For this reason, early in the process, personal contacts and interviews are critical to a smooth entry into the community and open access to informants and information sources.

A letter of introduction or a proposal for the assessment may be needed to gain access to formal community leaders, reports, and official data. The team needs to have a clear message that states the purpose of the investigation, what it will require of the community, and what benefits it will have to the people involved.

Will team members be participants in or observers of community life? If present, team members may be asked for their contributions to community decisions, may be requested for advance notice of the assessment findings, or made to feel somewhat uncomfortable. If any team members are "of" the community or population, they may be perceived to have a privileged position. Regardless, the presence of the assessment team will have an influence on the community; care must be taken to ensure ethical practice and minimize any potential for bias.

Inevitably, something will go wrong. When this happens, it is important to recognize it immediately and take action to rebuild relationships and re-establish the momentum of the assessment. Barton and colleagues (1993) suggest that a systematic analysis of issues related to assessment is needed to avoid pitfalls in the process, or to choose strategies that will minimize their impact. Issues related to data generation and strategies to address them are summarized in Table 9-1.

The team may encounter barriers during the entry phase (e.g., *resistance* to collecting or providing information and *impatience* about collecting information instead of "doing something"). It is important to cultivate relationships among key community stakeholders to ensure a smooth process.

TABLE 9-1 ◆ PROBLEMS COMMONLY ENCOUNTERED IN COMMUNITY ASSESSMENT WITH
SUGGESTED SOLUTIONS

Issue	Strategy
Boundaries for data sets do not match	Making inferences regarding the boundaries used for data and determining their accuracy by interview with key informants
Reluctance to report derogatory data	Emphasize the importance of veracity in the context of assessment
Conflicting opinions among vested-interest groups within the community	Ongoing sharing and analysis of information among team members so that all data are noted and discussed
Insider versus outsider views of various community issues	Make certain that various perspectives are obtained during data collection

To be useful for planning, intervention, and evaluation purposes, a community assessment must be based on the best data available—data that are reliable, accurate, and complete. Many methods can be used effectively to gather information; no single method is perfect, so a team will use a variety of means to get a complete picture of a community or an aggregate within the population.

McDevitt and Wilbur (2002) outline three main sources of community data:

1. Sociodemographic and vital statistics data (e.g., census reports, registry reports)
2. Archival materials (e.g., specific reports previously commissioned)
3. Original data collected specifically for the assessment (e.g., windshield surveys, key informant interviews, participant observation, questionnaire surveys)

Patton (1990) classifies data as numerical or nonnumerical. Numerical data can be analyzed statistically and displayed graphically. It can be used to calculate rates and other measures that have meaning to population health. Although numerical data have many advantages in terms of reliability, validity, understandability, and comparability over time, they do not provide a full picture of the community. Nonnumerical data provide depth and detail to statistics and allow us to interpret the beliefs, values, opinions, and culture of the community or population aggregate. They provide the context that situates the numerical data in its unique setting. Used together, both types of data provide a comprehensive community profile that can be used in planning health and social programs.

Edwards and Moyer (2000) provide a summary of health indicators, data sources, and health status reports that can be used in community assessments (p. 425–427). Depending on the purpose of your assessment and the nature of your information needs, the Internet can be an excellent resource along with the published literature and unpublished local reports.

Before actual data collection begins, the team must prepare itself. It is important that, early in the process, the team agrees on the purposes of the assessment, the goals it wants to achieve, and the framework it will use to organize the assessment. Often team members do not normally work together, so a purposeful team-building process is important to a successful process and outcome. Dimock and Devine (1994) have a series of booklets that suggest how a work team can make itself effective by setting standards of operation and behaviour that allow the group to operate and maintain itself. The team needs to determine how it will function: how often and where it will meet, who will chair or lead, how people will communicate, and how team members will divide the work. A work plan that sets the timelines, delineates responsibilities, and estimates resources required for each activity will guide the team and keep it on track. Minutes of meetings and decisions will remind people of commitments. Occasionally taking the "pulse" of the group in terms of self-reflection is helpful to minimize conflicts and ensure member satisfaction and enthusiasm.

It is essential in community work that members of the population group of interest are included in the process. Efforts to recruit and retain community people on working teams may be challenging. Community work is not completed quickly, making time commitment, travel costs, childcare costs, and other considerations important to volunteers. The team must agree to commit resources to supporting and sustaining the involvement of community people in its efforts.

Parks and Straker (1996) caution that much of what is assessed in community work traditionally focuses on problems, barriers, needs, and weaknesses, rather than on the strengths or "assets" of a community or its aggregates. We need to be as aware of a community's "possibilities" as we are of its issues to avoid portraying a negative image that can, according to Kretzman and McKnight (1993), have devastating effects on the community.

Methods of Data Collection

Before you begin the community assessment, the team needs to know *what* information it needs to meet its objectives, *where* that information can be found, and *how* it will be collected and organized. All methods of collecting information have strengths and weaknesses. All involve some ethical issues that need to be considered. No one method will give complete information; therefore, multiple methods are recommended and triangulation of information from one source to another, one type of data to another, and from different methods is needed to ensure the veracity of any inferences or conclusions drawn. Assessment team members are cautioned about jumping to early conclusions without substantiating data. Additional information and specific instructions for each method presented here can be located in Gilmore and Campbell (1996) if the team wants to develop and practise the skills and competencies needed for complete community assessment.

Observation

Observation methods range from being totally unobtrusive to being a full participant in the community. The observer is trying to understand the social setting and lives of the people in the community by observing or participating in events that occur in everyday life. It is particularly effective if the team are outsiders and not familiar with the culture of the community or population group. Obviously, a combined approach allows trust and rapport to build, whereas full observation does not allow for data interpretation and full participation may not permit an objective distance from which to reflect on meanings. Regardless, preparation is necessary to carry out observational surveys:

1. Establish written guidelines about what to observe.
2. Determine the locations for observations.
3. Assess the length of observation periods.
4. Assess and determine the methods for recording observations (i.e., some are more obtrusive than others, but offer better opportunity for team analysis).
5. Gather equipment to record observations (e.g., audio recorder or video camera, tapes, extra batteries, checklist, writing tools and paper for field notes).
6. Ensure any required permissions have been obtained.
7. Plan for creating systematic field notes and for their transcription.
8. Plan debriefing sessions with the team.
9. Use an analytic journal for decision-making and interpretation.

Windshield or walking surveys are other observational techniques. In this method, the team members make use of a variety of physical senses to capture the essence of a community, determine areas for further investigation, and sense the tone of the community. It is also useful in observing the physical spaces where population groups of interest meet and interact. Table 9-2 provides a guide for undertaking a windshield survey. In the first column key points of interest are listed, with suggested questions to ask as you experience the community. Column 2 provides space to capture your observations and, in column 3, space is provided for you to take note of information as you gather it. This chart then becomes part of the raw data you will analyse in the next step of the process.

Preparation for a walking/windshield survey includes mapping out a route, having a checklist (e.g., Table 9-2) from which to work, finding a means to record findings and reactions (e.g., audiovisual recording), a map to chart locations and make reference to field recordings, and proper equipment for the outdoor conditions (e.g., walking shoes, hats, sunscreen, identification, etc.). It is

TABLE 9-2 ◆ LEARNING ABOUT THE COMMUNITY ON FOOT*

I. Community Core	Observations	Data
1. History—What can you glean by looking (e.g., old, established neighborhoods; new subdivision)? Ask people willing to talk: How long have you lived here? Has the area changed? As you talk, ask if there is an "old-timer" who knows the history of the area.		
2. Demographics—What sorts of people do you see? Young? Old? Homeless? Alone? Families? Is the population homogeneous?		
3. Ethnicity—Do you note indicators of different ethnic groups (e.g., restaurants, festivals)? What signs do you see of different cultural groups?		
4. Values and beliefs—Are there churches, mosques, temples? Does it appear homogeneous? Are the lawns cared for? With flowers? Gardens? Signs of art? Culture? Heritage? Historical markers?		
II. Subsystems		
1. Physical environment—How does the community look? What do you note about air quality, flora, housing, zoning, space, green areas, animals, people, human-made structures, natural beauty, water, climate? Can you find or develop a map of the area? What is the size (e.g., square miles, blocks)?		
2. Health and social services—Evidence of acute or chronic conditions? Shelters? Alternative therapists/healers? Are there clinics, hospitals, practitioners' offices, public health services, home health agencies, emergency centers, nursing homes, social service facilities, mental health services? Are there resources outside the community but readily accessible?		*(continued)*

TABLE 9-2 ◆ LEARNING ABOUT THE COMMUNITY ON FOOT* (*Continued*)

I. Community Core	Observations	Data
3. Economy—Is it a "thriving" community or does it feel "seedy?" Are there industries, stores, places for employment? Where do people shop? Are there signs that food stamps are used/accepted? What is the unemployment rate?		
4. Transportation and safety—How do people get around? What type of private and public transportation is available? Do you see buses, bicycles, taxis? Are there sidewalks, bike trails? Is getting around in the community possible for people with disabilities? What types of protective services are there (e.g., fire, police, sanitation)? Is air quality monitored? What types of crimes are committed? Do people feel safe?		
5. Politics and government—Are there signs of political activity (e.g., posters, meetings)? What party affiliation predominates? What is the governmental jurisdiction of the community (e.g., elected mayor, city council with single member districts)? Are people involved in decision making in their local governmental unit?		
6. Communication—Are there "common areas" where people gather? What newspapers do you see in the stands? Do people have TVs and radios? What do they watch/listen to? What are the formal and informal means of communication?		
7. Education—Are there schools in the area? How do they look? Are there libraries? Is there a local board of education? How does it function? What is the reputation of the school(s)? What are major educational issues? What are the dropout rates? Are extracurricular activities available? Are they used? Is there a school health service? A school nurse?		
8. Recreation—Where do children play? What are the major forms of recreation? Who participates? What facilities for recreation do you see?		(*continued*)

TABLE 9-2 ◆ LEARNING ABOUT THE COMMUNITY ON FOOT* (*Continued*)

III. Perceptions	Observations	Data
1. **The residents**—How do people feel about the community? What do they identify as its strengths? Problems? Ask several people from different groups (e.g., old, young, field worker, factory worker, professional, clergy, housewife) and keep track of who gives what answer.		
2. **Your perceptions**—General statements about the "health" of this community. What are its strengths? What problems or potential problems can you identify?		

Note: Supplement your impressions with information from the census, police records, school statistics, chamber of commerce data, health department reports, and so forth, to confirm or refute your conclusions. Tables, graphs, and maps are helpful and will aid in your analysis.
*Revised "Windshield Survey." Anderson, E. T. & McFarlane, J. M. (1988). *Community as client: Application of the nursing process* (pp.178–179). Philadelphia: Lippincott, which also incorporates all aspects of the assessment wheel from Anderson, E. T. & McFarlane, J. M. (1995). *Community as partner: Theory and practice in nursing.* (2nd ed., p. 178), Philadelphia: Lippincott.

advisable to conduct walking or windshield surveys in teams of two for safety purposes and to have mobile communication devices available. Refrain from taking pictures of people, particularly children. Observations need to be made at different times of the day and different days of the week to fully capture the life of the community. Be prepared to explain your presence to community residents if challenged—have your identification and a statement of your project with contact information available to hand out. And remember, use all five senses (and maybe also your sixth sense—intuition) as you observe (Box 9-1).

BOX 9-1. USING YOUR SENSES TO COLLECT INFORMATION ABOUT THE COMMUNITY

Sight—condition of streets, sidewalks, playgrounds; age, sex, racial distributions, clothing, general health condition of the people; housing and services (e.g., schools, businesses, churches) visible

Hearing—noise levels and sources of noise

Taste—types of food supply stores, variety and prices of foods, water quality

Smell—pollutants, odours, sanitation levels

Touch—climate, psychological sense of safety, feeling of openness or oppression, friendliness

Key Informant Interview

There are people in the community who have much to offer an assessment team. They have perhaps lived there or are members of an aggregate of interest. Others may be in leadership positions (e.g., community association executive) or may serve the community in some capacity (e.g., police, fire, health and social services personnel, business people, school personnel). Their insights can be helpful in interpreting statistical findings or in offering information that other methods cannot capture. A variety of views and opinions can be obtained through key informant interviews that can be considered to reflect the views of the community at large (Conway, Hu, & Harrington, 1997).

To prepare for interviews, the team should meet to:

1. Determine who are the key people/positions that should be included in interviews
2. Outline the focus of each informant's potential contribution
3. Determine the structure, timing, and recording methods
4. Outline the questions and prepare the interview guide
5. Create the invitation to participate and design the process
6. Set the times and venues for interviews
7. Invite the key informants to be interviewed
8. Send out confirmation letters with the 'rules of engagement' clearly specified
9. Send letters of thanks after the interviews

It is helpful to send the questions to interviewees in advance so they can prepare themselves. Be certain to outline the purpose of your assessment and the outcomes you hope to achieve. Send only the questions to which you want their specific responses, not the entire community assessment tool. Offer them something tangible in return for their participation (e.g., an Executive Summary of the final report, an invitation to a presentation). As with all inquiry methods that involve humans, you must be sensitive to ethical issues and ensure that no harm comes to your participants. Make sure they know in advance that the interview will be audiotaped or that you will be keeping notes or both.

Be certain to choose interview sites that are comfortable, confidential, and quiet. Make certain your equipment works and take notes as well in the event of an equipment failure. Respect when your interviewee wants to go "off the record." Telephone interviews or the use of electronic surveys may be preferable in some instances, particularly if the questions are very structured or a key informant is not able to attend an interview in person.

Analysis of key informant interviews entails teasing out the main themes and patterns in the responses, and capturing the essence of any discussion, debates, or differing opinions. If interviews are transcribed, software can help to identify themes, but in small samples this may not be necessary.

Focus Groups

Focus groups are not intended to be group interviews in which new data are collected. Instead, they are best used when data themes have emerged from other sources and the team wants to add to the understanding of each theme and determine if they include a complete and accurate picture of community perspectives. Hence, focus group participants are limited to 8 to 12 homogeneous people (i.e., they share certain characteristics) with a variety of perspectives to facilitate in-depth discussion in an informal atmosphere where participants are encouraged to explore issues and express opinions freely. Focus group participants build on the comments of others and come to conclusions not considered individually. Additionally, it is possible to reach consensus about key issues and rank-order issues in terms of priority for action.

Focus group interviews need similar preparation as the key informant process. As well, skilled and unobtrusive facilitators are required to elicit the best information, ask open-ended questions, draw out reticent people, and keep the meeting on track with the stated objectives. Focus group interviews are usually audiotaped for later analysis, but a note-taker is important as well to assess interactions and keep track of points raised. It is important that results not be generalized to the whole population because the participants are not selected to be representative of the population.

There is more information on conducting focus groups in the literature that the team may find helpful (Hawe, Degeling, & Hall, 1990; Morgan & Kreuger, 1997).

Surveys and Questionnaires

Surveys can be used to collect information from people to supplement data from other sources, update information (e.g., demographic), solicit opinions (e.g., satisfaction, beliefs), assess risks (e.g., behaviours), and document exposure to various hazards (e.g., sexual harassment, pollutants). Information may be collected from people by questionnaires or surveys. Surveys can be in person (e.g., door-to-door, telephone) or in writing (e.g., mail-in surveys). If administration methods are properly carried out and the instruments are valid, a survey can be relatively inexpensive in terms of the amount and quality of data collected for the expenditure of time and resources.

The following issues must be considered when planning to conduct a survey:

◆ **Purpose**. Knowing the goal of the survey will help to decide which format to use, the target for the survey, and how many people to include in the sample.

◆ **Resources**. Conducting a survey will use people, time, money, and support services to create the questionnaire, reproduce it, administer the questionnaire, and follow up, analyze and report the data.

◆ **Information needed**. Instruments to collect data need to be sensitive (i.e., not intrusive), reliable, and valid. Developing or choosing a questionnaire that consistently measures what it is supposed to measure takes time and expertise.

◆ **Format**. Open-ended questions will provide richer data (e.g., unique perspectives) than fixed response questions (e.g., true-false, multiple choice, 1-5 scale) but they are more difficult to analyze.

◆ **Response rate**. In certain cases, a representative sample whose responses can be generalized to a wider population is desirable. At other times the survey may need to reach everyone in a target group. Different methods to collect data and improve response rates may be used to ensure the findings are not biased.

◆ **Training**. People who administer the survey need to be trained so that there is consistency among them. Data need to be recorded and input appropriately to facilitate analysis.

◆ **Analysis**. Responses to open-ended questions are analyzed thematically, seeking patterns and themes in the data. Results of fixed-response surveys are easily put into electronic form and analyzed statistically.

It is beyond the scope of this text to teach survey research, but excellent references are available to support the assessment team. As well, you may want to seek out the expertise of a statistician and appropriate software programs to support both qualitative and quantitative analysis.

Population Data

Several forms of data are collected in the course of everyday life: census, vital statistics, morbidity and mortality statistics, population health surveys, records of community services and schools, clinic records, screening records, environmental information (e.g., air and water quality), and the like. Many of these are in the public domain, but issues like confidentiality, data access, and quality of data must be assessed.

Population data can be used to establish baselines for the purposes of making comparisons, determining which indicators have enough support for their use, and setting benchmarks for measuring progress on goals and objectives, and when combined with critical reviews of the literature, they can be used to make program-related decisions.

Local data are often available from the municipality, health and social services departments, chamber of commerce, and similar groups in reports and on websites. As well, government ministries at both the provincial and national levels release population status reports that are available in local libraries or on the Internet. Health Canada regularly conducts a National Population Health Survey and makes reports available to the public. Statistics Canada also releases reports on population issues that may be of interest to the team for comparison purposes.

Other Assessment Strategies

The preceding is not an exhaustive list of mechanisms that can be used to collect information about a population or community. Other methods can be found described in the literature. Additionally, the literature can be critically examined as issues arise and potential target populations surface. The team is encouraged to meet frequently during data collection to share information and determine the scope and depth needed for analysis. Community members can be helpful in suggesting sources for further information (particularly regarding historical or recent events) and in providing evidence of community capacity and assets.

Elements of a Community Assessment

The use of a model to guide the assessment of a community, neighbourhood, population, or an aggregate assists with the organization of the process and of the data collected. This section will examine the data that describes the core, the eight subsystems, and the functions of the community according to the Assessment Wheel in Figure 9-1. The team may want to create its own process for data management or refer to Gerberich, Stearns, and Dowd (1995), who offer an assessment instrument with key questions for each subsystem that can be adapted to the Community-as-Partner model used here.

Community Core

The definition of *core* is "that which is essential, basic, and enduring." The core of a community is its people—their history, characteristics, values, and beliefs. The first stage of assessing a community, then, is to learn about its people to gain insight into their life experience. In fact, partnering with people in the community is an integral part of working in the community. Table 9–3 lists the major components of the community core along with suggested locations and sources of information about each component. Because every community is different, information sources available to one community may not be available to another.

The community core is described through information on sociodemographic, economic, and cultural variables and factors that describe social support. Lifestyle factors, employment patterns, resource production and con-

TABLE 9-3 ◆ COMMUNITY CORE DATA

Components	Sources of Information
History	Library, historical society, museum, newpaper archives
	Interview "old-timers," town leaders
Demographics	Census of population and housing
Age and sex characteristics	Planning board (local, county, province)
Racial distribution	Chamber of commerce
Ethnic distribution	City hall, archives
	Observation
Household types by	Census (municipal, national)
Family	
Non family	
Group	
Marital status by	Census (municipal, national)
Single	
Separated	
Widowed	
Divorced	
Vital statistics	Local and provincial departments of health (distributed
Births	through health department reports and websites)
Deaths by	
Age	
Leading causes	
Values and beliefs	Personal contact
	Observation ("Learning About the Community on Foot)
	(To protect against stereotyping, avoid the literature
	for this portion of the assessment.)
Religion	Observation
	Telephone book

sumption, and personal health behaviours help to understand the people of the community and how their values influence the choices made.

In the summer of 1875, 50 members of the North West Mounted Police, sent to stop the whiskey trade and bring law and order to the west, arrived at the junction of the Bow and Elbow Rivers to establish a new fort. Fort Calgary, named by Colonel MacLeod, became the Town of Calgary (pop. 1000) in the Northwest Territories in 1884 and a city (pop. 3900) in 1894, predating the creation of Alberta as a province in 1905. Situated at the gateway to the Rockies, Calgary was changed by the Canadian Pacific Railway from a frontier town to a major supply station. Although its beginnings were in fur trade, farming, and ranching, Calgary later became the hub of the petroleum industry and is famous for the Calgary Stampede "The Greatest Outdoor Show on Earth." Today it is a thriving and vibrant city of nearly 1 million people.

Throughout its history, health and social services developed along with the city. As presented in Chapter 2, federal and provincial jurisdictions governed how human services were delivered, and municipalities filled complementary roles to protect the health and well-being of their residents. Over time, the organization of the systems of health and social services delivery became cumbersome, and in 1995, the province of Alberta restructured its health care delivery system, and created 17 regional health authorities from over 200 separate boards that managed hospital, health units, and long-term care settings. Each health authority was responsible for amalgamating hospital, long-term care, emergency services, and community health and home care. Social services, children's services, mental health services, and other provincial services (e.g., tuberculosis and sexually transmitted infections) were also realigned over time to match health authority boundaries. In anticipation of this reorganization, a community needs assessment was carried out in 1994.

In this example, 5 of 15 inner-city communities will be described and used to illustrate an application of the Community-as-Partner model. Fifteen communities were selected for the initial study, representing approximately 51,380 residents (7.2% of the city's total population of 713, 610). An estimated 86,000 additional people come to the downtown area every day to work or to use services, and day care is provided to 2500 children. The unique profile of each neighbourhood was obscured when the downtown area as a whole was considered. The five communities that will be described and compared in this example are: Bankview, Connaught, Victoria Park, Bridgeland, and Inglewood. Data from the most recent years from the following sources were used: Census Canada, City of Calgary, Alberta Environment, and Alberta Health. More complete and recent reports are available from the Calgary Health Region.

To begin the process, experienced community workers find it helpful to write thumbnail sketches that succinctly describe the community or communities of interest. In this case, we are assessing geopolitical communities (or neighbourhoods); their descriptions are found in Table 9-4.

TABLE 9-4 ◆ COMMUNITY DESCRIPTIONS

Community	Description
Bankview (BNK)	In 1882, the land that became Bankview was purchased by an English immigrant for farming and ranching. In the early 1900s, the land was subdivided along a traditional grid pattern for housing development. Its character changed from low density in the 1950s to allow walk-up apartment buildings, and now offers a diversity of housing units and an inner-city lifestyle. There are no schools in this community.
Connaught (CON)	In 1893, the city limits included the Connaught district that encompassed large estates of prominent citizens. By 1912, development had extended south and west with 2- and 3-story homes, treed boulevards, and large open spaces. Many of the city's first fine institutions (religious, educational, cultural) were located here. The character of the area has changed dramatically through the years, with the addition of many medium- and high-density commercial office buildings, apartments, and condominiums. There is one community elementary school (public).
Victoria Park (VIC)	This community predates Calgary's incorporation as a town. Named after Queen Victoria, the community prospered in its early days because of its proximity to Fort Calgary, the railroad station, and the developing downtown. By 1902, 83% of the existing structures had been built, and by the 1950s and 1960s found itself hemmed in by transportation corridors and the community began to lose its appeal as a residential community. With the expansion of the Calgary Stampede and Exhibition in the 1970s, the construction of the Saddledome in the 1980s, and continuing rumours of further expansion, the community is under significant threat and even a neighbourhood improvement program has failed to revitalize the community. There is one public charter school.
Bridgeland (BRD)	This area, located across the Bow River, was enhanced in 1885 with the construction of the Langevin Bridge. It was annexed to the city in 1910. For many new Canadians, Bridgeland became their first home, originally Germans and Italians, and more recently Vietnamese. There are two public schools (elementary and junior) and one separate school (elementary).
Inglewood (ING)	Calgary's oldest community, dating back to the late 1800s, located where the Bow and Elbow Rivers join. People were attracted to the community by its industry (Burns Stockyards and Cross Brewery) and its proximity to the Fort. One environmentally sensitive industrial site (refinery) is located away from the residential area but could affect future development. Its residential community is low to medium density, and many projects are under way to restore its historical landmarks. It has one community elementary school.

Population Description

TOTAL POPULATION

Knowing the total number of people living in a neighbourhood or in a group of neighbourhoods allows the community worker to make certain judgements and comparisons between and among communities. Information that allows us to understand the elements of the community core is found in sociodemographic data that are often captured in the census. Table 9-5 provides an overview of the number of people residing in each of the communities we are discussing.

The five example communities have a population of 29,758 or 58% of the 15 downtown communities described in the initial study and 4.2% of the total population of the city. The communities are geographically arranged from west to east, with natural boundaries of the two rivers (Fig. 9-2). Description of the 5 communities will be compared with the "downtown" 15 (DT15) communities and to the city as a whole for the purposes of analysis (see Chap. 10).

AGE DISTRIBUTION

How a population is apportioned by age often provides important clues to potential issues that might be faced. For example, a neighbourhood with a high proportion of seniors will need different services and resources than a neighbourhood where young children predominate. In Table 9-6 the percent of age groups in each of the five communities of interest is presented and compared with the population distribution in the DT15 communities.

Further, knowing about some characteristics that can have an effect on health and well-being is important. The following information is presented to examine certain determinants of health and to further describe the community core for the five communities in which we are interested (Table 9-7). The data for the DT15 communities is also presented for comparison purposes. The raw data as well as the *rates* are provided to facilitate comparisons between and among neighbourhoods. Where rates are high, or higher in comparison to other

TABLE 9-5 ◆ NUMBER OF PEOPLE RESIDING IN EACH COMMUNITY

Neighbourhood	Population
BNK	5,175
CON	11,115
VIC	4,755
BRD	4,685
ING	4,028

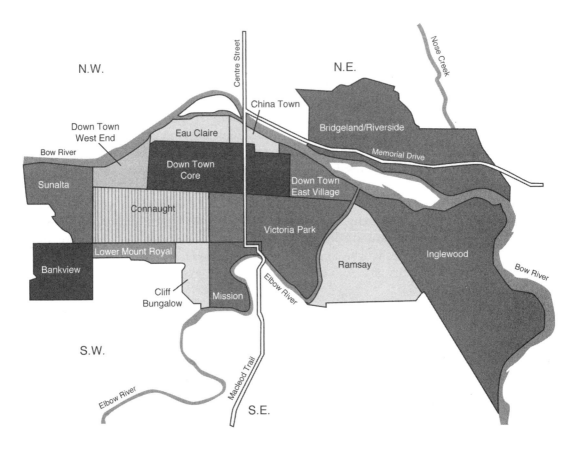

Figure 9-2 ◆ Map of 15 downtown Calgary communities (DT15).

TABLE 9-6 ◆ PERCENT OF COMMUNITY POPULATION BY AGE GROUP						
	BNK	**CON**	**VIC**	**BRD**	**ING**	**DT15**
0–4 y	5.7	2.7	4.5	6.3	5.7	3.8
5–14 y	4.4	2.8	4.1	5.7	8.0	3.6
15–19 y	3.9	3.2	5.0	3.6	5.1	3.7
20–24 y	18.1	15.7	14.6	8.9	8.2	14.1
25–44 y	52.2	48.7	44.0	38.0	41.0	46.7
45–64 y	10.3	15.0	15.5	13.2	18.6	15.1
65+ y	5.4	11.8	12.3	24.3	13.3	13.6

TABLE 9-7 ◆ SELECTED SOCIODEMOGRAPHIC CHARACTERISTICS

	BNK	CON	VIC	BRD	ING	DT15
Seniors living alone	125	685	365	285	125	3435
(rate per 100 seniors)	(44.6)	(52.3)	(62.4)	(25.0)	(38.5)	(49.7)
Unemployed youth	110	190	115	70	85	930
(rate per 100 youth)	(9.7)	(9.2)	(11.4)	(1.3)	(22.7)	(11.5)
Unemployed adults (>25 y)	285	500	350	235	115	2855
(rate per 100 adults 25+)	(8.0)	(6.0)	(10.5)	(7.9)	(6.5)	(7.4)
Lone-parent families	230	265	175	235	100	1670
(rate per 100 families)	(49.5)	(45.2)	(44.9)	(45.6)	(32.8)	(45.5)
Persons in low-income households	1750	3870	2365	1595	840	19020
(rate per 100 total population)	(34.0)	(35.6)	(51.6)	(39.6)	(43.4)	(40.6)
Home language not English	400	1505	1110	460	150	7165
(rate per 100 total population)	(7.8)	(13.9)	(23.9)	(11.5)	(6.1)	(18.4)
Recent immigrants (past 5 y)	270	1005	595	120	55	3625
(rate per 100 immigrants)	(24.9)	(37.0)	(37.2)	(11.3)	(15.1)	(24.1)
Persons moved in past year	2350	4915	1970	1215	620	20,155
(rate per 100 population >1 y)	(45.9)	(45.3)	(43.1)	(30.7)	(25.5)	(37.0)
Persons moved in past 5 y	3965	8835	3435	2360	1230	36,425
(rate per 100 population >5 y)	(76.5)	(79.5)	(72.1)	(50.4)	(50.1)	(70.9)
Education <secondary certificate (16+)	1190	2505	1885	1355	1000	14,340
(rate per 100 population 16+)	(25.4)	(24.2)	(43.6)	(38.4)	(46.4)	(34.8)
Median household income	23,824	27,054	15,980	23,419	27,644	

Note: The city median household income was $44,064.

neighbourhoods, it could indicate a concern; for instance, the youth unemployment rate in Inglewood is double that of the downtown and three other communities. However, Bridgeland is markedly less (one tenth of the downtown rate). Before taking action, however, more data are needed to analyze and interpret the meaning of these numbers.

Subsystems

A review of a community's subsystems tell us about the context in which people live, work, play, pray, and go to school. It provides insights into factors that influence how people live, what choices they make, and why. A subsystems analysis focuses on the external environment such as the sociopolitical and economic contexts and the infrastructures of the community and how these have an impact on the population.

PHYSICAL ENVIRONMENT

Just as the physical examination is a critical component of assessing an individual patient, so it is in the assessment of a community. And just as the five senses of the clinician are called into play in the physical examination of a patient, so, too, are they needed at the community level. Table 9-8 provides the components of the physical examination, both of an individual and a community, and compares tools and sources of data for each.

It is important to collect information about where and how the community/population is situated within the physical space to understand how the various elements have an impact on community life (e.g., weather, terrain, placement of services, population density, diversity). Such information allows us to assess availability, affordability, adequacy and access to services, housing, green space, and so forth and associated issues of safety, utilization, and community capacity.

Centre Street is the major north-south thoroughfare, and Memorial Drive on the north side of the Bow River and 9th Avenue on the south side are the major east-west routes. The railway traverses the borders of Inglewood, Victoria Park, and Connaught. The Exhibition Grounds are located in Victoria Park, the Bird Sanctuary and Fort Calgary Historic Site in Inglewood, and the Zoo in Bridgeland. In all areas there are businesses along main streets and a mix of housing options. Inglewood and Bridgeland have a lower population density than the others; Connaught, with its large number of high- and low-rise apartments, has the highest density. Victoria Park is in a state of decay as the Stampede and the City pursue urban renewal options. Inglewood is undergoing a renaissance, with an active main street revitalization program that is giving rise to quaint bistros, antique shops, art galleries, and specialty boutiques.

TABLE 9-8 ◆ PHYSICAL EXAMINATION COMPONENTS AND SOURCES OF DATA

	Sources of Data	
Components*	Individual	Community
Inspection	All senses	All senses
	Otoscope	Windshield survey
	Ophthalmoscope	Walk through community
Auscultation	Stethoscope	Listen to community sounds/residents
Vital signs	Thermometer	Observe climate, terrain, natural boundaries, and resources
	Sphygmomanometer	"Life" signs such as notices of community meetings; density
Systems review	Head-to-toe	Observe social systems, including housing, businesses, churches, and hangouts
Laboratory studies	Blood tests	Almanac; census data
	X-rays	Chamber of commerce planning
	Scans, other tests	studies and surveys

*Carried out at different times of the day, week, month, and/or year to determine the flow of community life

Because parking is at a premium in the downtown, residential streets are crowded, and through streets are often jammed during rush hours.

The climate is mild, with sunny summer days and cool evenings. Chinooks (http://www.nucleus.com/~cowboy/Misc/Chinooks.html) temper the winter chill, and the mountain playgrounds are nearby for hiking, skiing, high-country sports, and artistic pursuits. The Calgary climate is termed "moderate"; descriptive statistics are located in Box 9-2.

There are bike and jogging trails throughout the downtown and along the scenic riverbanks. Stately trees planted to remember the soldiers of the two world wars shade Memorial Drive; small parks dot the downtown with green space. The Alexandra Community Centre is a gathering place for the community of Inglewood. Connaught has a public pool. Downtown residents are served by churches of a variety of denominations, public and separate schools, museums, galleries, fire and police services, banks, supermarkets, and a large library. The downtown also contains services for the homeless (Drop-In Centre, Calgary Urban Projects Society, Mustard Seed, EXIT Outreach for street youth, among others). In some areas, particularly Victoria Park, yellow mailboxes are placed around the neighbourhoods to serve as receptacles for used needles. In this area, prostitution has been an ongoing problem, accompanied by drug trafficking, crime, and alcohol abuse. Residents complain that because of the proximity to the light rail transit system, events at the Exhibition Grounds, and downtown bars, prostitutes use the area to attract men from other parts of the city, disrupting community life and making the community unsafe in the evenings. The condition of houses in a neighbourhood is a physical sign that indicates community

---

BOX 9-2. CLIMATE DESCRIPTION FOR CALGARY, ALBERTA

Moderate Climate

Mean rain fall per year: 30.1 cm (11.8")

Mean snowfall per year: 152.5 cm (60.0")

Days with measurable snowfall: 62

Seasonal Temperatures

Summer (June–August): 20°C (68°F)

Fall (September–November): 11°C (52°F)

Winter (December–February): −11°C (10°F)

Spring (March–May): 9°C (42°F)

well-being. If people are not putting effort into home maintenance, it may be a symptom of concern when considered with other information during the analysis process (Table 9-9). The following information is available from the census.

HEALTH AND SOCIAL SERVICES

A review of this subsystem allows an assessment of the "social safety net" infrastructure and provides insight as to how basic needs are met in the community. The focus is on need and utilization—how is it met (availability, access, affordability) by services within and outside the community. Various sectors that provide health and services are included in the assessment (e.g., formal [government] and informal [volunteer], publicly funded and private).

One method of classifying health and social services is to differentiate between facilities located outside the community (*extracommunity*) versus those within the community (*intracommunity*). Once the health and social service facilities are identified, group them into categories, perhaps by type of service offered (e.g., hospitals, clinics, extended care), by size, or by public versus private usage. Table 9–10 suggests a classification system as well as possible major components of each facility requiring assessment.

DOWNTOWN HEALTH FACILITIES AND SOCIAL SERVICES

At the time of the community assessment, there were two acute care hospitals in the downtown area, two large long-term care facilities, and a veterans' facility. The Alexandra Health Centre is located in Inglewood, the Children's Hospital in Scarboro (next to Bankview), and the District Public Health serves the downtown from City Hall. Home care is provided from the Central Office in the downtown area. Several general practice, walk-in clinics, and specialists have offices in the downtown communities. Pharmacies, laboratory and radiology services, dental offices, and vision care centres are located throughout the inner-city area. The food bank and a thrift store are sited in the downtown core near the housing shelters and other social services. The Victorian Order of

TABLE 9-9 ◆ HOME MAINTENANCE						
	BNK	**CON**	**VIC**	**BRD**	**ING**	**DT15**
Homes needing major repairs (rate per 100 of all homes)	300 (9.8)	395 (5.6)	360 (12.9)	250 (11.6)	165 (13.9)	2305 (11.2)

TABLE 9-10 ◆ HEALTH AND SOCIAL SERVICES

Component	Sources of Information
Health Services Extracommunity or intracommunity facilities. Once identified, group into categories (e.g., hospitals and clinics, home health care, extended care facilities, public health services, emergency care). For each facility, collect data on 1. Services (fees, hours, and new services planned and those discontinued) 2. Resources (personnel, space, budget, and record system) 3. Characteristics of users (geographic distribution, demographic profile, and transportation source) 4. Statistics (number of persons served daily, weekly, and monthly) 5. Adequacy, accessibility, and acceptability of facility according to users and providers	Chamber of commerce Planning board (district, county, city) Phone directory Talk to residents Interview administrator or someone on the staff Facility annual report and websites
Social Services Extracommunity or intracommunity facilities. Once identified, group into categories (e.g., counseling and support, clothing, food, shelter, and special needs). For each facility, collect data on areas 1–5 listed above.	Chamber of commerce United Way directory Phone directory Municipality Nongovernmental agencies and associations

Nurses provides wellness services in seniors' housing apartments and a foot clinic out of the veterans' hospital.

Also located in the downtown are the Sexually Transmitted Disease Clinic, Southern Alberta Clinic (HIV/AIDS), Family Planning Clinic, Travel Clinic, Communicable Diseases Unit, Salvation Army Mission, YWCA, Crisis Services (violence, mental health), along with churches and community schools that offer social outreach programs, "Inn from the Cold" emergency shelter, hot meals, and clothing programs. Vans roam the streets in the evenings to provide needle exchange services, hot beverages and sandwiches, minor health care, and counselling services to street-involved people. In total, 54 health-related services are located in the downtown area (Fig. 9-3).

Family physician locations and ambulatory care centres are shown on Figures 9-4 and 9-5, respectively. Maps are provided to demonstrate different ways of displaying the information gathered by the assessment team. A map provides a visual picture that cannot be illustrated by lists of addresses. As geographic information systems (GIS) become more readily available, mapping will become increasingly important to illustrate distributions across territory.

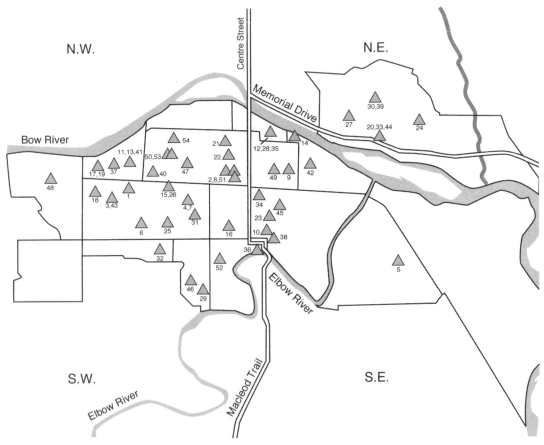

Figure 9-3 ◆ Map showing the location of health services in the 15 downtown Calgary communities (DT15).

Other services in the DT15 include:

Aboriginal services	Food bank
Anger management	Housing agencies
Before/after school programs	Immigrant agencies
Child welfare	Information/referral/advocacy agencies
Clothing exchange	Job search/training
Community kitchen	Language training
Counselling	Library
Day care	Parent support groups
Emergency shelters	Places of worship

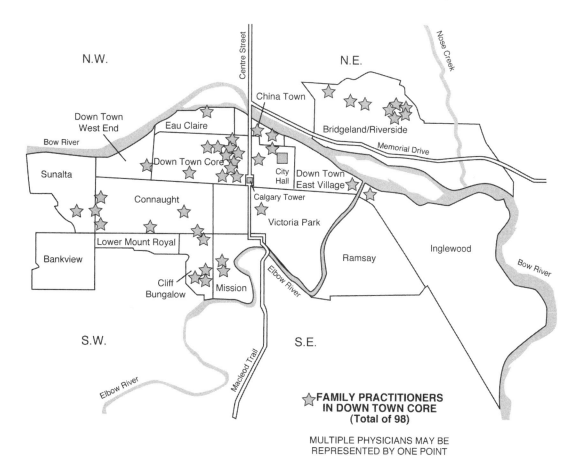

Figure 9-4 ◆ Map showing the location of family physicians in the 15 downtown Calgary communities (DT15).

Public health	Social events/activities
Recreation/leisure programs	Special needs program
School/education	Teen drop-in centre
Seniors club	Youth leadership

It is important to collect information not only about what services are available in the community itself, but also about what services exist in the immediate area that people would access. In this instance, the DT15 communities share a number of services. Planners need to know this information if they are going to avoid duplication, facilitate access, and remove barriers or obstacles to utilization.

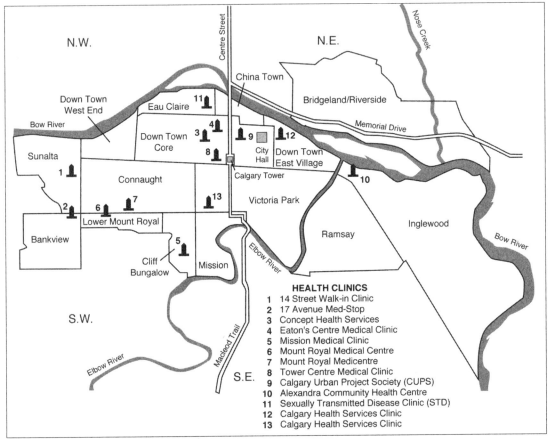

Figure 9-5 ◆ Ambulatory care centre locations in the 15 downtown communities (DT15).

ECONOMICS

The economic subsystem includes the "wealth" of a community—that is, the goods and services available to the community—as well as the costs and benefits of improving patterns of resource allocation. It should be evident that extracommunity factors, such as the state of the national and world economies, affect in great measure the local economy. Nevertheless, intracommunity economic factors impinge on all other subsystems, so they must be included in the assessment.

The economy affects household finances through employment, business, productivity, and measures that describe the labour force (e.g., employment rate, occupations) give insight into the "morale" of a population and the vitality of a community.

Table 9-11 lists the suggested areas for studying a community's economy, along with sources of the data. The census data can be used to summarize most of these economic indicators. Two key indicators of a community's economic "health" are the percentage of households below the poverty level and the unemployment rate.

People who live in poverty are unable to afford adequate housing, purchase enough food to satisfy hunger and nutritional requirements, and hence rely on social services for supplementary income, food banks for food, and thrift stores for clothing. When poverty becomes chronic, quality of life suffers and in the long term, psychological consequences can have adverse effects on people, especially children and seniors. Seniors face a greater poverty risk because of their reliance on fixed incomes and the lack of employment opportunity. Seniors can receive a guaranteed income supplement (GIS) and families living in poverty may receive support for independence (SFI) (Table 9-12).

TABLE 9-11 ◆ INDICATORS AND SOURCES OF INFORMATION

Indicators	Source
Financial Characteristics	
Households	
Median household income	
% households below poverty level	
% households receiving public assistance	
% households headed by females	Census records
Monthly costs for owner-occupied	
households and renter-occupied households	
Individuals	
Per capita income	
% of persons who live in poverty	Census records
Labor Force Characteristics	
Employment Status	
General population (age 18+)	
% employed	
% unemployed	Chamber of commerce
% not participating in employment (retired)	Department of Labour
Special groups	Census records
% women working with children under age 6	
Occupational Categories and Number (%) of Persons Employed	
Managerial	
Technical	
Service	
Farming	Census records
Production	
Operator/laborer	
Union Activity and Membership	Local union(s) office

TABLE 9-12 ◆ ECONOMIC INDICATORS FOR FIVE COMMUNITIES AND THE DOWNTOWN						
	BNK	CON	VIC	BRD	ING	DT15
Percent of seniors receiving GIS	44.7	36.3	66.3	55.2	41.7	30.9
Children living in SFI households (%)	17.6	14.9	13.7	15.1	12.2	5.1

BUSINESS

Since the discovery of oil and gas in nearby Turner Valley in 1914, Calgary has become known as the energy capital of Canada. Building on that strength the city's economy has diversified to include major activity in manufacturing, transportation, logistics, hi-tech, construction, tourism, and financial services. It is this diversity that has kept the city growing steadily and makes for a positive future of opportunity and prosperity. Calgary's traditional oil industry's cycle of boom and bust has given way to the modern, international, technology-intensive operations of today. The city has diversified its business to the point that in the late 1990s when the price of oil was down dramatically Calgary's economy was still moving forward and growing. This stability prompted analysts to refer to Calgary's economy as "bullet-proof." The city is maintaining that reputation with forecasts indicating Calgary will continue to lead the country in economic growth. Figures 9-6 and 9-7 present indicators of the economic subsystem. These data will become important as teams analyze data (see Chap. 10) and plan interventions (see Chap. 11).

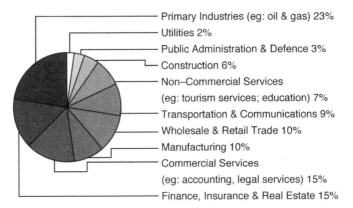

Figure 9-6 ◆ Calgary GDP by industry (% contribution to total, 2001). (Source: Conference Board of Canada.)

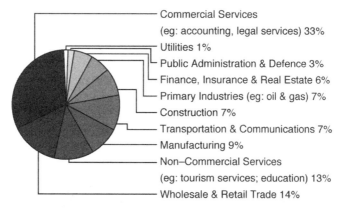

Figure 9-7 ◆ Calgary employment by industry (% contribution to total, 2001). (Source: Conference Board of Canada.)

LABOUR FORCE

The labour force includes all persons over the age of 15 who were either employed or unemployed in the week prior to Census Day. Persons not in the labour force "refers to persons 15 years of age and over, excluding institutional residents, who ... did not work for pay or in self-employment in the week prior to enumeration and (a) did not look for paid work in the four weeks prior to enumeration, (b) were not on temporary lay-off and (c) did not have a new job to start in four weeks or less. It also includes persons who looked for work during the last four weeks but were not available to start work in the week prior to enumeration." (Statistics Canada, 1997).

Work activity (number of hours and weeks worked per year) is related to income adequacy. People who work full time for less than a year, or part time, are almost three times as likely to have incomes below the low-income cutoff (LICO) than fulltime workers who worked for the full year. Particularly disadvantaged by earning inequality are women and youth workers.

Educational attainment of the work force tends to be related to income adequacy and employment opportunity. Rates of low income are highest for those workers with low education levels (i.e., less than high school certificate).

HOUSEHOLD STRUCTURE

The rate of lone-parent families in the downtown is about twice that of the city average. In families that are headed by single parents, one parent carries the full burden of finances and nurturing, increasing the risk of social and emotional stress and vulnerability. Of the 82% of lone-parent households in Canada headed by women, 57% were living in poverty.

TABLE 9-13 ◆ PERCENTAGE OF INCOME DEVOTED TO SHELTER IN CALGARY AND DOWNTOWN COMMUNITIES

	BNK	CON	VIC	BRD	ING	City
Percent of renters spending >30% income on housing	42.7	36.8	43.1	42.0	50.9	37.8
Percent of families below the ownership affordability threshold	59.7	58.5	72.6	61.1	35.0	43.1

SHELTER

The majority (83%) of people living in the DT15 communities live in apartments; in contrast, only 22% of Calgarians live in apartments. In Calgary, 53% of the population lives in one-family dwellings, but in the downtown, only 7% reside in single-family dwellings. The ability to afford adequate housing contributes to the health of individuals, families, and communities. Families with low incomes may divert money from other necessities to cover shelter costs or may become homeless. The percentage of income devoted to shelter is a useful measure of housing affordability; this information is located in Tables 9-13 and 9-14 for the communities of interest and the downtown area.

SAFETY AND TRANSPORTATION

Without a safe and secure environment based on public order and respect for property, people will be fearful of participation in community events. Structures in this subsystem exist to reduce fear or anxiety and promote a sense of safety in a community or population. Hence, the availability of fire, police, sanitation, sewage, recycling, and solid waste services, as well as those that protect air quality, monitor dangerous goods, and protect us from animals are assessed. Public and community services that offer health promotion, injury and disease prevention, and health protection services are important to the health and well-being of a community. Transportation safety measures (i.e., roads and road maintenance, private vehicle safety regulations, public transit, air, and rail safety measures, lighting of public places and roads) protect the public from hazards.

TABLE 9-14 ◆ AVERAGE HOUSING VALUES 2002 (IN $100,000) ACCORDING TO SALES RECORDS

	BNK	CON	VIC	BRD	ING	City
Condominium	140.6	165.9	169.8	118.3	138.6	150.0
Residential	274.1	288.5	165.0	202.5	263.0	196.0

Table 9-15 lists the major components of safety and transportation that affect the community.

PROTECTION SERVICES

Fire, police, waste disposal, and sanitation services are provided by the City and paid for by property taxes. Crime rates are higher in the inner city than the Calgary average, ranging from 1.1 to 2.7 times the rate for the city as a whole (Table 9-16). Police patrol the areas by car, on foot, and with bicycles. For the park areas, horse patrols are also used.

There are Neighbourhood Watch programs in the communities, and by-law enforcement officers pick up stray animals.

WATER AND SANITATION

Water supplies for the downtown area are from the Glenmore Reservoir; chlorine and fluoride are added at the source. There is no heavy industry in the area with the closure of the brewery and stockyards, so industrial pollution is min-

TABLE 9-15 ◆ SAFETY AND TRANSPORTATION

Indicators	Sources of Information
Safety	
Protection services	Planning office (municipality)
Fire	Fire department (local)
Police	Police department (municipality)
Sanitation	
Waste sources and treatment	Waste and water treatment plants
Solid waste	
Air quality	Environment department
Transportation	
Private	
Transportation sources	
Number of persons with a transportation disability	Census data: population and housing characteristics
Public	
Bus, subway, and light rail services (routes, schedules, and fares)	Local and city transportation authorities
Roads (number and condition; primary, secondary, and farm-to-market roads)	Provincial highway department
Interstate highways	
Freeway system	
Air service (private and publicly owned)	Local airports (*Note:* Local airports are frequently owned and operated by city government.)
Intercity rail service	CP Rail
	VIA Rail

imal. Trains make some noise and traffic creates some air pollution. Occasionally during the spring people with respiratory disorders are advised to stay indoors because of the cottonwood pollen in the air.

TRANSPORTATION

Calgary is on the Trans Canada Highway and on the north-south truck route from Mexico to Alaska. An international airport in the northeast provides access to air travel. The Canadian Pacific Railway goes through the city, and Greyhound has a large terminal for passenger and freight service. Several smaller commercial airlines operate out of the airport in Calgary, and other bus services provide local access to the mountains and along the north-south corridor. There is a light rail transit system and regular bus service. A hazardous chemicals route goes through the city to the east of downtown. Traffic is heavy with people moving into and out of the downtown for employment and services. Parking is expensive, and people are encouraged to "Park'n Ride." There are no special privileges for carpools on the many trails that move traffic around the city and few dedicated bike lanes on the major streets.

SOCIAL INCLUSION

Geopolitical communities provide opportunity for the development of informal and formal social ties. Communities with people who are interested in their neighbourhoods, aware of resources available, and involved in the safety and health of the community are strong communities. Those communities that lack connection to the people risk social isolation and underutilization of available resources to prevent negative physical and economic outcomes. It takes time to develop an attachment to a community; hence, those communities with high mobility and recent in-migration may have lower participation rates in community life. Individuals who lack fluency in the official languages of the country face further risk of social or economic isolation. People who live alone (e.g., seniors) or in a household where they are not related to any other people who live there must bear social and financial stress on their own. Furthermore, they are more likely to have incomes below the LICO. Seniors and those with disabilities may also face difficulties accessing services due to their frailty. In

TABLE 9-16 ◆ CRIME RATES IN THE DOWNTOWN COMMUNITIES						
	BNK	CON	VIC	BRD	ING	DT15
Reported crime (rate per 1000 population)	856 (178.2)	3742 (342.7)	2237 (472.7)	762 (165.8)	600 (241.3)	20,376 (399.1)

TABLE 9-17 ◆ PERCENT OF PEOPLE LIVING ALONE IN THE DOWNTOWN AREA						
	BNK	**CON**	**VIC**	**BRD**	**ING**	**City**
Percent of unattached individuals	51.5	53.1	53.4	36.6	34.4	14.9

Table 9-17, the percent of people who live on their own in the five downtown communities of Calgary is presented, compared to the percent of people who live alone in the city as a whole.

POLITICS AND GOVERNMENT

The various forms and levels of government are responsible for public policy-making through legislation. We need to understand which government is responsible for the portfolios that influence healthy public policy, how special interest groups can influence policy, and how to gain access to these resources with the communities and population aggregates with which we are working. We must be aware of the influential people in positions of power to influence the health and well-being of people: mayor and alderpersons, school board and other trustees, provincial premier, key ministers in provincial government, leader of the provincial opposition, local medical officer of health, and heads of social and community agencies. On a national level, we must know who the persons of influence are with respect to issues of federal jurisdiction, including local members of parliament. Within the disciplines that are involved in community work, there are opportunities to bring issues and resolutions forward for action locally, provincially, and on the national scene. For instance, the Canadian Public Health Association (CPHA) has worked successfully with the various provincial branches and associations to influence public policy on gun control, home care, clean air, homelessness, and unemployment issues, among others.

The five example communities are situated within the downtown area of Calgary. Calgary has a mayor-council form of government with 14 aldermen elected every 2 years. City Council meets weekly and has several standing committees. The list of alderman is available on the City website (http://calgary.foundlocally.com/Local/Gov-CityAldermen.htm) and residents are encouraged to telephone, mail, or e-mail their representatives on a wide array of issues. There are seven trustees elected to both the public and separate school boards; the chairpersons are elected from among them (http://calgary.foundlocally.com/Local/Gov-SchoolTrustees.htm). In 2001, nine elected and six appointed board members governed the local health region; the Alberta Minister of Health and Wellness appointed the chairperson.

In 2003 the Province once again reorganized health regions, cutting the number of regions to nine and eliminating elected members to regional boards. Now the health region has a chair and 13 members. Several members are from former rural boards now amalgamated into the expanded Calgary Health Region (www.calgaryhealthregion.ca/board/listing/htm). Twenty-one Members of the Legislative Assembly (MLAs) represent Calgary in the provincial government, and Calgary sends eight Members of Parliament to Ottawa. Each of these has an office in their home area, and residents are welcome to bring concerns to the staff.

COMMUNICATION

This subsystem details how people communicate within the target population and the broad community on an every day basis and also how emergency messages are conveyed. Access to communication links determines how well people are informed. Because information is key to awareness of goods and services, lack of a satisfactory means of gathering information can adversely affect access and utilization of needed services.

Communication may be formal or informal. Formal communication usually originates outside the community (extracommunity) as opposed to informal communication, which almost always originates and is disseminated within the community. Salient components of formal and informal communication, as well as sources of data, are presented in Table 9-18.

Two major papers serve Calgary, along with 7 AM and 13 FM radio stations and 8 television stations. Cable and satellite services are available. Every neigh-

---

TABLE 9-18 ◆ COMMUNICATIONS

Components	Sources of Information
Formal	
Newspaper (number, circulation, frequency, and scope of news)	Chamber of commerce
Radio and television (number of stations, commercial versus educational, and audience)	Newspaper office
	Telephone company
Postal service	Yellow Pages
Telephone status (number of residents with service)	Telephone book
	Canada Post, courier services
Informal	
Sources: bulletin boards; posters; hand-delivered flyers; and church, civic, and school newsletters	Learning about the community on foot
Dissemination (How do people receive information?)	Talking to residents
Word of mouth	Survey
Mail	
Radio, television	Reports, surveys

bourhood has a community association that is funded on a per capita basis by the city and association executives are important routes of communication to aldermen. In the downtown, postal service is provided door-to-door, unlike in the suburbs, where super boxes are the norm.

EDUCATION

Education is closely linked with employment and economic status of a community and population aggregate. The general educational status of a community can be summarized using census data. Census information lists the number of residents attending schools, years of schooling completed, and percentage of residents who speak English. This information describes the community core, but the infrastructure for learning—basic, specialized, literacy—is what comprises the subsystem.

To supplement this broad assessment, information is needed about major educational sources (e.g., schools, colleges, and libraries) located both inside and outside the community that people use for formal as well as continuing education and personal interest purposes. Table 9-19 is a suggested guide for assessing a community's educational sources.

It is sometimes difficult to decide which educational sources to include in the assessment. Community usage is probably the single most important indicator. Primary and secondary schools attended by the majority of youngsters in a community, regardless of intra- or extracommunity location, are major educational sources and require a thorough assessment, whereas schools composed

TABLE 9-19 ◆ EDUCATION

Components	Sources of Information
Educational Status	
Years of school completed	Census data
School enrollment by type of school	Census data
Language spoken	Census data
Educational Sources	
Intracommunity or extracommunity (collect data for each facility)	Local board of education reports and websites
Services (educational, recreational, communication, and health)	School administrator (such as the principal or director) and school nurse
Resources (personnel, space, budget, and record system)	School administrator
Characteristics of users (geographic distribution and demographic profile)	Teachers and staff
Adequacy, accessibility, and acceptability of education to students and staff	Students and staff

primarily of students from outside the community do not require such an extensive appraisal.

The Calgary Board of Education has elementary and junior high schools in the downtown communities that feed into the high school system. Similarly the separate school system offers facilities throughout the downtown. Children can take the bus to school if they live a certain distance away, and parents can opt into lunch programs if the children stay at school over the noon hour. Calgary also offers religious schools (Jewish, Christian), schools for special needs children, and charter schools in addition to an array of private schools. Public postsecondary education in Calgary is provided from several institutions: University of Calgary, Mount Royal College, Southern Alberta Institute of Technology, Alberta College of Art and Design, and Bow Valley College. All but Mount Royal are accessible by light rail transit; public transportation is readily available at reduced rates for those who attend school in the city. Private postsecondary education can be accessed from DeVry Institute, Columbia Business College, and Rocky Mountain Bible College, among others.

RECREATION

The recreation subsystem allows us to focus on assessing the degree of lifestyle support in the community. We will want to link recreation information with the data on physical environment and safety subsystems for a complete picture but collecting information on parks, sports facilities, jogging and bicycle paths, as well as resources for social interaction (e.g., special interest clubs, seniors' centres, theatres, art galleries, restaurants, bars, festivals, zoo, museums, teams) offers insight into access, affordability, and use patterns that can suggest opportunities for community capacity building and help to determine activity and social needs of the population.

Summary

The community assessment is never complete; however, we must pause at some point. Because we have addressed all parts of the model, this is where we will stop. A description of each community subsystem has been recorded. Note that at every step of the assessment, people in the community were included. Not only did we interview the "professionals" (e.g., school nurses, social workers, physicians, principal, police chief, alderman, and so on), but also individuals within the subsystems were also included (parents, shoppers, patients, and people on the street). The assessment, like all steps in the process, is carried out *in partnership with the community.* The next step is analysis, a process that synthesizes the assessment information and derives from it diagnoses specific to the community.

Crucial to community assessment is a model, or map, to direct and guide that process. The model (community assessment wheel) shown in Figure 9-1 provided a framework, and the tool, "Learning About the Community on Foot" (see Table 9-2), guided the assessment of the neighbourhoods of the downtown area of Calgary, Alberta. In the Suggested Readings list, several other approaches to community assessment are presented. As you are aware, there are other models you may wish to consider as you continue your practice of community health assessment. Workbooks to facilitate the process of community assessment are frequently available from local social planning departments. For instance the Edmonton Social Planning Council (1988) offers "Doing it right! A needs assessment workbook" for sale ($5). See www.edmspc.com for information.

References

Barton, J. A., Smith, M. C., Brown, N. J., & Supples, J. M. (1993). Methodological issues in a team approach to community health needs assessment. *Nursing Outlook, 41*(6), 253–261.

Conway, T., Hu, T., & Harrington, T. (1997). Setting health priorities: Community boards accurately reflect the preferences of the community's residents. *Journal of Community Health, 22*(1), 57–68.

Dimock. H. G., & Devine, I. (1994). *Making workgroups effective* (3rd ed.). North York, ON: Captus Press.

Edmonton Social Planning Council. (1988). *Doing it right! A needs assessment workbook.* Edmonton: Author.

Edwards, N. C., & Moyer, A. (2000). Community needs and capacity assessment: Critical components of program planning. In M. J. Stewart (Ed.), *Community nursing: Promoting Canadians' health* (pp. 420–442). Toronto: Saunders.

Gerberich, S. S., Stearns, S. J., & Dowd, T. (1995). A critical skill for the future: Community assessment. *Journal of Community Health Nursing, 12*(4), 239–250.

Gilmore, G. D., & Campbell, M. D. (1996). *Needs assessment strategies for health education and health promotion* (pp. 51–61, 73–87). Dubuque, IA: Brown & Benchmark.

Haglund, B., Weisbrod, R., & Bracht, N. (1990). Assessing the community: Its services, needs, leadership and readiness. In N. Bracht (Ed.), *Health promotion at the community level* (pp.99–108). Newbury Park, CA: Sage.

Hancock, T., & Minkler, M. (1997). Community health assessment or healthy community assessment: Whose community? Whose health? Whose assessment? In M. Minkler (Ed.), *Community organizing and community building for health* (pp. 139–156). New Brunswick, NJ: Rutgers University Press.

Hawe, P., Degeling, D., & Hall, J. (1990). *Evaluating health promotion.* Sydney, Australia: MacLennan & Petty.

Kretzman, J. P., & McKnight, J. L. (1993). *Building communities from the inside out: A path toward finding and mobilizing a community's assets.* Chicago: ACTA Publications.

McDevitt, J., & Wilbur, J. E. (2002) Locating sources of data. In N. E. Ervin (Ed.),

Advanced community health nursing practice (pp. 109–141). Upper Saddle River, NJ: Prentice Hall.

Morgan, D. L., & Kreuger, R. A. (1997). *The focus group kit.* (Vol. 1-6). Thousand Oaks, CA: Sage.

Parks, C. P. & Straker, H. O. (1996). Community assets mapping: Community health assessment with a different twist. *Journal of Health Education, 27,* 321–323.

Patton, M. Q. (1990). *Qualitative evaluation and research methods* (2nd ed.). Newbury Park, CA: Sage.

Suggested Readings

Bennett, E. J. (1993). Health needs assessment of a rural county: Impact evaluation of a student project. *Family & Community Health, 16*(1), 28–35.

Gregor, S., & Galazka, S. S. (1990). The use of key informant networks in assessment of community health. *Family Medicine, 22*(2), 118–121.

Keppel, K. G., & Freedman, M. A. (1995). What is assessment? *Journal of Public Health Management, 1*(2), 1–7.

Lindell, D. H. (1997). Community assessment for the home health nurse. *Home Healthcare Nurse, 15*(1), 618–626.

Palfrey, J. S. (1994). *Community child health: An action plan for today.* Westport, CT: Praeger.

Ruth, J., Eliason, K., & Schultz, P. R. (1992). Community assessment: A process of learning. *Journal of Nursing Education, 31*(4), 181–183.

Schultz, P. R. & Magilvy, J. K. (1988). Assessing community health needs of elderly populations: Comparisons of three strategies. *Journal of Advanced Nursing, 13,* 193–202.

Serafini, P. (1976). Nursing assessment in industry: A model. *American Journal of Public Health, 66*(8), 755–760.

Statistics Canada. (1997). *Guide to the Labour Force Survey.* Catalogue no. 71-528-PB. Ottawa, ON: Author.

Urrutia-Rojas, X., & Aday, L. A. (1991). A framework for community assessment: Designing and conducting a survey in a Hispanic immigrant and refugee community. *Public Health Nursing, 8*(1), 20–26.

White, J. E., & Valentine, V. L. (1993). Computer assisted video instruction and community assessment. *Nursing and Health Care, 14*(7), 349–353.

Internet Resources

Canadian Consortium of Health Promotion Research Centres: **www.utoronto.ca/chp/chp/consort/index.htm**

Canadian Institute for Child Health: **www.cich.ca**

Canadian Institute for Health Information: **www.cihi.ca**

Canadian Institutes for Health Research: **www.cihr.ca**

Canadian Public Health Association: **www.cpha.ca**

City of Calgary Communities: **www.gov.calgary.ab.ca**

Health Canada: **www.hc-sc.gc.ca**

Social Sciences and Humanities Research Council: **www.sshrc.ca**

Statistics Canada: **www.statcan.ca**

United States Centers for Disease Control and Prevention: **www.cdc.gov**

10

Community Analysis and Diagnosis

OBJECTIVES

This chapter is focused on the second phase of the community process, analysis, and the associated task of forming community diagnoses.

After studying the chapter, you should be able to:

◆ Practise within a team environment to critically analyze and synthesize data collected

◆ Classify community assessment data into the categories of the community-as-partner model

◆ Create summary statements and note aspects of incomplete or contradictory information

◆ Interpret summary statements in comparison with benchmark data and trends

◆ Generate inferences and formulate community diagnoses

◆ Validate information and inferences

Introduction

Analysis is the study and examination of data by the processes of classification, summarization, interpretation, and validation of information in order to write community diagnoses and establish priorities (Helvie, 1998). These data may be quantitative (numerical) as well as qualitative. All aspects need to be considered. Analysis is necessary to determine community health needs and community strengths as well as to identify patterns of health responses and trends in health care use. During analysis, any need for further data collection is revealed as gaps and incongruities in the community assessment data. The end point of analysis is the community diagnosis.

Community Analysis

Analysis, like so many procedures we perform, may be viewed as a process with multiple steps. The phases we will use to help in the analysis are classification, summarization, interpretation, and validation. Each is described and illustrated below.

Classify

To analyze community assessment data, it is helpful to first classify the data. Data can be classified into categories in a variety of ways. Traditional categories of community assessment data include:

◆ Demographic characteristics (family size, age, sex, and ethnic and racial groupings)
◆ Geographic characteristics (area boundaries; number and size of neighbourhoods, public spaces, and roads)
◆ Socioeconomic characteristics (occupation and income categories, educational attainment, and rental or home ownership patterns)
◆ Health and social resources and services (hospitals, clinics, mental health centres, etc.)

However, models are being used increasingly in the organization and analysis of community health data because they provide a framework for data collection and a map to guide analysis. Because the community assessment wheel (see Fig. 9-1) was used to direct the community assessment, that same model can be used to guide analysis. Each of the community subsystems will be analyzed, and the smaller components within each subsystem will help to describe the categories by which information is sorted.

Ultimately, we want to describe the community's normal line of defence (NLD), that is, the health status of the community. We also want to locate sources of risk or hazard (stressors) and identify the flexible lines of defence (FLD) that are in place, and the lines of resistance (LR) that represent the community's strengths and assets.

Summarize

Once a classification method has been selected, the next task is to summarize the data within each category. Both summary statements and summary measures, such as rates, charts, and graphs, are required.

✎ TAKE NOTE

Many health care agencies and educational institutions have access to computerized information systems—a system through which formatted data can be retrieved in a variety of forms—including summary health statistics. For example, data entered into a computer system as census figures can be configured into population pyramids, and census and vital statistics information can be programmed to calculate birth, death, and fertility rates. Calculations that previously required hours to complete are now computed in seconds. In your practice, make it a point to inquire as to the availability of computer systems and, if possible, use computer processes to carry out quantitative data analysis. In addition, your local health department may be able to furnish the rates for you (e.g., the infant mortality rate [IMR]). Note, however, that the denominator used to calculate this rate may not be the community as you have defined it.

Interpret

To interpret data often requires comparison to established standards or benchmarks, provincial and national statistics, and the community's own statistics for previous years (Helvie, 1998). Outcomes of data analysis include the identification of data gaps, inconsistencies, or omissions and the generation of inferences or hypotheses about the findings. Frequently, comparative data are needed to determine if a pattern or trend exists or if data do not seem correct and the need for revalidation of original information is required. Data gaps are inevitable, as are mistakes in recording data; the important task is to analyze data critically and be aware of the potential for gaps and omissions. To have professional colleagues as well as community residents review the analysis is helpful. Every person has a unique perspective; it is only through the sharing of views that a whole and comprehensive picture of community assessment data can evolve.

Using the data from your community, compare them with other similar data to determine the size of the problem. For instance, you calculate (or discover) an IMR of 12/1000 live births—how does this compare with other communities? The province? The nation? Is it for the entire infant population of your community or are there differences among structural or demographic factors? Is the IMR different for different ethic groups, ages and marital status of mothers, or geographic parts of the community? Have there been any changes for the better or worse in recent years or the past decade? (Note: This is a good time to review Chap. 2 to assist you with epidemiologic reasoning as you try to make sense of your data.)

Other resources for comparison are the documents produced as health report cards by regional health authorities, provinces, and Health Canada (and other federal departments such as Environment, Immigration and Citizenship, Human Resources Development). The *Report on the Health of Canadians* (2000) presents national figures, such as incidence and prevalence when available, for our major health concerns. Although Canada does not yet have a specific document regarding population health goals, *Healthy People 2010* (U.S. Department of Health and Human Services, 1997), though not Canadian, can be invaluable to you because it contains goals and objectives that help in both data analysis and planning.

Having classified, summarized, and compared the data you have collected, the final phase is to draw logical conclusions from the evidence, that is, to draw inferences that will lead to the statement of a community diagnosis. This is where you synthesize what you know about the community, that is, what do these data *mean*? Synthesis is the linking of the summary statements from the classification process and formulating hypotheses about the connections among them.

Validate

It is a common complaint of communities that "experts" come in and collect data, make judgments, then leave. It is important to validate the conclusions you reach and the hypotheses you generate to ensure they are correct and reflect the community accurately. This requires the team to confirm their information and its interpretation by returning to sources for confirmation or additional data. Solicit feedback and check with key sources (e.g., community informants, external experts) to verify that your findings are appropriate. Validation can be carried out by town hall or focus group meetings, purposive surveys, or interviews.

Barton and coworkers (1993) discuss the issues that may face the team during its analytic process and offer suggestions to address them (Table 10-1).

The remainder of this chapter will walk you through analysis of the data we collected in the community assessment of five downtown Calgary communities.

Sample Community Analysis

After the analysis examples (Table 10-2), information on how to form community diagnoses is presented (see the Community Diagnosis section later in this chapter). The analysis of the five-community (DT5) assessment data, as in the assessment process, begins with the community core, because it is the core (the people and their health) that is of interest to the community health professional. Recall that the core is affected by (and affects) all of the subsystems depicted in the model surrounding it. Some subsystems will influence certain problems more than others, but it is important to assess the subsystems because of their contribution to the causes and alleviation of problems in the core.

Community Core

An analysis of the core of the five communities (DT5) is presented in Table 10-2. Community core data include many sociodemographic measures, data that

TABLE 10-1 ◆ TEAM ANALYSIS ISSUES AND STRATEGIES FOR SOLUTION

Issues	Strategies
Coordinating the sharing of volumes of data	Using electronic tools; sharing information during team meetings
Disagreement in interpretations of data	Ensure the data are broadly representative of key community perspectives. If gaps exist, seek to fill them with further information.
Community-team disagreement on the meaning of data	Include community members in all aspects of analysis.
Contradictory data from different sources	Seek further data or clarification; report with recommendations for further exploration.

TABLE 10-2 ◆ AN ANALYSIS OF THE CORE OF FIVE DOWNTOWN COMMUNITIES (DT5)

Data Category	Summary Statements	Inferences
History	• Inglewood is the historic site of Fort Calgary. Being revitalized. • Victoria Park grew around the Stampede grounds; very run down. • Bridgeland, originally called "Little Italy" now has a large immigrant population of Vietnamese. Borders the zoo. • Connaught has many highrise apartment buildings. • Bankview is the newest of the five communities.	The downtown communities are not homogeneous; there is a great deal of variation in terms of neighbourhood history, pride, and attractions.

Demographics	• Connaught has the largest population of the five communities.
	• More than 43% of the residents over 1 y of age from Bankview, Connaught, and Victoria Park moved in the past year, above the downtown (DT15) average of 37%.
	• Inglewood and Bridgeland residents were less mobile than average downtown residents in the past year.
	• A similar pattern exists for 5-year mobility.
	• Immigrants comprise approximately 25% of the downtown population.
	• Connaught and Victoria Park have 37% new (past 3 y) immigrants among their residents; Bankview matches the downtown average, and Inglewood and Bridgeland are below the average at < 15%.
	• Victoria Park has the highest proportion of people not speaking English as their first language at home (24%), compared to the average for downtown (10%).
	• Combined, the downtown communities (DT15) have a dependency ratio of 33. However, this obscures the differences among the 5 example communities:
	    Bankview 24
	    Connaught 26
	    Victoria Park 37
	    Bridgeland 67 (seniors)
	    Inglewood 47
		The five downtown communities have high mobility rates. A significant proportion of immigrants have settled in Vicoria Park, accounting for the higher proportion of residents/homes that speak a language other than English in the home.
		Bridgeland has the highest dependency ratio, due largely to the number of seniors living there. The other four communities are more evenly balanced between children and seniors.

Vital Statistics	• Data gap: Unable to disaggregate the DT15 vital statistics data by neighbourhood. • In the period 1990-1992, there were 1901 births in DT15. • Crude birth rate DT15: 12.3/1000 population: Calgary: 15.6 • Proportion of births to women 15-19 in DT15: 11.3%; in Calgary: 5.1% • Teen birth rate DT15 is twice the Alberta rate; Calgary is half the Alberta rate. • DT15 low-birth-weight rate: 8.6%; Calgary: 6.1% • In the period 1990-1992, 688 DT15 residents died. The standardized mortality ratio = 0.9, not significantly different from the rest of the city.	DT15 women are at higher perinatal risk than other city women as a result of youth, immigration, mobility, and language.

(continued)

TABLE 10-2 ◆ AN ANALYSIS OF THE CORE OF FIVE DOWNTOWN COMMUNITIES (DT5)
(*Continued*)

Data Category	Summary Statements	Inferences
Health Status	• Causes of death: Cancer (28%) Ischemic heart disease (20%) Respiratory disease (20%) Cerebrovascular disease (8%) Injury (8%) • The most frequent reason for emergency room visits is injury (30%). Of these, falls account for the largest proportion. • DT15 accounts for 6.5% of the population of the health region, but 8.5% of inpatient services, 6.7% of day procedures, and 10.5% of emergency room visits. • Bridgeland residents used all services more often than other communities. • DT15 patients aged 20-64 received 39.2% of home care service. In Alberta, patients 75 and older receive the largest percentage of care. • Infectious disease rates do not differ between DT15 and the city.	Bridgeland seniors are a risk group. Injuries (e.g., from falls) are a concern, particularly in Bridgeland where the senior population is high.

are especially amenable to graphs and charts. The adage "one picture is worth a thousand words" is particularly meaningful for demographic characteristics. The population (by age) of the five downtown communities in which we are interested is located in Table 10-3.

You will notice a data gap in Table 10-3; we cannot determine the sex composition of the population of these DT5 communities from this table. Perhaps the most representative illustration of the age and sex composition of a population is the population pyramid. In Table 10-4 the sex and age distribution of males and females are separately listed for the group of 15 downtown commu-

TABLE 10-3 ◆ AGE DISTRIBUTION BY DT5 COMMUNITY

	BNK	CON	VIC	BRD	ING	DT15
0–4	295	300	214	295	230	1952
5–14	228	311	195	267	322	1850
15–19	202	356	238	169	205	1901
20–24	937	1745	694	417	330	7245
25–44	2701	5413	2092	1780	1651	23,994
45–64	533	1667	737	618	749	7758
65+	279	1312	585	1139	536	6988

BNK, Bankview; BRD, Bridgeland; CON, Connaught; ING, Inglewood; VIC, Victoria Park.

	Males		Females	
TABLE 10-4 ◆ PERCENT POPULATION BY SEX AND AGE GROUP FOR 15 DOWNTOWN COMMUNITIES (DT15) AND CITY				
Ages (y)	DT15	City	DT15	City
<5	2.5	2.9	2.3	2.9
5-19	6.3	10.3	6.2	9.8
20-24	3.8	4.0	3.9	3.8
25-34	12.3	8.5	10.4	8.3
35-44	10.5	9.7	8.7	9.5
45-54	6.5	7.4	5.8	6.9
55-64	4.1	3.6	3.9	3.6
65-74	3.2	2.5	3.7	2.8
75+	2.2	1.4	3.9	2.3

nities (DT15) and city of Calgary. They are further illustrated as a population pyramid in Figure 10-1. Which of these best illustrates how the population of DT15 compares with the entire city on age and sex distribution?

The population pyramid is formed of bars; each bar represents an age group. Usually 5- or 10-year age groups are used, although adaptations can be made for smaller or larger age ranges. Bars are stacked horizontally, one on another, with bars for males on the left of a central axis and those for females on the right. The percentage of males and females in a particular age group is indicat-

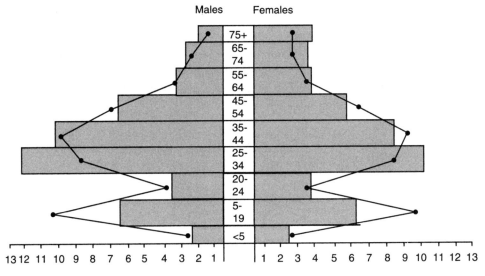

Figure 10-1 ◆ Population pyramid for DT15 (bars) with city superimposed (lines).

ed by the length of the bars, as measured from the central axis. All age groups in a pyramid should be the same interval.

To construct a population pyramid, use Table 10-5 to calculate the percentage contribution of each age and sex group and Table 10-6 for actual pyramid construction. Note that parts of the population pyramids in Figure 10-1, those depicting people younger than 20 years and older than 65, are shaded; this was done to denote the dependent portions of the population. A dependency ratio (Table 10-7) can be calculated when we have this information.

TABLE 10-5 ◆ CALCULATIONS FOR A POPULATION PYRAMID

Community Name, Census Tract, or Geographic Boundaries: _____

Total Population: _____

Ages (Years)	Males		Females	
	Number	% of Total Population	Number	% of Total Population
Total				
< 5				
5–9				
10–14				
15–19				
20–24				
25–29				
30–34				
35–39				
40–44				
45–49				
50–54				
55–59				
60–64				
65–69				
70–74				
75 +				

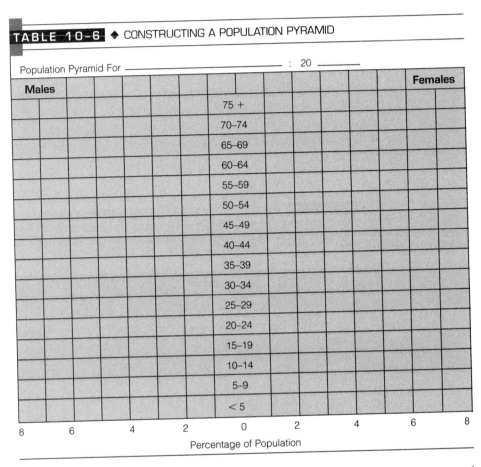

TABLE 10-6 ◆ CONSTRUCTING A POPULATION PYRAMID

Population Pyramid For ———————————————— : 20 ———

The dependency ratio describes the potentially self-supporting portion of the population and the dependent portions at the extremes of age. It is usually calculated as follows:

$$DR = \frac{\text{population under 20 + population 65 and over}}{\text{population 20 to 64 years of age}} \times 100$$

TABLE 10-7 ◆ DATA FOR CALCULATING THE DEPENDENCY RATIOS OF DT5 AND DT15

	BNK	CON	VIC	BRD	ING	DT15
Total population	5175	11,115	4755	4685	4028	51,380
Dependents	1004	2279	1232	1870	1293	12,691
Working	4171	8825	3523	2815	2730	38,897
Ratio	24	26	35	67	47	33

The dependency ratio is interpreted as the number of persons under age 20 and over age 65 needing support (because of age) for every 100 persons aged 20 to 65 years.

Studying the population pyramids for DT15 and the city reveals striking age and sex differences, and this illustrates an important lesson. If the demographics of the downtown had been presented as one population pyramid as depicted by city statistics, important age and sex differences might have been minimized or have gone unrecognized, and their associated age- and sex-related health needs would be left unmet. Similarly, if the demographics of each of the five communities were analyzed, significant differences may be detected between each community and the downtown data. This hazard in data analysis is referred to as aggregating or pooling the data. It is important to divide data along all possibly meaningful lines so important information is not overlooked. Be alert to this problem as you proceed with your analysis.

Studying the data presented in conjunction with the population pyramids the following summary statements can be made about DT5's core.

◆ The DT5 population is more mobile than the general city population.
◆ Immigrants comprise one quarter of the DT5 population compared with 20% for the city.
◆ Compared to the city as a whole, DT5 has a higher proportion of recent immigrants.
◆ Young adults and seniors are in higher proportions in the downtown than in the city.
◆ DT5 has a smaller proportion of school-age children than the city.
◆ The vast majority of DT5 residents live in apartments compared with 22% of city residents.
◆ In DT5, 62% of the senior population lives alone, more than double the proportion of seniors living alone in the city as a whole.

Physical Environment

To study the physical components, data were collected by inspection (i.e., windshield survey) and from written reports prepared by City Hall, Social Services, the Chamber of Commerce, and the regional health authority.

Rental accommodations are scarce with less than 1% vacancy rate. There is a waiting list of 1400 compared to 1000 in 1996 for public housing; no new public housing units are under construction. Average rent in Calgary, highest of prairie cities, is $511 for one-bedroom and $635 for two-bedrooms. For someone working full-time at minimum wage affordable housing would have to be in the $250/month range. New arrivals are at high risk of being homeless or inadequately housed because the first month's rent, damage deposits, and utility hook-up fees often cost up to $2000. Homelessness is increasingly severe with 615 observed in one night in May 1996 and 3800 individuals identified over 4 months in 1997, and 4 in 10 people are turned away from shelters. Traditionally most are men but there are increasing numbers of women and families. Many are educated (20% with postsecondary education) and 45% are employed with average earnings of $7.40/hr. Half have never been homeless before; the majority have been on the street less than 3 months. One third have mental health problems and addictions; 30% to 40% have serious mental health problems and 34% are involved in substance abuse.

Summary statements include:

◆ DT5 are communities of contrast and diversity, both intracommunity and among them.
◆ There are many historical sites throughout the DT5 communities.
◆ Population density is the highest in the westernmost communities of Bankview and Connaught.
◆ There is little or no heavy industry in DT5; commercial enterprises, professional offices, and small businesses are common along main thoroughfares and in strip malls.
◆ Housing values are higher in the westernmost communities, but Inglewood is undergoing significant revitalization. With the land available for development on the Bow Valley Centre site, Bridgeland will soon experience a construction boom.
◆ Victoria Park is a community in decline with many abandoned buildings and property in disrepair. There is concern over homeless squatters, prostitution, and drug use in the area.
◆ Major transportation routes transect the DT5 communities, including trains that may carry hazardous materials.
◆ The proportion of good air quality samples for downtown DT15 is 95% compared with 87% in the industrial area and only slightly lower than suburban residential areas.

From this, it can be inferred that the different communities will have different health and social needs and concerns, varying capacities to address issues, and different levels of motivation to develop a sense of community.

Health and Social Services

Summary statements regarding the use of health and social services include:

◆ There is variation among the rates of day procedures by residents of DT5, with Bridgeland the highest at 108.4/1000.

◆ The top day procedure for Inglewood and Bridgeland is lens removal/replacement.

◆ Connaught and Bankview have higher rates of utilization for gynecologic services than the other communities.

◆ The utilization rates for in-patient services were higher for DT15 residents (152.9/1000) than for the region (112.0/1000), but hospital day procedures were used at the same rate as region residents. Bridgeland residents used all services more often than residents of other communities.

◆ Inglewood youth have a 22.7% unemployment rate compared with 1.3% in Bridgeland and around 10% in the remaining three communities.

◆ For adults over the age of 25, Victoria Park has the highest unemployment rate at 10.5%.

◆ Bridgeland has the lowest proportion of single-parent families, lower than the DT15 rate of 45.5/100 families. Still, this is double the city average.

◆ Over half the residents of Victoria Park live in low-income households. In DT15 the rate of persons living in low-income households is more than 2.5 times that of the rest of the city.

Inferences we can draw are:

◆ Bridgeland residents account for a high use of health facilities because of the proportion and frailty of seniors in the community.

◆ Bankview and Connaught residents account for a significant use of reproductive health services, likely due to their age and lifestyle.

◆ Many residents of the DT5 communities are living with low incomes; a high proportion are living in poverty, hence are at high risk for health-related problems due to socioeconomic status.

◆ Homelessness is an issue in the DT15, and particularly in Victoria Park, where crime levels are high. The reasons that create homelessness and the health threats of homelessness are enormous.

◆ With the high proportion of new immigrants, English as second language services will likely be required, as will translators and interpreters at health and social service agencies.

Economics

The city has strong population growth with high net migration, a large proportion of which settle in the downtown area because of the proximity to resettlement and social services such as employment and second language training, and proximity to established communities of immigrants from their country of origin.

The city had the lowest unemployment rate (4.7%) in the province (5.4%) and Canada (8.6%) in 1998. There is a resurgence of construction because of the rising demand for office, warehouse, and residential space. Wages and prices are rising more quickly in Calgary than in the rest of Canada even though Alberta has the lowest minimum wage in the country at $4.90/hr. Calgary's inflation rate is at 2.2% versus 1.6% in Canada. Purchasing power has been eroded; price increases affect low-income budgets largely in food and shelter costs. The combined effect of inflation for basic needs and the reduction in Alberta's social assistance benefits amounts to a 19% decrease in purchasing power for single employable persons.

The "low income cutoff" (LICO) is used in Canada as a measure of the "poverty line." A household is poor if it spends at least 20% more than the average household on the basic necessities (food, shelter, clothing). It has been determined that the average Canadian household spends 34.7% of its income on the basic necessities; therefore, a family is considered to be poor if it spends 54.7% of its income (or more) on food, shelter, and clothing (Statistics Canada, 1998).

The causes of poverty are many: prolonged periods of unemployment, employment that is part-time or that provides inadequate wages for the household, and inability to work because of disability, lack of skill, or lack of opportunity. Youth, seniors, single parents, single women, immigrants, persons who are visible minorities, Aboriginal people, and individuals with disabilities are more likely to experience unemployment.

Households with low incomes tend to be more vulnerable to the fluctuating costs of goods and services and may not be able to afford basic needs (Box 10-1). This may be a threat to both the physical and mental well-being of those who live in low-income households.

Summary statements:

◆ The rate of people living in low-income households is 2.3 times higher in the downtown than in the city as a whole. In Victoria Park, it is nearly three times higher.
◆ In Victoria Park the median household income is one third that of the city; in the four remaining DT5 communities, the median income is half that of the city.

BOX 10-1. A DAY IN THE LIFE OF POVERTY

Monthly family income $1666.00
Basic shelter, food, clothing $1596.00
Balance remaining $70.00

A family of four with both parents working full-time (2000 hrs/yr each) at minimum wage would have $13.69 available per family member per day. The daily cost of the bare essentials of shelter, food, and clothing are estimated to be $13.13 per day per family member, leaving only 56 cents a day per person to pay for child care, personal care items, household needs, furniture, telephone, transportation, school supplies, and health care. Because grocery money is more discretionary than other fixed expenses, poor families often run out of food before month's end. The impact of this is seen at food banks and in the nutritional health of families who are poor. www.gov.calgary.ab.ca

---

◆ Unemployment for youth is very high in Inglewood.

The overall well-being of a community is determined by both the volume (number of people in need) and risk (percentage of the population in need). One can infer the following about the downtown communities:

◆ All DT5 communities have social, economic, and health risks because of income, employment, education, and education.
◆ Those who are young, elderly, immigrants, and women are at increased risk because of inequalities in employment, income, and independence.
◆ Because all communities have different risk factors, a single program will not serve all communities equally; Bridgeland is more in need of seniors' services, Victoria Park is in more need of community safety services; single-parent families in several neighbourhoods may benefit from parenting programs to reduce their stress levels.

Community Diagnosis

In the preceding pages, each subsystem of five downtown communities has been analyzed in relation to its effect on the core (the people), and inferences have been drawn. The final task of analysis is the synthesis of the inference statements into community diagnoses (Neufeld & Harrison, 2000).

A *diagnosis* is a statement that synthesizes assessment data. A diagnosis is a label that both *describes a situation* (or state) and *implies an etiology* (reason) and gives evidence to support the inference.

A *nursing diagnosis* limits the diagnostic process to those diagnoses that represent human responses to actual or potential health problems nurses are licensed to treat. A *medical diagnosis* includes those issues a doctor is licensed to treat. A *community* diagnosis differs, however, in that it is focused on an aggregate or a community (rather than individuals), it requires multidisciplinary action to address (treat), multiple determinants must be considered when planning interventions, and outcomes of action may not be visible in the short term.

Although no standard format exists, most community diagnoses have four parts:

1. A *description* of the problem, response, or state
2. A statement of the aggregate, population, community of *focus*
3. Identification of factors *etiologically* (causally) related to the problem
4. Signs and symptoms (*manifestations*) that are characteristic of the problem

A *community diagnosis* focuses the diagnosis on a *community*—usually defined as a *group, population, or cluster of people with at least one common characteristic* (such as geographic location, occupation, ethnicity, or housing condition). To derive a community diagnosis, community assessment data are analyzed and inferences are presented. Inference statements shape community diagnoses. Some inference statements form the *descriptive* part of the diagnosis; that is, they testify to a *potential or actual community problem* (risk, hazard, or concern) to a particular segment of the population (i.e., *among*).

For instance, health status data (normal line of defence) may indicate the low-birth-weight rate is higher than a comparison standard (stressor). Literature provides information regarding the causes of low birth weight, and these are compared to the data collected, the conclusions drawn about their applicability to the community of interest, and community resources available to address the issue (lines of resistance), and any flexible lines of defence (temporary responses to the situation) in place.

Finally, the *signs and symptoms* of the community diagnosis are the inference statements that *document the duration or magnitude of the problem*. Examples of documentation include data from record accounts, census reports, and vital statistics. This final piece of the community diagnosis establishes the relevant data and is linked to the first two parts with an *"as manifested by"* clause (Box 10-2). In Box 10-3, an example of a community diagnosis for an aggregate of adolescent pregnant women who reside in the downtown area is presented.

BOX 10–2. TEMPLATE FOR A COMMUNITY DIAGNOSIS

Issue description (risk, concern, issue, state, i.e., potential/actual)	Focus (boundaries of the population segment of interest)	Etiology/causal factors (signs and symptoms)	Manifestations (data in support of the etiologic inference)

In comparison to taking a "problem" approach (Box 10-3), there are many strengths exhibited by this community and the focus population that offer the opportunity to reframe the issue as a wellness or positive diagnosis. For instance:

There is opportunity to improve the health status (issue description) of adolescent pregnant women in the downtown (focus) by maintaining presence at school, receiving social assistance, enroling in the Best Beginning program, and providing support (manifestations) for effective parenting, stress reduction, and smoking cessation (etiology).

Although a single problem is stated, the causes and signs and symptoms may be multiple. Also notice that, although the problem inferences are drawn from the analysis of one subsystem (such as the health and social services sub-

---

BOX 10–3. AN EXAMPLE OF A COMMUNITY DIAGNOSIS

Issue description	Focus	Etiology	Manifestations
Risk of low birth weight	*Among* teen pregnant women living in the downtown area	*Related to* a) inadequate income	*as manifested by* insecure housing, use of the food bank, unemployment rates among
		b) use of tobacco	*as manifested by* smoking rates among pregnant teens

system or the educational subsystem), the causation may be, and usually is, drawn from several subsystems. For example, regarding the issue of low birth weight, etiologic inferences can be derived from four subsystems—educational, health and social services, safety and transportation, and economic.

This example sums up the most important lesson of community health practice: *All community factors (subsystems) join to determine the health status of a community. No one subsystem is more important or crucial than any other in determining a community's health.* Every subsystem has a role in addressing community issues.

Some community diagnoses for the five downtown communities are:

◆ Lack of safety for residents of Victoria Park due to crime after dark related to prostitution, drug use, burglary and vandalism as manifested by Police Service statistics, incidence of used needles and condoms found in vacant lots near school grounds and parks, rate of break and enter crimes, and gang tagging graffiti on vacant buildings
◆ Lack of adequate affordable housing for the residents of Connaught related to single-parent families headed by women living in poverty, as manifested by the percent of single-parent families spending more than 30% on housing, number of children living in homes receiving support for independence, and the volume of Connaught single mothers using food bank, thrift stores, and other community services before month's end
◆ Perceived stress of lone women heading families in Connaught related to lack of social support, isolation, and parenting stress as manifested by reports from Family Social Services
◆ Poor nutritional status among female seniors in Bridgeland related to social isolation and inability to obtain food as manifested by reports of home care nurses and parish-based social workers

The process of deriving community diagnoses always remains the same. First, assessment data are classified and studied for inferences that are descriptive of potential or actual problems (stressors that have penetrated the NLD or FLD); next, associated inferences are identified that explain the derivation or continuation of the problem and the community assets or strengths available to address the issue (lines of resistance); and last, documentation (data) is presented to support the inferences. Several community diagnoses may be stipulated; determining the order of priority among them is part of program planning and depends on existing community goals and resources. This important skill is discussed in the next chapter.

Deriving community diagnoses requires critical thinking, decision-making, and astute study; it is a challenging and vital task. The completeness and validity of the diagnoses that have been derived will be tested during the next stage of the community process and will form the foundation of that stage—the planning of a health program.

This is an excellent time to share your assessment data with colleagues and people in the community to solicit their analysis. Because we all have opinions and values that colour our perceptions, group critique and analysis of assessment data are ways to foster objectivity. Validating your community diagnoses with the community residents is an important step for establishing and maintaining the partnership. Equally important are the rights of community leaders, organizations, and residents to confidentiality of privileged information and to choose not to participate in health planning. Communities have the right to identify their own health needs and to negotiate with the community health team with regard to interventions and specific programs. In turn, the community health team has the responsibility to provide or assist with the development of information needed for this process.

In the mid-1990s Alberta was reorganizing its delivery of health, children's, and mental health services. As a result, Calgary service providers and concerned citizens met to discuss how they could best serve Calgary's inner city communities and formally established itself in 1999 as the Inner City Family Resource Centre Network (ICFRN). The network was formed to coordinate resources and services to meet the needs of the residents (families and individuals) of Calgary's inner city communities. Its goal was to form one or more Community Coordinating Councils (CCCs) that would facilitate both community and service agency input into the planning and delivery of services.

One of the network's first initiatives was to conduct a survey to confirm the findings of the community assessment report. The purpose of the "Inner City Survey" was to give community members a voice into services needed to address their concerns.

Before we continue, a few words are needed about composing questionnaires. Everyone is confronted daily with people who are asking questions. Questionnaires arrive in the mail, and people call on the phone. Frequently, the interviewees learn neither the purpose of the questionnaire nor how the information will be used. When you draft a questionnaire, begin with introductory information that states who you are and what the purpose of the questionnaire is. Emphasize that participation is voluntary and that the information given will be confidential. Sign your name and, if the questionnaire is to be mailed, include a phone number where you can be contacted. Write questions that can be answered quickly (the whole questionnaire should not take longer than 10 minutes to complete). Ideally, place all questions on one side of a standard 8½-inch by 11-inch piece of paper that, if it is to be mailed, can be refolded so that a return address shows. Before sharing the questionnaire with agencies or community residents, administer it informally to friends and family; any comments made (such as "What do you mean by...?" or "I don't understand...") signal the need for further rewriting and clarification. The same references used for the development of surveys in the assessment phase will be helpful as you plan a survey for this phase. Remember to check the reading level and language of the questions and allow for costs of translation as needed.

✎ TAKE NOTE

How should the questionnaire be administered? Should the questionnaire be mailed to all households? Should the questionnaire be given to a specific group only? Or should the questionnaire be used as an interview and given to a selected number of participants at a specific site? (Recall from research that people who have been randomly selected can be considered representative of the total population.) What would you recommend? Before making a decision, list each option and consider the benefits and drawbacks of each. Here is some information for your decision-making: Mailed questionnaires have about a 50% return rate that can be increased somewhat with a reminder postcard or telephone call, whereas questionnaires administered as an interview potentially have a 100% return rate. However, interviews require trained people and about 5 minutes per person per page of the survey, whereas mailed questionnaires require less labour but have the financial cost of postage. Decisions...decisions...

The "Inner City Survey" questionnaire consisted of 15 open- and close-ended questions and was produced in October 1999 in English and four other languages: Chinese, Serbo-Croatian, Tagalog (Filipino), and Polish. Convenience sampling procedures were used to obtain participants; the survey was distributed over 20 weeks through inner city service agencies, schools, and recreational facilities in the downtown area. Three convenient downtown locations were designated as drop-off points for completed questionnaires. To encourage participation, those who submitted the survey were eligible to enter a contest. Two thousand forms were printed and distributed, with a return rate of 470 (23.5%); 43 responses were in languages other than English. It was recognized that limitations from the low response rate, the fact that respondents had to be literate, and the sampling process interfered with the ability to generalize across communities. Nevertheless, the findings were robust enough to be used to supplement the community diagnoses from the assessment phase and to begin the planning process. The details regarding the topics included in the survey are listed in Box 10-4.

BOX 10–4. INNER CITY SURVEY CONTENT

Which community the respondent lives in and for how long
Challenges faced and their importance
Service utilization
Service needs
Reasons that prevent use of community programs
Preferred location for services
Demographic information

Then, once the surveys were returned, the information was classified, analyzed, and summarized for the use of the steering committee. Next, the Health
Department held meetings with the downtown community associations to set
priorities among the issues identified and to begin the process of brainstorming ways of meeting the needs of downtown residents. In the next chapter, the
planning process will be detailed.

Summary

Critical analysis of five downtown communities has been completed using the
community assessment wheel as a guide. Subsequently, community diagnoses
were formulated, based on the inferences from the analysis. Although community diagnoses are relatively new to practice, community health workers have,
since the inception of community development and advocacy work, derived
inferences from assessment data and have acted on those data. However, the
terminology and format that have surrounded these informally produced inferences (diagnoses) have been inconsistent. There is considerable discussion, and
some controversy, regarding the structure and terminology that would be optimal for community-focused diagnoses. In your practice, you will be exposed to
various formats for making community diagnoses—evaluate and test the usefulness of each. It is only through collaboration and vigorous testing that a standard format will evolve. In the Suggested Readings list, there are additional
sources to help you as you develop community diagnoses.

References

Ervin, N. E. (2002). *Advanced community health nursing practice*. Upper Saddle River, NJ: Prentice Hall.

Health Canada. (2000). *Second report on the health of Canadians*. Ottawa: Author.

Helvie, C. O. (1998). *Advanced practice nursing in the community*. Thousand Oaks, CA: Sage

Neufeld, A., & Harrison, M. J. (2000). Nursing diagnosis for aggregates and groups. In M. J. Stewart (Ed.), *Community nursing: Promoting Canadians' health* (pp. 370-385). Toronto: Saunders.

Statistics Canada. (1998). *Low income cut-offs*. Ottawa: Author.

U.S. Department of Health and Human Services. Office of Disease Prevention and Health Promotion. (1997). *Developing objectives for Healthy People 2010*. Washington, DC: US Government Printing Office.

Suggested Readings

Allor, M. T. (1983). The "community profile." *Journal of Nursing Education, 22,* 12–16.

Anderson, E. T. (1990, Fall). Community diagnosis: A guide for planning. *Visions* (A publication of Population-Focused Community Health Nursing Education at Pacific Lutheran University, Tacoma, WA), 8–10.

Barton, J. A., Smith, M. C., Brown, N. J., & Supples, J. M. (1993). Methodological issues in a team approach to community health needs assessment. *Nursing Outlook, 41*(6), 253–261.

Bjaras, G. (1993). The potential of community diagnosis as a tool in planning an intervention programme aimed at preventing injuries. *Accident Analysis & Prevention, 25,* 3–10.

Stoner, M. H., Magilvy, J. K., & Schultz, P. R. (1992). Community analysis in community health nursing practice: The GENESIS Model. *Public Health Nursing, 9,* 223–227.

U.S. Department of Health and Human Services. Public Health Service. (1990). *Healthy People 2000: National health promotion and disease prevention objectives.* Washington, DC: U.S. Government Printing Office.

11

Planning a Community Health Program

OBJECTIVES

This chapter covers the planning of actions to promote the health of a community.

After studying this chapter, you should be able to:

◆ Use principles of change theory to direct the planning process
◆ In partnership with the community, plan a community-focused health program that includes
   ◆ A process for priority setting
   ◆ Development of a program logic model
   ◆ A sequence of actions and a time schedule for achieving goals
   ◆ Resources needed to accomplish the plan
   ◆ Potential obstacles to planned actions and revised actions
   ◆ Revisions to the plan as goals and objectives are achieved or changed
   ◆ Recording the plan in a concise, standardized, and retrievable form

Introduction

Once a community has been assessed, the data analyzed, and community diagnoses derived, it is time to consider interventions that will promote the community's health—to formulate a community-focused plan. Each of the three parts of the diagnosis statement—the descriptions of the actual or potential problem, its causes, and its signs and symptoms—directs planning efforts for the community team. All three provide equally important information from which to plan. Figure 11-1 displays the process for deriving a community diagnosis and summarizes how the parts of the diagnosis both describe the community assessment and give direction for program planning, intervention, and evaluation. Community-focused plans are based on the community diagnoses and contain specific goals and interventions for achieving

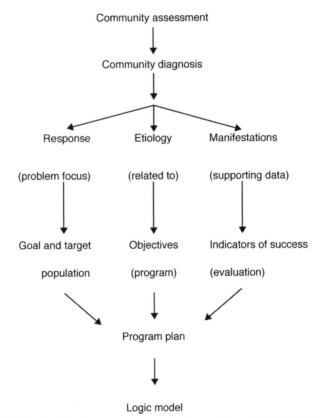

Figure 11-1 ◆ Relationship of assessment, analysis, and diagnosis with program planning.

desired outcomes. Planning, like assessment and analysis, is a systematic process completed in partnership with the community.

✎ TAKE NOTE

Before proceeding, let's stop and consider the word *partnership* and its implications for community health. Recall that a community is a social group determined by geographic boundaries and common values and interests. Community members function and interact within a particular social structure that both creates and exhibits behaviours and values. The normative behaviours and value systems of individuals, families, groups, and the community that you have assessed may be very different from your own individual and family behaviours and values as well as the shared values of the community in which you reside. This creates a potential conflict. What may appear to you as a primary health problem of the community may not hold the same importance for the community's residents. They may be far more concerned about another possibility. Hence, there is a real need to prioritize community diagnoses *with* the community. There is one question to ask: Are the community diagnoses of importance to community residents? Methods of setting priorities among community diagnoses will be presented in this chapter.

Planning in Partnership With the Community

It is important to validate community diagnoses with the residents and leadership of the community; it is their right to participate in decisions that affect them. The validation process can serve as an important trust-building activity in maintaining the partnership, and it is the role of the community worker to ensure they have all the information they need on which to base their choices.

In addition to forming a partnership with the community, the community worker must consider the influences of social, economic, ecological, and political issues. Larger policy issues directly and profoundly affect many (if not all) community issues. For instance, the number of injuries due to falls by seniors living in Bridgeland is related as much to the age and frailty of the people as it is to the condition of the sidewalks, the knowledge of seniors about home safety, the lack of seniors' programs in the community, social isolation, and the nutrition levels of seniors and their access to adequate food. Each of these causes is related to municipal, provincial, and federal policies and legislation. None of the diagnoses can be considered separate from others; all must be considered when doing community-focused planning.

The team involved in community-focused health planning must also consider the needs of populations at risk. Special at-risk groups reside in all communities—the homeless, the poor, new immigrants, pregnant women, infants, children, and the elderly are groups at increased risk for decreased health status. The health needs of at-risk groups must be considered as part of all community health plans.

As is obvious from the assessment phase, resources exist within the downtown to serve the needs of residents. However, utilization was "spotty" at best—some services were appropriately and effectively utilized; others were underutilized or used by a population that was not its primary target, and others were overutilized because the demand for service was far greater than the resources available. The following reasons for not using available services were included on the Inner City Survey to assist in planning services that would be acceptable and accessible to the residents of the inner city:

◆ I don't have any way to get there.
◆ It is too far from home.
◆ It is not a convenient time.
◆ It is too expensive.
◆ I don't know what programs exist.
◆ Do not offer the programs I want.
◆ I don't know how to apply for the programs.
◆ Nobody to look after my children.
◆ Access issues for special needs.
◆ I have difficulties speaking/understanding English.
◆ The programs offered conflict with my cultural values.
◆ Other _____

The community's planning needs must be assessed when determining the membership of the planning team. It may be that the community team formed for assessment purposes and the team pulled together for the planning process will be somewhat different, depending on the nature and priority of the community diagnoses and the scope of the issues of concern. Smith and Maurer (2000) offer the following guidelines for those who should be represented on a planning team, keeping in mind that the team should be neither too large nor cumbersome to manage (p. 391):

◆ Broad segments of the community to provide wide base of support to the program
◆ Leaders with financial and legal authority for the problem
◆ People in a position to promote acceptance of the program (e.g., media, community leaders)

- Those who will implement the program
- Those who will be affected by the program (i.e., the target group)
- Those who will most likely offer resistance (i.e., the opposition)
- Specialists in the field who can contribute to understanding and offer alternative solutions

Last, community-focused planning involves an awareness and application of planned change—a process of well-thought-out actions to make something happen. Planned change is discussed in detail later in this chapter.

Prioritizing Community Diagnoses

Not all issues can be addressed at the same time, so priorities must be determined. Many factors can influence the priority of an issue—a life-threatening emergency will take priority over everything else. Other factors are the seriousness of a concern, the desires of the community or aggregate, time, cost, and availability of resources. Five factors to consider are:

1. Magnitude of concern expressed by members of the community
2. Extent of existing resources to deal with the concern (e.g., knowledge, time, money, equipment, supplies, facilities, personnel)
3. Potential for success in solving the problem with existing resources
4. Need for special education or training
5. Extent of additional resources and policies needed for equitable, cost-effective, and efficient response

Several processes can be used to determine which issue or concern is the highest priority. For instance, each concern identified can be listed and posted around a meeting room. Members of the community team could be given a means to "vote" on their top three priorities (e.g., three coloured dots, three post-it notes) and those concerns that receive no "votes" are first removed from the list of priority issues.

In the next step, those that receive the most votes are assessed, one by one, according to a predetermined set of criteria, rated on a scale of 1 to 5, on which the team again "votes" or comes to consensus. The team may decide that community motivation is the most important criterion, and if that is not present to a high degree, action on the issue will fail. Or, the team may decide that quick success is most important, rating the speed criterion the highest. In any event, decisions about how to rate each criterion must be made in advance by the team, before the rating exercise begins.

- How aware is the community of the issue?
- How motivated is the community to resolve the issue?

♦ How able is the team to influence the resolution of the issue?

♦ How available is the needed expertise to address the issue?

♦ How severe are the consequences if the issue remains unresolved?

♦ How quickly can the team achieve resolution?

As each member rates each criterion for each issue, scores will indicate the order in which the community ranks its priorities. Discussions can then proceed regarding approaches to addressing the priority issue(s). So, for the first issue, compare the agreed-on issue weighting criteria with the average of the individual team members' ratings on each criterion by averaging the ratings, then multiplying them by the weighting. The sum of the ranking provides an overall assessment of the priority of the issue. This ranking process is detailed in Table 11-1.

In this way, issues can be examined and compared horizontally (across the row) to determine which criterion has the highest ranking overall, and vertically (down the column) to determine which issue is the highest priority for action. In the instance illustrated below, the severity of the issue if left unresolved is clearly at a maximum. However, the speed with which the team can address it is at the minimum in the context of relatively low community motivation even though there is relatively high availability of expertise to address the concern. The team can discuss the meaning and interpretation of scores, and effective priorities can be set with efficiency.

The top issues in the five downtown Calgary communities in the example, as prioritized through the inner city survey and community meetings, are summarized in Table 11-2.

Planned Change

We all experience change. As you read these words, your knowledge level is changing. Yet planned change differs from change in that actions occur in a def-

TABLE 11-1 ♦ RANKING EACH ISSUE BY CRITERION WEIGHT

Criteria	Criterion Weight	Average Rating	Ranking (weight × rating)	Total Possible Score
1 Awareness	4	5	20	20
2 Motivation	5	2	10	25
3 Influence	3	4	12	15
4 Expertise	4	3	12	20
5 Severity	5	5	25	25
6 Speed	1	1	1	5
	Maximum (6×5)=30	Maximum (6×5)=30	Actual score=80	Maximum score=110

TABLE 11-2 ◆ PRIORITY OF COMMUNITY ISSUES	
Theme	**Rank**
Crime and safety	
In the neighbourhood	1
Break-ins/robbery	5
Vandalism	10
Prostitution	6
Teen gangs	9
Parenting issues	4
Access to services	7
Housing	
Cost	2
Homelessness	9
Having enough money	3
Literacy and training	
Cost of programs	11
Reading and writing skills	8
Job training	12

inite sequence, with each one serving as preparation for the next. Planned change is a well-thought-out effort designed to make something happen; all efforts are directed and targeted to produce change. (Many theorists have written about planned change; several works are listed at the end of this chapter.) Reinkemeyer's stages of planned change are presented in Box 11-1. The stages are like a recipe in that to produce the intended outcome, it is helpful to follow them strictly and completely to reach the intended outcomes.

BOX 11-1. REINKEMEYER'S STAGES OF PLANNED CHANGE

Stage 1	Development of a felt need and desire for the change
Stage 2	Development of a change relationship between the agent and the client system
Stage 3	Clarification or diagnosis of the client system's problem, need, or objective
Stage 4	Examination of alternative routes and tentative goals and intentions of actions
Stage 5	Transformation of intentions into actual change
Stage 6	Stabilization
Stage 7	Termination of the relationship between the change agent and the client system

Reinkemeyer, A. (1970). Nursing's need: Commitment to an ideology and change. *Nursing Forum, 9*(4), 340–355.

One theorist, Kurt Lewin (1958), described three stages of planned change: unfreezing, moving, and refreezing, as shown in (Box 11-2). It is during the *unfreezing* stage that the client system (in other words, the organization, community, or at-risk population) becomes aware of a problem and the need for change. Then the problem is diagnosed, and solutions to the problem are identified. From these alternative solutions, one is chosen that seems most appropriate for the situation. In the *moving* stage, the change actually occurs. The problem is clarified, and the program for solving the problem is planned in detail and begun. Finally, the *refreezing* stage consists of the accomplished changes becoming integrated into the values of the client system. In this stage, the idea is established and continues to be influential. Lewin also addressed forces that help or hinder change to occur, labelling them the *driving forces* and the *restraining forces*, respectively

Theories of planned change are important because they can be used to guide and direct the planning process. Conceptual frameworks that suggest how individuals change their behaviour also inform the planning process. Table 11-3 details the key components of the transtheoretical (stages of change) model (Prochaska et al., 1995). The *processes* of change addressed by the trans-

---

BOX 11-2. LEWIN'S STAGES OF PLANNED CHANGE AND THEIR APPLICATION TO THE PLANNING PROCESS

Lewin's Stages of Planned Change	Application to the Planning Process
>> ◆ Unfreezing	◆ Unfreezing ● Identification of a need for change
>> >> ◆ Moving process	◆ Moving process ● Presence of a change agent ● Identification of problems ● Consideration of alternatives ● Adaptation of plan to circumstances
>> >> >> ◆ Refreezing	◆ Refreezing ● Implementation of the plan ● Stabilization of the situation

Lewin, K. (1958). Group decision and social change. In E. Maccoby (Ed.), *Readings in social psychology* (3rd ed.). New York: Holt, Rinehart and Winston.

TABLE 11-3 ◆ STAGES OF CHANGE OF THE TRANSTHEORETICAL MODEL

Stage of Change	Characteristics
Precontemplation (PC)	Still engages in risky behaviour
	Has no intention of changing within the next 6 months
	May be uninformed, in denial, or demoralized from previous failures
	Defensive and resistant to change, avoids addressing risky behaviour
Contemplation (C)	Engages in the risky behaviour but is aware of problem
	Seriously considering change within 6 months, but has not yet made a commitment to take action
	Indecisive, lacks commitment to enact significant change in high-risk behaviour
Preparation (P)	Still engages in high-risk behaviour, but intends to take action within the next month
	Has typically taken some significant action in the past year
	Is on the verge of taking action and needs to set goals
Action (A)	Has modified behaviour, experiences, or environment within the last 6 months
	Involves overt behavioural changes and requires considerable commitment of time and energy
Maintenance (M)	Works to prevent relapse and consolidate the gains attained during action
	Is less tempted to relapse and has become increasingly more confident to continue changes
	A continuation, not an absence of change
Termination (T)	Feels zero temptation and complete confidence
	New, healthier behaviour has become second nature
	Unlikely for most behaviours

theoretical model are located in Table 11-4 (Prochaska et al., 1995). Other models of change are described in the suggested readings.

Applying Change Theory to Community Planning

To validate the priorities and initiate the planning process, Reinkemeyer's stages of planned change (see Box 11-1) have been chosen as a guide.

STAGE 1: DEVELOPMENT OF A FELT NEED AND DESIRE FOR THE CHANGE

To initiate a felt need and desire for change within a community, those people and organizations that were involved in the assessment phase can be contacted and invited to a meeting to receive a report of the community assessment findings and proposed community health diagnoses, and to engage in an exercise to validate the findings and discuss priorities.

TABLE 11-4 ◆ PROCESSES OF CHANGE OF THE TRANSTHEORETICAL MODEL

Process of Change	Characteristic
Consciousness raising	Individuals need to raise their awareness of the negative consequences of their behaviour.
Dramatic relief	Individuals need to release and express emotions related to their high-risk behaviour. Life events, such as the death of a close friend or family member, can move people into precontemplation emotionally, especially if the death was related to the high-risk behaviour.
Environmental reevaluation	In precontemplation, individuals need to recognize how the presence or absence of a personal habit affects one's social environment.
Self-reevaluation	This process is most important when the individual is moving from contemplation to preparation, when people assess how they feel and think about the behaviour. People may become aware of their guilt about a particular behaviour.
Self-liberation	While preparing for action, individuals need self-liberation, that is, the belief that they can change and the commitment to act on that belief.
Reinforcement management	During action, individuals need to provide consequences for taking steps in a particular direction, including the use of punishments for slips, or rewards for making positive changes.
Helping relationships	Helping relationships can include those with health professionals who are actively involved in assisting the person to change or supportive members of a social network.
Counterconditioning	During the action and maintenance stages, individuals need to substitute healthier behaviours for the high-risk behaviours.
Stimulus control	People in action or maintenance need to remove stimuli that were associated with the unhealthy behaviour, and add stimuli that signal the new behaviour.
Social liberation	Social liberation requires an increase in social opportunities or alternatives, especially for people who are relatively deprived or oppressed.

STAGE 2: DEVELOPMENT OF A CHANGE RELATIONSHIP BETWEEN THE AGENT AND THE CLIENT (PARTNER) SYSTEM

Both stages 1 and 2 are often completed during the assessment and analysis phases and the presentation of the report to stakeholders because the team has entered the community and begun to establish connections with it. At this point, stakeholders express a desire to become involved in the planning process to address the priority concerns. To preserve momentum and to expedite the planning processes, agencies/groups delegate a representative to the planning committee. At this point, a member of the community team is usually named to function as a change agent to guide and facilitate, but not to direct, the planning process. Sometimes a co-chair is elected from the community, the committee is given a mandate to plan, reporting measures are determined, and initial meetings are set.

STAGE 3: CLARIFICATION OR DIAGNOSIS OF THE CLIENT SYSTEM'S PROBLEM, NEED, OR OBJECTIVE

Now the time has arrived for the planning team to confirm the community diagnoses and compare interpretations of the data with the perceptions of the selected target population. This process can be done by a questionnaire focused on a particular population or neighbourhood; it can be designed as a mail-out or completed as an interview. For instance, single parents who live in the target neighbourhoods and are receiving social assistance can be invited by social workers to provide information about the appropriateness of inferences drawn from the data about the need for parenting classes. Single parents can be approached by public health nurses when they bring their children for immunization to make suggestions about what services might meet their child-rearing needs. On the other hand, if you are planning to intervene at a community level with a community development project, you may choose to interview community leaders and civic groups (key informants) that are representative of the target population. The word *representative* is very important; the team needs to ensure that they are including the appropriate people in the validation process. For instance, if you are concerned about issues relevant to the well-being of a particular neighbourhood, people from a variety of walks of life, ethnic backgrounds, ages, religions, sex, marital status, and family structure, and so forth should be included. Otherwise, a complete picture of life in the community will not be drawn. Validation from professionals and business owners, though informative, will not necessarily provide the most reliable perspective.

STAGE 4: EXAMINATION OF ALTERNATIVE ROUTES AND TENTATIVE GOALS AND INTENTION OF ACTIONS

At this stage, as the results are examined, planning committee members make suggestions about how to address the issues. Inventories of services, resources, and funding already available are compiled. Literature about successful programs in other jurisdictions is examined, program evaluation findings are analyzed, and decisions are made about a preferred approach to the issues.

As details emerge about how to address the issues, the planning committee must make decisions among suggested strategies based on the resources available, likelihood of success, acceptability to the community, and the time it will take to meet the goals.

> ✎ **TAKE NOTE**
> Each stakeholder will consider how information and suggested routes can be assimilated into existing or planned programs. All agencies have budgets and a set number of staff members to deliver services. Agencies must be as cost efficient as possible and will want to consider how to include new services into an existing program or whether new funding will be needed. Community workers can facilitate this process by becoming familiar with the organizational structure and purpose of each stakeholder to learn as much as possible about their services and decision-making processes to facilitate the planned change interventions.

Developing a Program Logic Model

Now is the time to transform the ideas and proposals of each stakeholder into a community-focused goal and concrete intentions for action. A logic model is a diagrammatic representation of a program (Dwyer & Makin, 1997) that depicts the relationships among program goals, objectives, activities, indicators, and resources. It shows how different facets of a program are related and helps to integrate the program planning function with evaluation. The logic model also links back to the data collected in the community assessment phase and the diagnosis formulated in the analysis (see Fig. 11-1).

What is a program? It is an organized set of activities intended to meet specific goals and objectives (outcomes). A program may have a broad series of activities (e.g., a national tobacco reduction program) or it may be smaller and more specifically targeted (e.g., a pre-lunch hand washing program for kindergarten students at a local school).

The program goal is a directional statement that specifies the desired outcome of the intervention. The *target group* is, as specified in the community diagnosis, the recipient of the program. This recipient group may be defined by age, sex, income level, ethnicity, health characteristics, or geographic location. Groups of activities that go together are called *components* and given a descriptive label. Then, for each component, *outcome objectives* are written using the SMART formula (i.e., specific, measurable, action-oriented, realistic, and time specific). Outcome objectives can be short term or long term and represent the desired end results of the intervention. Process objectives specify the activities that are needed to achieve the outcome objectives. Indicators based on the wording of the objectives need to be specified for each objective. Resources needed to successfully carry out the intervention should be listed; they might include personnel, funding, materials, training, and promotional expenses.

Program Goals

The *goal* is stated as a long-term future condition, situation, or status (Ervin, 2002) of a particular population group that clearly identifies what outcome the intervention is designed to achieve or what change is expected in the target population.

From the setting of the goal, the target of an intervention becomes evident. The focus may be individuals, a group, or the community. When the focus is on individuals, their unique perspectives will govern the level of success attained. For instance, according to the Health Belief Model, the degree of behaviour change achieved may be related to the individual's perceived susceptibility to the condition, severity of the threat to personal health, benefits of acting, barriers to action and cues to action (Rosenstock, Strecher, & Becker, 1988). Social support is a factor in how people adapt to situations, and other models (e.g., transtheoretical [stages of change] model [TTM]) define the stages people pass through as they go through the change process.

When the focus of an intervention is a group, we find that people in the group fall into five categories: innovators, early adopters, early majority adopters, late majority adopters, and laggards. The focus on a larger community requires different approaches such as those described by Lewin and Reikenmeyer (see Boxes 11-1 and 11-2). Understanding the processes of change is important for the team when making decisions about what activities to undertake to meet the stated goal.

Program Activities

Program activities map out the actions necessary to deliver the program and thereby reach the goal(s). Choosing an activity requires knowledge of a broad range of intervention strategies. Strategies can be classified as promotion, prevention, or protection and are aimed at education, engineering, or enforcement. Not all strategies are effective on all groups. For instance, an awareness program may be sufficient for action among innovators and early adopters, but personal contact may be needed for laggards. In many instances a combination of education, policy change, and enforcement may be needed to help populations adopt healthy behaviours (e.g., seatbelt campaigns).

In our Calgary example, the downtown Health Department office had many pamphlets and resource materials for parents with advice about common parenting issues (e.g., toilet training, sibling rivalry, sleep patterns, nutrition, etc.) and also offered "Baby and You" classes to new parents. The recreation/pool centres offered "parent and me" swim and gym classes. The library had weekly story sessions for preschoolers. Yet, many parents still felt stressed and isolated. Based on this information it was logical for community workers to suggest "Nobody's Perfect" parenting classes be held in the downtown area. But in which neighbourhood? Where was the easiest access for the most people? Where was the highest need for this activity?

Calendar charts are an effective means of planning and documenting program activities. An example is located in Figure 11-2. Note that the activities are sequenced in a stepwise manner with start and completion months specified along with the initials of the person responsible to carry out the activity. Such charts are versatile and can show weekly or daily progress, depending on the needs of the project. They may be more or less detailed as required by funding agencies, administration, or working groups.

	J	F	M	A	M	J	J	A	S	O	N	D
1. Invite partners to participate (AA)	0	X										
2. Create steering committee (AA)		0	X									
3. Develop logic model and work plans (ALL)				0	X							
4. Budget planning (CA)				0	X							
5. Protocols and policy development (DD)					0	X						
6. Develop program materials (CC)					0	→	X					
6. Hiring program staff (AA)						0	X					
7.Training staff (DD)						0	X					
8. Pilot test (CC)							0	X				
9. Evaluate pilot and revise (CC)									0X			
10. Set up demonstration site (DD)										0X		
11. Official launch (AA)											0X	
12. All sites participating (AA)												→

0= Begin task, X= End task (Initials of person responsible)

Figure 11-2 ♦ A calendar chart for coordinating and tracking planning activities.

Program Objectives

Objectives are measurable and describe the behaviour expected in a specific time frame. They describe the step-by-step outcomes that are required to meet the long-term goal and specify who will perform the behaviour, under what conditions, how well they must perform (standard to be met), and how performance will be measured. The literature relevant to the health issue, population, group, and performance targets will need to be reviewed to ensure the objectives are realistic in the time allotted.

✎ TAKE NOTE

The planning team must make every effort to involve community partners in the writing of outcome objectives if the program is to be acceptable to the target group. The team must also weigh the costs of intervention against the outcomes so that the most people can benefit at affordable cost.

Once program activities have been established, objectives are written. Outcome objectives focus on the client and are derived from a goal and describe the precise behaviour or changes that will be required to achieve the goal. Whereas process objectives map out the actions necessary to deliver the program, outcome objectives specify what changes in knowledge, behaviours, or attitudes are expected as a result of program activities.

If the activity chosen is health education, the objectives ought to detail the knowledge changes anticipated, e.g., awareness, understanding, application, or evaluation. If the team is planning to engineer the environment to make the healthy choice the easy choice, it is the environment that must change. If the activity is to change policy, create new policy, or enhance the enforcement of policy, the objectives must reflect those elements that support this activity.

Both process and outcome objectives can be written in sequential steps that are required to reach the goal, or each objective may have different aspects that, when combined, achieve the goal.

Objectives need to be stated in measurable terms. To make statements measurable, use precise words. Examples of precise terms and less precise terms appear below:

Less Precise Terms (Many Interpretations)
◆ To know
◆ To understand

◆ To realize
◆ To appreciate
◆ To be aware
◆ To lower

More Precise Terms (Fewer Interpretations)
◆ To identify
◆ To discuss
◆ To list
◆ To compare and contrast
◆ To state
◆ To decrease by 20%

In addition, strive for each objective to include:

◆ A time frame for attaining the change (e.g., "By June 15th...")
◆ The direction and magnitude of the change (e.g., "Immunization levels at school entry will increase to 95%")
◆ The method of measuring the change (e.g., "After the session, each participant will demonstrate...")

Goals and objectives help to clarify a program and establish the expected changes that will result from the program. Although much has been written on the mechanics of writing goals and objectives (several such texts are listed at the conclusion of this chapter), little information exists on the collaborative relationship that must exist between the community team and community agencies before meaningful goals and objectives can result.

Interviews with single parents in the downtown underscored the stress they experienced particularly with decisions about raising children. When asked about what could help, they suggested opportunities for parents to get together to learn from each other how to handle things, especially child (mis)behaviour; day programs to keep young children occupied while parents carried out activities such as food shopping, appointments with agencies; adopt-a-grandparent or Big Brother/Big Sister programs for positive role modelling, and so forth.

Action on access to day care was being lead by a social service agency, and the Boys and Girls Clubs were sponsoring Big Brothers and Big Sisters, so the community planning team felt the implementation of a Health Canada parenting support program called "Nobody's Perfect" would benefit the community in several ways. First, people in similar situations (single parents of young children) would have the opportunity to meet in a central location with day care on site to learn effective parenting. Second, connecting in this way would serve to form connections and attachments that could provide social support and reduce isolation. Third, as parents became less stressed and more confident, they would have more energy to devote to the demands of being a single parent and a community member. The logic model for the program is provided in Table 11-5.

TABLE 11-5 ◆ "NOBODY'S PERFECT" PROGRAM LOGIC MODEL

Overall goal: Parents will be capable of obtaining the support and information they need to maintain and promote the health of their children 0-5 years of age.

Target group: Parents who are young, single, socially or geographically isolated, or who have low income or limited formal education. Participation is voluntary and free of charge. The program is not intended for families in crisis.

Program Components	Support	Education
Short-term objectives	Establish a group for mutual support development. Increase self-help knowledge and skill	Increased knowledge and understanding of children's health, safety, and behaviour Increased coping skills
Long-term objectives	Increased opportunities to offer aid to other parents in "Nobody's Perfect" Improved self-help, information, and assistance seeking behaviour Decreased sense of isolation in parenting	Positive change in parenting knowledge and actions re: children's health, safety, and behaviour Improved self-image as a parent Increased confidence in parenting skill and ability
Short-term indicators	Referred parents will enrol in "Nobody's Perfect." Parents will attend 75% of sessions. Parents will be engaged in session activities. Parents will be satisfied with group process. Parents will be able to articulate sources for self-help and mutual aid.	Able to demonstrate learning from each session. Posttest scores greater than pretest scores Appropriate responses to case study examples Reported use of coping techniques at home
Long-term indicators	Accepts assistance/advice from group members and facilitators. Provides examples, ideas to group. Actively seeks and accepts support and information from community resources Feels more connected to the community	Consistently displays positive responses re: children's health, safety, and behaviour Views self as a good parent Is confident in ability to deal with new situations as children grow and develop
Program/facilitator activities	Recruitment of parents Facilitation of sessions Encouragement of parents Environmental support for learning	Teach, using adult education principles Facilitate session discussions and problem-solving
Resources	Infrastructure for recruitment and registration Physical facility Child care Finances Refreshments "Nobody's Perfect" materials	"Nobody's Perfect" materials Supplies Telephone and other contact resources

Based on the logic model for the parenting program and with contributions from several service agencies, the planning team recommended this program be implemented in the community of Connaught, where the highest number and proportion of parents resided. A program steering committee that consisted of the facilitator, partners, and community members (single parents) was formed and met regularly to carry out the details for implementation.

COLLABORATION

What is meant by a collaborative relationship? Could several community concerns be addressed in the same program? If they could, what would be the program goal? The objectives? This process is an example of collaborative planning and is the essence of community health practice. You may be wondering how to establish collaborative planning and inform agencies about the usefulness of goals and objectives. Although you may be convinced of the value of planned change, how do you convince others to agree, especially because planned change is not commonly practised in agencies? Role modeling is probably the best strategy. After reviewing the community diagnoses and validating data with an agency, propose goals and objectives that are congruent with the agency's purpose and organizational structure. Solicit input from the group and continue to revise the goals and objectives until a group consensus is reached.

The advantages of collaboration include preventing duplication of effort, pooling resources for maximum impact, creating more publicity and credibility than any stakeholder partner could accomplish alone, and increasing opportunities for sharing information.

To be effective, each objective needs to be supported by a clear work plan that details the specific steps to be taken in each facet of the planned program. What actions need to be done? How will they be accomplished? For instance, protocols and policies may need to be written to ensure that activities are carried out as designed by front-line workers. What resources are needed? A detailed purchasing or refurbishing plan may need to be developed, in-kind contributions tracked, and training programs developed and undertaken. Who is responsible for each action, when it is to begin, and by when is it to be completed can be detailed using a calendar chart such as in Figure 11-2. The work plan must consider communication methods to ensure each working group is in concert with every other one. Coordination meetings must be held regularly with full attendance to ensure the plan runs smoothly and the program is implemented on time. Be sure to keep stakeholder agencies informed of progress along the way.

Resources, Constraints, and Revised Plans

Once goals and objectives are written, the next step is to identify available resources and any constraints to the plan. These are analogous to Lewin's driving and restraining forces. Last, revised plans are proposed to the planning group. *Resources* are all the available means for accomplishing a task, including staff and budget as well as physical space and equipment. Recall that part of your community assessment included the identification of strengths. As you consider resources, include those strengths that may facilitate meeting program goals and objectives. For program planning, it is important to identify the resources needed as well as the resources available. *Constraints* are obstacles that restrict or limit actions and can include a lack of staff, budget, physical space, and equipment. Constraints may be thought of as the difference between needs and resources. Revised plans are actions that are proposed based on the knowledge of resources and constraint.

Universal constraints are staff and money—agencies never have enough. An additional constraint is resistance to change. All people are reluctant to change existing routines and patterns of behaviour. Initially, change is uncomfortable, and until new roles are learned, there is anxiety. Making people aware of the natural discomfort associated with change can build rapport and establish a collaborative relationship.

When each agency had shared its program goals, objectives, and activities, along with resources and constraints, several alternative actions became apparent. Therefore, the following revised plan was proposed.

Classes will be held at the Connaught community school at 6:30 PM on Tuesdays because no early evenings were available at the community centre. Social workers, public health nurses, and teachers will place posters prominently in their offices, clinics, and classrooms. Professional partners also committed to inviting people to register. Registration will be done by the health clinic. The community police office will supply refreshments for three sessions; the seniors' group will alternate with them for the remaining 3 weeks. The health department will supply the books and a nurse to facilitate the sessions. Grade 7 student volunteers will baby-sit in the child care room, and community volunteers from the steering committee will be present at the classes to welcome the participants and provide support to the sessions.

As word spread, the Vietnamese community in Bridgeland asked to be next on the schedule. To facilitate this, a Vietnamese-speaking community worker from Bridgeland was invited to attend the Connaught sessions to learn the facilitation techniques with the mentorship of the nurse, social worker, teacher, and peace officer involved. She also received advice and support from the community members on the steering committee about how to set up a similar process in Bridgeland. One woman even offered to go to the community association meeting with the facilitator to celebrate the Connaught success and encourage Bridgeland to get behind the project.

For each constraint identified, a revised plan was proposed, discussed, and adopted. This is a period of intense collaboration between the community team and community agencies, and only at the completion of this stage is the community ready for stage 5 of planned change—transformation of intentions into actual change behaviour. This transformation of intentions is the actual program implementation (which is covered in the next chapter). However, before the plan is implemented costs must be calculated and the plan recorded.

BUDGETING

Several general areas require financing in any program. It is helpful to managers and funding agencies if you use a balance-sheet format and specify sources of funds (e.g., new grants, in-kind contributions, funds already dedicated or earmarked for the intervention, donations) as well as the cost centres (e.g., personnel, supplies), staff expenses (e.g., travel, parking), operating costs (e.g., office administration, phone, fax, postage), and meeting expenses (e.g., refreshments, rent). Indicate how anticipated shortfalls or revenues will be managed. Budgets need not be overly detailed at this stage. As the plan progresses, financial expertise may need to be sought to prepare the accounting methods to ensure accountability.

RECORDING

Community plans must be recorded in standardized, systematic, and concise forms that clearly communicate to others the purpose and actions of the plan as well as the rationale for revisions and deletions of actions. Discuss with each agency its present recording system and decide on a format and system for recording the plan. The format need not be elaborate; a short written memorandum is a key component in the explicit agreement among people and agencies about what was agreed on. The memo should include a *background* statement that details the key community assessment findings, the diagnosis, a description of the target population, and the model used for program planning. The components of the *logic model* should be clearly articulated (goals, objectives, indicators, etc.) along with a description of the program and its related activities. A separate section should present the *intervention* itself and the details relevant to the *delivery* of the program. A statement of the available and needed *resources*, along with the current and anticipated *constraints*, will set the stage for the budget proposal. It is also a good idea to articulate the anticipated outcomes and impacts of the program without overstating your case and creating expectations the program cannot be expected to achieve.

Summary

The planning process begins with validation of the community diagnoses—a process that establishes the community's perception and value of community health needs. Next, using theories of planned change, the planning team and the community form a collaborative partnership to establish program goals, objectives, and the program logic model. Then, based on resources and constraints, intervention plans are proposed and revised, work plans and critical paths are recorded, and a final plan is adopted. Although only one example is offered here, the process of community planning is essentially the same for all programs that are developed. To create programs that are acceptable to the target population, the program planning and steering committees must encourage active participation by community representatives.

References

Dwyer, J. J. M., & Makin, S. (1997). Using a program logic model that focuses on performance measurement to develop a program. *Canadian Journal of Public Health, 88*(6), 421–425.

Ervin, N. E. (2002). *Advanced community health nursing practice.* Upper Saddle River, NJ: Prentice Hall.

Prochaska, J., Norcross, J., & DiClemente, C. (1995). *Changing for good.* New York: Avon Books.

Reinkemeyer, A. (1970). Nursing's need: Commitment to an ideology & change. *Nursing Forum, 9*(4), 340–355.

Rosenstock, I. M., Strecher, V. J., & Becker, M. H. (1988). Social learning theory and the health belief model. *Health Education Quarterly, 15*(2);175–183.

Smith, C. M., & Maurer, F. A. (2000). Community diagnosis, planning and intervention. In C. M. Smith & F. A. Maurer (Eds.), *Community health nursing: Theory and practice* (pp. 381–406). Philadelphia: Saunders.

Suggested Readings

Bertera, R. L. (1990). Planning and implementing health promotion in the workplace: A case study of the DuPont Company experience. *Health Education Quarterly, 17*(3), 307–327.

deVries, H., Weijts, W., Dijkstra, M., & Kok, G. (1992). The utilization of qualitative and quantitative data for health education program planning, implementation, and evaluation: A spiral approach. *Health Education Quarterly, 19*(1), 101–115.

Dignan, M. B., & Carr, P. A. (1992). *Program planning for health education and promotion* (2nd ed.). Malvern, PA: Lea & Febiger.

Ervin, N. E., & Kuehnert, P. L. (1993). Application of a model for public health nursing program planning. *Public Health Nursing, 10*(1), 25–30.

Gold, R. S., Green, L. W., Kreuter, M. W. (1998). *EMPOWER: Enabling methods of planning and organizing within everyone's reach.* London, England: Jones & Bartlett. (Workbook with CD-ROM from www.jbpub.com).

Health Canada. (2000). *Second report on the health of Canadians.* Ottawa: Author.

Helvie, C. O. (1998). *Advanced practice nursing in the community.* Thousand Oaks, CA: Sage.

Lewin, K. (1958). Group decision and social change. In E. Maccoby (Ed.), *Readings in social psychology* (3rd ed.). New York: Holt, Rinehart and Winston.

Patten, S., Vollman, A. R., & Thurston, W. E. (2000). The utility of the transtheoretical model of behavior change for HIV risk reduction in injection drug users. *Journal of the Association of Nurses in AIDS Care, 11*(1), 57–66.

Salazar, M. K. (1991) Comparison of four behavioral theories: A literature review. *AAOHN Journal, 39*(3), 128–135.

Shuster, G., & Goeppinger, J. (2000). Community as client: Using the nursing process to promote health. In M. Stanhope & J. Lancaster (Eds.), *Community and public health nursing* (pp. 306–329). St Louis, MO: Mosby.

Wong-Rieger, D. (n.d.). *A hands-on guide to planning and evaluation.* Canadian Hemophilia Society: Ottawa (Available from CPHA www.cpha.ca).

12

Implementing a Community Health Program

OBJECTIVES

Implementation is the action phase of the community process; it is carrying out the plan. Implementation is necessary to achieve goals and objectives, but, more importantly, the implementation of interventions acts to promote, maintain, or restore population health and community well-being.

In this chapter we discuss the process of implementing a community- or population-focused program. Intervention strategies are presented as well as resources that are helpful in program implementation.

After studying this chapter, you should be able to:

◆ Suggest strategies to the community for implementation of health programs

◆ Working in partnership with the community:

◆ Implement planned programs

◆ Review and revise interventions based on community responses

◆ Use interventions to formulate and influence health and social policies that have an impact on the health of the community

Introduction

Once goals and objectives have been agreed on and recorded during the planning stage, all that remains for implementation is to actually carry out the activities to meet those objectives. This probably seems straightforward and simple. Indeed, at this point, you will have spent considerable time assessing, analyzing, and planning a program. You will be ready and eager to begin. But this very eagerness (and the associated impatience of the intervention stage) is a danger. You must take time to consider how you can promote community ownership, create a unified program that respects the overall goals of the community, and maintain a clear focus on your target population and the activities planned.

> ✎ **TAKE NOTE**
>
> This chapter focuses on the *process* of intervention and provides you with some general resources that may prove helpful in your community work. Many excellent examples of interventions in which community teams work as partners with the community are included in Part III.

Community Ownership

Essential to achieving the desired outcomes of an intervention is the active participation of the community. The meaning of partnership and collaboration was discussed in the preceding chapter, but the present concern is ownership. The people of the community need to feel a sense of ownership of the program or event, which can only come with their full participation in the decisions regarding planning as well as their assuming some responsibility for implementation. Herein lies a potential conflict. The human service professions are dedicated to nurturing, sustaining, and caring for others. It is part of our professions to do *for* others what they would do for themselves if they were able. Indeed, many human service disciplines interact professionally with people during an altered state (crisis) that requires professionals to do for others; but this is not true in community practice. Stepping into the community requires an attitude of doing *with* the people, not doing things to them or for them. When things are done to us or for us, our emotional commitment remains limited.

How might you ensure community ownership for a proposed program and planned interventions? How can you facilitate involvement? In Calgary, an inner city network functioned to coordinate interagency planning for community-focused programming. When the university students doing a course practicum completed the community assessment phase and submitted their report, community meetings had been held by the health department to determine priority issues, and planning was undertaken with community members on the various interagency planning teams. Once funding was located to support programming, the inner city network directed its attention to the coordination of activities for implementation. The important point in this example is that a coordinating or "umbrella" group was already in place (the network). A separate working group within the network planned the "Nobody's Perfect" program and will be continuing to lead its implementation in the Connaught community.

The working group returned to the assessment data and learned that the United Way listed 14 agencies that served Connaught children and families in some capacity. The planning group decided to contact each of these agencies to inform them about the "Nobody's Perfect" program, enlist their support, inform them how parents were referred to the program, and invite them to provide speakers, audiovisual resources, and contributions to support refreshments and cover babysitting costs.

✎ TAKE NOTE

Do not panic at this point and feel that you must be knowledgeable about all agencies and their programs in the community that you have assessed. At the implementation stage, refer back to your initial assessment and consider logically which service agencies may have resources helpful to the planned program(s). Then contact selected agencies, request information on their purpose and current programs, share with the agency your community-focused program plans, and solicit recommendations with regard to materials and resources. Many voluntary and nongovernmental organizations (NGOs) have professional staff at the national and provincial levels and an affiliated or community linkage structure. These voluntary organizations have ongoing programs for a wide variety of issues, and most acknowledge health promotion as a vital part of their mission. The Internet is a good way to locate such resources in your community.

Health Canada publishes a tremendous amount of information that is designed to promote health among Canadians. Special attention is given to facilitating prevention activities. In addition, provincial health and social service ministries, Canadian Institutes for Health Research, the Canadian Consortium for Health Promotion Research, and other national and provincial departments (e.g., environment, education, justice, housing, transportation) have publications and initiatives that support population health.

Several national or provincial libraries are designated as government depositories or information clearinghouses and, therefore, have many government publications. And do not ignore publications from other countries (such as the U.S. Centers for Disease Control and Prevention, World Health Organization).

Having discussed the importance of community participation and ownership of the program, the remaining issues to consider are a unified presentation of the program and an emphasis on community outcomes.

Unified Program

Because of limited resources, staff constraints, and other situations beyond the control of the planners, many good programs are implemented in a piecemeal fashion that minimizes their impact. A unified program requires collaboration and coordination among the agency personnel who will implement the program, the program's recipients (the target population), and the community. Allowing plenty of time for publicizing the program (and how you perform the mechanics of publicity—the how, where, and to whom) can make a crucial difference in whether people attend and what the subsequent impact will be.

After a time and place have been selected (based on initial input from the survey questionnaires), how might you publicize a program? Public service announcements, notification in the newspapers, bulletin inserts for civic and religious associations, flyers sent home with school-aged children, and posters and notices in community service buildings and local shopping centres are some of the methods to consider.

In the Connaught community, elementary teachers placed articles in the school newsletter so that interested parents would know about the program, who was leading it, what costs were involved, that child care would be provided, and how to get a referral to participate. The Community Association put a notice on its electronic bulletin board and placed posters in the pool and recreation centres. Social workers and public health nurses responded to requests from parents, suggestions from teachers and community workers, and registered parents into the program. A junior high teacher used the opportunity in a social studies course to offer class credits for those students who volunteered for the program in some capacity (e.g., child care).

Report on the Health of Canadians

The first *Report on the Health of Canadians* was released in 1996, and the second report *Towards a Healthy Future* in 1999. These reports summarize the current information available and comment on the state of the nation's health from a population health promotion perspective; they can be used as tools in identifying actions that can be taken to improve the health of Canadians, the residents of a province, city, or neighbourhood. The implicit goals of population health promotion is to reduce or eliminate disparities in health experienced by different groups of people, improve quality of life, and add years to life expectancy by strengthening communities and community action on the determinants of health. Provincial ministries of health and regional health authorities use these goals to establish performance objectives and determine funding priorities.

✎ TAKE NOTE

Are the goals and objectives for your community realistic in terms of its past history, current context, and in relation to trends over time? Do the goals and objectives for your community-focused program further regional and provincial goals and objectives?

When the "Nobody's Perfect" working group examined its logic model and implementation plans, it was noted that its work was consistent with the overall purpose of the Network and the mandate of the Parent Advisory Committee, and was congruent with the health ministry's children's initiative.

Community Health Focus

There is one remaining question to ask before initiating the program: Does it focus on community health? This may seem to be a strange question. You might wonder, do not all health programs focus on maintaining, restoring, or promoting health of the community? Frequently, the answer is no. Some *community-based* programs (i.e., located in the community, not in an acute care institution) focus on individuals and do not take the larger systems of family and community into context. *Community-oriented* and *community-focused* programs seek to improve the health of groups of people to benefit the quality of life and well-being of the community at large.

In the Inner City Project, the Network and designated staff had become very involved in planning specific activities and information modules associated with the various community projects. Several programs had been enlarged to include screening and health fairs (e.g., the seniors' health fair in Bridgeland and the community kitchen in Victoria Park); and additional activities were suggested at each meeting of the Network. The initial goal of promoting the health of downtown (DT15) residents had seemingly changed to providing lots of activities and information about health to individuals. Carrying out activities, going after every competitive funding opportunity announced, and being visibly "involved" had taken precedence over strategic planning, community participation, and collaborative coordination of activities to meet the needs of the community *as expressed by* the residents of that community and carried out *in collaboration with* community stakeholders. What had happened? Remember, we discussed the impatience and eagerness that are often associated with new programs. This situation is normal. Committees tend to overemphasize activities and knowledge and forget the initial reason for the program—to improve *community* health and quality of life. As activities were successful, more and more people approached the Network with more and more ideas and requests. In an effort to do as much as possible for as many people as possible, Network members found themselves in a state of burnout, community representatives felt burdened, and programs began, were carried out once, then fizzled.

It must be remembered that it is the sustained day-to-day use of knowledge and lifestyle practices that improve quality of life. Frequently, a program begins with enthusiastic momentum; media publicity attracts people to screening and information sessions—and then the program is over. Objectives are evaluated as having been achieved successfully, and another program is planned and implemented. But was there any real improvement in health? Was there any impact on participants' lifestyle practices? Will the changes be maintained and continued for a week? A month? A year? Most importantly, are the changed lifestyle or health practices supported by the surrounding environment and culture? Without sustained program activity and improvement over time, public policy that supports healthy choices, and social support networks that create a positive environment, population behaviour change and long-term impact on a community's health status will not be achieved.

Environmental and Cultural Support

Many parents in the downtown communities responded affirmatively to survey questions about child discipline. These parents believed that they or another person had hurt a child when the child was punished; parents wanted to learn ways to keep from hurting children when adults were angry. The Inner City Network responded with a series of programs on effective parenting that included information on various nonphysical strategies for disciplining youngsters as well as role-playing and open-discussion periods. However, as part of the community assessment, the school nurse recorded that the community school had a history of bullying and that no protocol for addressing it was in place because the Parent Advisory Committee had decided to focus instead on an antiracism initiative. School children were experiencing harassment and bullying, but if it was not racial in nature, it often went unreported. The conflict between the effective parenting programs and the bullying at the school was obvious. What could be done? What would you suggest?

In Connaught, part of the planned "Nobody's Perfect" classes included discussion sessions on the difference between discipline and punishment and the importance of inquiring as to disciplinary techniques used by caregivers when parents left their children in someone else's care (e.g., at child care facilities, at schools, or with babysitters). During this discussion, parents with school-aged children expressed their concerns about bullying on the school grounds. How, they wondered, could they deal with children who had to "fight back" at school and were acting the same way at home with younger siblings? Although some parents were unaware that the school board has an anti-bullying policy, most were aware of the reputation of the school as "tough" and believed that environment could not be changed. Following a discussion of parental rights and responsibilities, one parent raised the issue with the community association president. A group of equally concerned parents subsequently came together to generate action against school violence; they made an appointment with the principal to discuss the situation. (After additional meetings with Parent Advisory Committee members and an open public meeting on school violence, the school changed its procedures regarding how it dealt with bullying, harassment, and racism. The process took 2 years, but resulted in a parent-supported peer anti-bullying program that created a positive school environment where children flourished in a context that valued diversity, leadership and achievement.)

✎ TAKE NOTE

Countless such incongruities exist between healthy lifestyles and environmental and cultural practices and policies. Here is one additional example: A school nurse taught hygiene to the elementary grades, emphasizing the importance of washing hands before meals and after using the toilet. However, the school did not provide soap in the washrooms and, for safety purposes, all taps ran with cold water. Additionally, those students who ate lunch at school were not allowed to go to the washroom to wash their hands before going to the lunch room. The reason? It was too disruptive and students did not finish lunch soon enough. How would you approach this issue?

Identify the environmental and cultural practices and policies that are in conflict with the proposed community-focused health program that resulted from your community assessment. What can be done to increase community awareness of these conflicts, and how can change begin? To focus on health and the maintenance of healthy lifestyles, all of the community must be involved.

The best way to maintain a focus on health and not on the activities of the program is to use your practice model as a guide. The community practice model built and described in Chapter 8 (see Fig. 8-2) defines intervention as primary, secondary, and tertiary levels of prevention. Does the program proposed for Connaught address these three levels of prevention?

Levels of Prevention

Recall that *primary prevention* improves the health and well-being of the community, making it less vulnerable to stressors. Health promotion programs are primary prevention, as are programs that focus on protection from specific problems. Usually health promotion is nonspecific and directed toward raising the general health of the total community (e.g., teaching youngsters about nutritious foods or conducting adult exercise/fitness and stress-reduction sessions). Primary prevention can also be very specific, such as providing immunization against certain diseases, wearing seatbelts in cars, and purifying public water supplies. The Connaught peer leadership initiative that prevented school bullying by embracing diversity and teaching positive communication and conflict resolution strategies is an example of primary prevention.

Secondary prevention begins after a disease or condition is present (although there may be no symptoms). Emphasis is on screening, early diagnosis, and treatment of possible stressors that may adversely affect the community's health. The Mantoux test for tuberculosis, the Denver Developmental Screening Test for developmental delays, blood pressure assessments, and breast self-examinations are secondary prevention interventions to which we are accustomed. At a community level, Block Watch or Block Parent programs are often initiated after problems arise. Similarly, requests for services such as Boys and Girls Clubs escalate when local youth begin to get involved with vandalism and petty crime. A community kitchen or "Wheels to Meals" program might be offered as a remedy to poor nutritional status of certain populations (e.g., immigrants, seniors).

Tertiary prevention focuses on restoration and rehabilitation. Tertiary prevention programs act to return the community to an optimum level of functioning. Adequate shelters for battered women and counselling and therapy programs for sexually abused youngsters are examples of tertiary prevention. The Exit

Outreach program is an example of a tertiary level preventive program intended to assist street youth. The Children's Cottage is another example, providing shelter for children when parents are experiencing a temporary crisis. The Calgary Drop-in Centre, Urban Projects Society, and Mustard Seed offer support for rehabilitation and recovery, advocacy for housing and employment, and assistance for street-involved people to gain access to treatment for financial, physical, and mental health issues.

The distinction between prevention levels is not always clear. Is a program on the assessment of fever in children (and the prevention of febrile convulsions and dehydration through use of tepid baths and extra fluids) secondary or tertiary prevention? How would you classify an effective parenting program? Support groups for single parents? A crime prevention program? Workshops on stress reduction and physical fitness? Can some programs be primary, secondary, and tertiary depending on the needs of the persons who attend? Certainly effective parenting classes for the parent with a child who has a behaviour problem will have a different purpose than classes designed for expectant parents of a first child. Likewise, the corporate executive who has been diagnosed with cardiovascular disease and placed on a low-cholesterol diet and activity program has very different learning needs from those of the senior citizen on a fixed income. Few programs are purely at one level of prevention. The important point is to assess your programs (the implementation phase of the community process) and ask if the interventions are consistent with the community practice model.

Community Interventions

As discussed previously, there are three types of interventions: education, engineering, and enforcement. In this next section, we will briefly discuss each, with the focus of interventions being the group/aggregate or population.

Education

HEALTH EDUCATION

Learning can be defined as a measurable change in knowledge, attitude, or behaviour that persists over time. Learning occurs in three different domains: cognitive (memory, recognition, understanding, and application), affective (attitudes and values), and psychomotor (using the muscles and nervous system). For learning to be effective, learners must have the ability to perform and opportunities to practice. The environment needs to be supportive and the teaching format and communication process adapted to the needs of the group.

The health education literature is replete with helpful suggestions for teaching adults. For instance, Onega (2000) has adapted an acronym to describe the process of health education:

T—Tune in. Listen before you start teaching. Client needs should direct the content.
E—Edit information. Teach necessary information first. Be specific.
A—Act on each teaching moment. Teach whenever possible. Develop a good relationship.
C—Clarify often. Make sure your assumptions are correct. Seek feedback.
H—Honour the clients as partners. Build on clients' experiences. Share responsibility with the client group.

Knowles (1998), a scholar in adult education, offers six principles to guide adult learning:

Message—Send a clear message to the group. Avoid jargon. Select issues that are meaningful to the community.
Format—Select the most appropriate learning format. Begin where people are. Use learning aids judiciously.
Environment—Create the best possible learning environment including physical space, interpersonal connections, and administrative aspects.
Experience—Organize positive and meaningful learning experiences—continuous, sequenced, integrated, and relevant to the group/community.
Participation—Engage learners in participatory learning. Encourage activity —discussion, role play—so people learn by doing.
Evaluation—Evaluate and give objective feedback to learners, and receive feedback from them to modify the teaching process. (Meade, 1997, p.168)

The educational process uses the same steps as the community process, making it very straightforward for community educators to assess learner needs, plan and implement teaching interventions, and determine the effectiveness of the process.

Assessment	Identify the information needs and readiness, barriers to learning, and capacities of the target group.
Analysis and Diagnosis	State the educational goals and objectives.

Planning	Select methods, materials, site, time, and market the event.
Implementation	Carry out the sessions(s) as planned.
Evaluation	Assess the effectiveness of processes and achievement of outcomes.

Some formats for learning include brainstorming, demonstration, group discussion, lecture, role play, and panel discussion. Strategies to enhance learning may include printed material (bulletin boards, drawings, flashcards), audiovisual material (overhead transparencies, videotapes, photographs), computer-assisted software and on-line resources, guest speakers, peer presentations, and field trips. Care must be taken that materials are appropriate to the technology available, the culture, literacy and language levels of the participants, and the size of the group. Pretesting newly developed material is important, and critically assessing print resources for reading level, layout, type font and size, content (verbal and visual), and aesthetic quality is key to ensuring the resources are appropriate, culturally sensitive, and accurate.

SOCIAL MARKETING

In social marketing, mass media are used to "sell" health through particular behaviours or products. With its components of marketing and consumer research, advertising and promotion, social marketing clearly has a central role to play in health promotion (Mintz, 1989). Mintz views the social marketing process as developing the right product, backed by the right promotion, and put in the right place at the right price. Although a social marketing campaign on its own cannot be expected to change the behaviour of large populations, it can be a potent component in a comprehensive health promotion program.

The *product* is the message and how it is presented. The *price* is not only the cost of producing and publishing the message, but also the cost to the consumer of acting on it. *Promotion* is the means of persuasion or the communication function of marketing. *Place* respects adequate and suitable distribution as well as response channels or access to information. In other words, how can people who are motivated take follow up action?

Steps in preparing a social marketing campaign are:

1. Analyze the situation	Ensure that clear direction, expertise, and resources are in place.
	Do your homework. Use qualitative and quantitative methods to analyse the environment.

	Learn from others: analyze the competition, and review programs already in place for evidence of success.
	Locate community partners.
2. Target the market	Segment the market, isolating those that offer the greatest potential for success by using demographics, values, lifestyles, and personality variables.
	Concentrate on narrow population groups for maximum impact.
	Position the message and develop a distribution channel.
3. Set program elements	Develop processes to support advertising, public relations, access to information, creating networks, and measuring effectiveness.
4. Determine the message	Protect the integrity of information, ensuring it is accurate, timely, relevant, and culturally appropriate to the target group.

No education or social marketing intervention is effective if the environment erects barriers to people taking action. In this instance, the community team must act to effect change by creating conditions that support making the healthy choice the easy choice.

Engineering

MEDIA ADVOCACY

Media advocacy, based on the recognition that health is a result of the social and environmental conditions in which people live, uses the mass media to influence the development of healthy public policy through changing the nature of public debate on issues that affect health. It is a political tool in that it exerts pressure to influence decision-makers and legislators.

There are several components of media advocacy. Reframing the debate, or presenting the issue differently than it is usually discussed, results from setting the agenda, shaping the debate, and advancing policy. It involves capturing the attention of the media and demonstrating the newsworthiness of an issue. The next step is to tell the story from the perspective of the population, with emphasis on broad social issues rather than on individuals. The third step involves putting forward the policy solution you are aiming to achieve (Wass,

2000). Community participation plays a key role in media advocacy. To be effective, media advocacy relies on the formation of coalitions that are sustained over a long period of time so that a grassroots movement can gain enough momentum to maintain the issue in the public eye for more than a short time.

Advocacy campaigns consist of providing newsworthy items to the media, writing letters to the editor, preparing media releases, releasing photographs or providing photo opportunities, and doing media interviews (Wass, 2000). Be certain to follow the protocols of your organization before contacting the media, and be prepared for questions that generate controversy!

POLICY FORMULATION

Healthy public policy is chiefly concerned with creating a healthy society (Glass & Hicks, 2000). Healthy public policy is multisectoral; it explicitly recognizes the contributions from other sectors that influence the determinants of health. It is founded on public involvement and principles of primary health care (Glass & Hicks, 2000): population health focus, equity, multidisciplinary approaches, intersectoral collaboration, participation, information systems, and health system reform.

Stages of policy formulation are:

Policy analysis	Identification of issues, analysis of options, and a choice of an optimal policy
Policy design	Communication with all sectors, problem identification and definition
Policy development	Specification of goals and specific targets
Policy implementation	Deliberation on strategies and instruments that will incorporate policy into the system, funding models, legislation, and involvement of nongovernmental organizations
Policy evaluation	Monitoring the impact of policy on the population

Each stage is itself a political process (Helvie, 2000) and requires resource allocation, negotiation, conflict resolution, and compromise. Policy change takes a long time to occur, particularly because health and social policy are in provincial jurisdiction. Change challenges entrenched values and perceptions, requiring extensive consultation and development, and, because of the complexity of the social situation, skill and patience are keys to eventual success.

Enforcement

When legislation is in place to require people to act in a certain way, and there is resistance or lack of compliance, protection services (e.g., police, fire, food inspectors) may enter the community to enforce the law. If community workers can combine education and engineering with this approach, then enforcement can be most effective. For instance, many health departments collaborate with the police and transportation officials during seatbelt checkpoints. If children are unrestrained in a vehicle, or improperly restrained, professionals demonstrate proper restraint methods, provide information on purchasing appropriate restraints, and teach the parents the importance of restraints for child safety. The parents are given a "ticket" to attend a child safety workshop in their community, and when the parents attend they receive a coupon for restraints at a local store. If, however, parents are found on check-stop to be repeat offenders, they are levied a fine that can be "paid" not only by money, but also by attendance at the workshop. Notices regarding the check-stops are placed in community papers and school newsletters. If children are also taught car safety at school, they can be effective monitors of family vehicle safety, demonstrating the impact of multiple strategies on changing health behaviours.

Summary

Having considered the importance of community ownership of the program, the need to offer a unified program, and maintaining a focus on health and well-being, there remains one step in the process—evaluation. Before a program is implemented, the manner in which it is to be evaluated must be established, hence the importance of the logic model. The following chapter explains why this final stage of the community process is best considered before implementation begins.

References

Courtney, R., Ballard, E., Fauver, S., Gariota, M., & Holland, L. (1996). The partnership model: Working with individuals, families, and communities toward a new vision of health. *Public Health Nursing, 13*(3), 17–186.

Duncan, S. M. (1996). Empowerment strategies in nursing education: A foundation for population-focused clinical studies. *Public Health Nursing, 13*(5), 311–317.

Glass, H., & Hicks, S. (2000). Healthy public policy in health system reform. In M. J. Stewart (Ed.), *Community nursing: Promoting Canadians' health* (pp. 156–170). Toronto: Saunders.

Health Canada. (1999). *Toward a healthy future: Second report on the health of Canadians.* Ottawa: Health Canada. Available www.hc-sc.gc.ca.

Heiss, G. L. (2000). Health teaching. In C. M. Smith & F. A. Maurer (Eds.), *Community health nursing: Theory and practice* (pp. 498–519). Philadelphia: Saunders.

Helvie, C. O. (1998). *Advanced practice nursing in the community* (pp.287-313). Thousand Oaks, CA: Sage.

Knowles, M. (1998). *The adult learner: A neglected species.* Houston, TX: Gulf.

Meade, C. (1997). Community health education. In J. M. Swanson & M. A. Nies (Eds.), *Community health nursing: Promoting the health of aggregates* (pp. 155–192). Philadelphia: Saunders.

Mintz, J. (1989). Social marketing: New weapon in an old struggle. *Health Promotion, 28*(4), 6–12.

Mintz, J., & Steele, M. (1992). Marketing health information: The why and how of it. *Health Promotion, 31*(2), 2–5, 29.

Onega, L. L. (2000). Educational theories, models and principles applied to community and public health nursing. In M. Stanhope & J. Lancaster (Eds.), *Community and public health nursing* (pp. 266-283). St. Louis, MO: Mosby.

Wass, A. (2000). *Promoting health: The primary care approach.* Marrickville, AU: Harcourt.

Suggested Readings

Abraham, T., & Fallon, P.J. (1997). Caring for the community: Development of the advanced practice nurse role. *Clinical Nurse Specialist, 11*(5), 224–230.

Anderson, E. T., Gottschalk, J., & Martin, D. A. (1993). Contemporary issues in the community. In D. J. Mason, S. W. Talbott, & J. K. Leavitt (Eds.), *Policy and politics for nurses: Action and change in the workplace, government, organizations and community.* Philadelphia: Saunders.

Beddome, G., Clarke, H. F., & Whyte, N.B. (1993). Vision for the future of public health nursing: A case for primary health care. *Public Health Nursing, 1*(1), 13–18.

Chavis, D. M., & Florin, P. (1990). Nurturing grassroots initiatives for health and housing. *Bulletin of the New York Academy of Medicine, 66*(5), 558–572.

Dahl, S., Gustafson, C., & McCullagh, M. (1993). Collaborating to develop a community-based health service for rural homeless persons. *Journal of Nursing Administration, 23*(4), 41–45.

Durpa, K. C., Quick, M. M., Andrews, A., Engelke, M. K., & Vinvent, P. (1992). A collaborative health promotion effort: Nursing students and Wendy's team up. *Nurse Educator, 17*(6), 35–37.

El-Askari, G., Freestone, J., Irizarry, C., Mashiyama, S. T., Morgan, M. A., & Walton, S. (1998). The Healthy Neighborhoods Project: A local health department's role in catalyzing community development. *Health Education & Behavior, 25*(2), 146–159.

Farley, S. (1993). The community as partner in primary health care. *Nursing & Health Care, 14*(5), 244–249.

Flick, L. H., Reese, C., & Harris, A. (1996). Aggregate community-centered undergraduate community health nursing clinical experience. *Public Health Nursing, 13*(1), 36–41.

Flynn, B. C. (1997). Partnerships in healthy cities and communities: A social commitment for advanced practice nurses. *Advanced Practice Nursing Quarterly, 2*(4), 1–6.

Gamm, L. D. (1998). Advancing community health through community health partnerships. *Journal of Healthcare Management, 43*(1), 51–66.

Hawe, P., King, L., Noort, M., Gifford, S. M., & Lloyd, B. (1998). Working invisibly: Health workers talk about capacity-building in health promotion. *Health Promotion International, 13*(4), 285–295.

Hollinger-Smith, L. (1998). Partners in collaboration: The Homan Square Project. *Journal of Professional Nursing, 14*(6), 344–349.

Jenkins, S. (1991). Community wellness: A group empowerment model for rural America. *Journal of Health Care for the Poor and Underserved, 1*(4), 388–404.

Kinne, A., Thompson, B., Chrisman, N. J., & Hanley, J. R. (1989). Community organization to enhance the delivery of preventive health services. *American Journal of Preventive Medicine, 5*(4), 225–229.

Labonte, R. (1993). Community development and partnerships. *Canadian Journal of Public Health, 84*(4), 237–240.

Murashima, S., Hatono, Y., Whyte, N., & Asahara, K. (1999). Public health nursing in Japan: New opportunities for health promotion. *Public Health Nursing, 16*(2), 133–139.

Perino, S. S. (1992). Nike-footed health workers deal with the problems of adolescent pregnancy. *Public Health Reports, 107*(2), 208–212.

Primomo, J. (1990). Diapering decisions: A community education project. In H. Tilson (Ed.), Notes from the field. *American Journal of Public Health, 80*(6), 743–744.

Rutherford, G. S., & Campbell, D. (1993). Helping people help themselves. *Canadian Nurse, 89*(10), 25–28.

Scott, S. (1990). *Promoting healthy traditions workbook: A guide to the Healthy People Campaign.* St. Paul, MN: American Indian Health Care Association.

Wardrop, K. (1993). A framework for health promotion. *Canadian Journal of Public Health, 84*(Suppl. l), S9–S13.

Woodard, G. R., & Edouard, L. (1992). Reaching out: A community initiative for disadvantaged pregnant women. *Canadian Journal of Public Health, 83*(3), 188–190.

13

Evaluating a Community Health Program

CHAPTER OUTLINE

Introduction
Evaluation Principles
The Evaluation Process
Components of Evaluation

Evaluation Strategies
Selected Methods of Data
    Collection
Summary

OBJECTIVES

Evaluation is determining the worth (or value) of something. During the evaluation process, information is collected and analyzed to determine its significance and worth. Changes are appraised, and progress is documented. This chapter discusses evaluation and the professional practices that are necessary to plan and implement it.

After studying this chapter, you should be able to act in partnership with the community to:

◆ Establish evaluation criteria that are timely and comprehensive

◆ Use baseline and current data to measure progress toward goals and objectives

◆ Validate observations, insights, and new data with colleagues and the community

◆ Revise priorities, goals, and interventions based on evaluation data

◆ Document and record evaluation results and revisions of the plan

◆ Participate in evaluation research with appropriate consultation

◆ Appreciate the complexity of program evaluation as well as the multiple paradigms that affect its implementation

Introduction

The community health team evaluates the responses of the community to a program to measure progress that is being made toward the program's goals and objectives. Evaluation data are also crucial for revision of the assessment database and the community diagnoses that were developed from analysis of the community assessment data.

Do you feel as if we are talking in circles? Evaluation is the "final" step of the community process, but it is linked to assessment, which is the first step. Professional practice is cyclic as well as dynamic, and for community-focused interventions to be timely and relevant, the community assessment database, community diagnoses, and program plans must be evaluated routinely. The effectiveness of community interventions depends on continuous reassessment of the community and on appropriate revisions of planned interventions.

Reflecting on the community-as-partner model (see Fig. 8-2), the purpose of evaluation is to determine if stressors have been repelled or minimized, if the normal line of defence (health status of the population) is stronger, and if the community's capacity (lines of resistance) is strengthened as a result of the intervention.

Evaluation is important to community practice, but of equal importance is its crucial role in the functioning of human service agencies. Staffing and funding are frequently based on evaluation findings, and existing programs are subject to termination unless evaluation evidence can be produced that answers this question: What has been the program's impact on the community? Recent years have witnessed a growing focus on program evaluation; training programs on evaluation have become common, and evaluation has become big business. Unfortunately, evaluation is sometimes practised separately from program planning. It may even be tacked onto the end of a program just to satisfy funding sources or agency administration. The problems of such an approach are evident. Effective community practice requires an integrated approach to evaluation; it is a unique aspect of the field.

Evaluation Principles

Congruent with the theoretical foundations of working with the community as partner, we base our program evaluation on principles explicated by the W. K. Kellogg Foundation (1998). These principles are summarized below.

1. *Strengthen programs.* Our goal is health promotion and improving a community's self-reliance. Evaluation assists in attaining this goal by providing an ongoing and systematic process for assessing the program, its impact, and its outcomes.
2. *Use multiple approaches.* In addition to multidisciplinary approaches, evaluation methods may be numerous and varied. No one, single approach is favoured, but the method chosen must be congruent with the purposes of the program.
3. *Design evaluation to address real issues.* Community-based and community-focused programs, rooted in the "real" community and based on an assessment of that community, must design an evaluation to measure those criteria of importance to the community.
4. *Create a participatory process.* Just as the community members were part of assessment, analysis, planning, and implementation, so too, they must be partners in evaluation.
5. *Allow for flexibility.* "Evaluation approaches must not be rigid and prescriptive, or it will be difficult to document the incremental, complex, and often subtle changes that occur..."(W.K. Kellogg Foundation, 1998, p 3).
6. *Build capacity.* The process of evaluation, in addition to measuring outcomes, should enhance the skills, knowledge, and attitudes of those engaged in it. This includes both professionals and nonprofessionals alike.

The Evaluation Process

There is a burgeoning literature on evaluation (see the references and suggested readings at the end of this chapter). Program or project evaluation has become a specialty with whole departments and consulting firms focused on measurement and evaluation.

For our purposes (i.e., to provide an introduction to program evaluation), we will use a three-part model (Table 13-1). In this model, we look at the process of implementing the program, the program's impact, and the outcome of the program.

Our focus in this text is on health promotion, and health promotion programs are designed to "... influence target populations through planned activities (process) that may have immediate effects (impact) as well as more long-term effects (outcomes)" (Dignan & Carr, 1992, p. 153). Program evaluation is the systematic gathering, analysis, and reporting of data about a program to assist in making decisions (Porteous, Sheldrick, & Stewart, 1997).

TABLE 13-1 ◆ A MODEL FOR PROGRAM EVALUATION

	Process (formative)	Impact (summative; short-term outcome)	Outcome (longer-term)
Information to collect	Program implementation, including • Site response • Recipient response • Practitioner response • Competencies of personnel	Immediate effects of program on, for example: • Knowledge • Attitudes • Perceptions • Skills • Beliefs • Access to resources • Social support	Incidence and prevalence of risk factors, morbidity, and mortality
When to apply	Initial implementation of a program or when changes are made in a developed program (eg, moved to a new site, provided to a different population)	To determine if factors that affect health—both within the individual and in the environment—have changed. For example did the person's behavior change? Was the new policy implemented?	To measure if incidence and prevalence have been altered. For example, has the immunization rate of 2 year olds increased? Did the rate of admissions for illnesses decrease? Did the industry filter its polluting smoke stack?

Adapted from Green, L. W. & Lewis, F. M. (1986). *Measurement and evaluation in health education and health promotion.* Palo Alto, CA: Mayfield.

The steps in the evaluation process (adapted from Porteous, Sheldrick, & Stewart, 1997) are:

1. Focus the evaluation

   ◆ Identify the purpose
   ◆ Review the logic model
   ◆ Consult with stakeholders
   ◆ Determine evaluation questions

2. Select evaluation methods

   ◆ Establish or clarify program expectations
   ◆ Develop a data collection plan based on the indicators specified the logic model
      ◆ Select the type of tool
      ◆ Determine the source of data
      ◆ Determine the data collector
      ◆ Set the design, number of participants, and time frame

◆ Develop the logistics plan and assess its feasibility
  ◆ Consider the resources required

3. Develop measurement tools

  ◆ Find existing measures and tools
  ◆ Develop data collection measures and tools
    ◆ Draft questions
    ◆ Determine types of responses and response categories
    ◆ Put the tool together
  ◆ Assess the quality of the data collection tool
    ◆ Content and clarity
    ◆ Stability and reliability

4. Gather and analyze data

  ◆ Gather data
    ◆ Select data collectors
    ◆ Prepare instructions for data collection
    ◆ Train data collectors
    ◆ Pretest the method
    ◆ Assess the data collectors
    ◆ Monitor data collection activities
  ◆ Analyze the data (refer to Chap. 10 for methods)
    ◆ Organize the data by classifying and categorizing
    ◆ Analyze by finding patterns of evidence, discrepancies
    ◆ Perform calculations
    ◆ Examine internal and external contexts for interpretation

5. Report on your evaluation

  ◆ Consider the audience
  ◆ Determine how the report will be disseminated

Process or formative evaluation is intended to improve the operation of an existing program. It answers the question: Are we doing what we said we would do? That is, did we deliver the program, provide a place to meet, include handouts at our meeting, and so forth? For example, when the pilot for the "Nobody's Perfect" program was offered in another Calgary community from 8 to 9 PM, very few parents attended regularly. They stated that the time was too late for them to return home and complete homework, family, and bedtime activities for their school-aged children. As a result of this formative evaluation, the time chosen for the Connaught program was 6:30 to 8 PM to allow for refreshments and socializing; student volunteers provided babysitting on site. Participants were satisfied with this time frame and there were few absences during the 6 weeks of the program. Some authors (Green & Lewis, 1986) make a distinction between formative and process evaluation by using 'process' to denote evaluation conducted during the program and 'formative' (as the name implies) at the program formation or preprogram stages.

Outcome (or summative) evaluation is concerned with the immediate impact of a program on a target group. It answers the question: Is our program effective? If your program is aimed at changing a group's knowledge and behaviour relating to sexually transmitted disease, for instance, you might build in a test to find out what they learned and what their intent is about modifying behaviour. In the case of the "Nobody's Perfect" program in Connaught, summative evaluation criteria might include parental self-reports that they have increased their knowledge about children's health, safety, and behaviour, and that they have improved their coping skills with stressors related to child growth and developmental stages and needs. In addition, parents can provide feedback in terms of whether or not they feel they have had the opportunity to develop some supportive community connections.

It is in the long-term outcome evaluation, however, that you find out if the changes had a lasting and real effect. That is, did the incidence of child abuse drop in this population group? Because we are getting closer to the cause-and-effect question, careful evaluative research is needed to determine the actual contribution of the program to the outcome being measured.

✎ TAKE NOTE

An in-depth review of evaluation research is beyond the scope of this text. There are several excellent texts that focus on evaluation research, and two examples of evaluation research are included later in this chapter.

Before considering specific evaluation strategies, it is important to consider the "evaluability" of the program. To do this, review the program plan and ask yourself the following questions:

◆ Are program activities stated in precise words whose concepts can be measured?
◆ Is a time frame for attaining the change included?
◆ Are the direction and magnitude of the change included?

◆ Is a method of measuring the change included?
◆ Are the data that will be needed to measure the objectives available at a reasonable cost?
◆ Are the program activities that are designed to meet the objectives plausible?

If you find that any of these questions cannot be answered in the affirmative regarding your plan, review Chapter 11 and amend the plan and logic model to make them as concise and complete as possible. The plan for process and outcome evaluation should be built into your overall plan prior to its launch. Early planning ensures that you will be able to collect baseline data (how things were before you implemented your program) and collect the right data at the right time, from the right sources, using the appropriate methods. When the above factors are considered, evaluation becomes a part of everyday program activities, not a burdensome add-on to program staff.

✎ **TAKE NOTE**

A positive response to each of the above questions would be an ideal state that few programs attain. Therefore, do not despair if your program is less than perfect but rather strive to increase your sensitivity to the issues that need to be considered in program planning to achieve optimum program evaluation.

Components of Evaluation

Why collect evaluation data? To whom will the evaluation data be given, and for what purpose will it be used? What programs or activities will result from or be discontinued as a result of evaluation data? Before a strategy or method of evaluation can be selected, the reasons for and uses of the evaluation data must be established. An evaluation strategy appropriate for answering one type of evaluative question would not be useful for another. For example, if a Health Promotion Council wanted to know the relevancy to community needs of a program on crime prevention, then questions would be asked of the participants concerning the usefulness and adequacy of the information that was given. Possible questions would cover a range of topics:

◆ Did the information make a difference as to how residents protect themselves from crime?

◆ What protective behaviours do the residents practise now that were not practised before the program?
◆ Did the program answer the residents' questions?
◆ Did the program meet perceived needs?

However, if the Council wanted to know the outcome of the crime prevention program (such as if the program decreased the incidence of crime experienced by the participants), then self-reports and community crime statistics would be monitored. Usually questions of evaluation focus on the areas of relevancy, progress, cost efficiency, effectiveness, and outcome.

Relevancy

Is there a need for the program? Relevancy determines the reasons for having a program or set of activities. Questions of relevancy may be more important for existing programs than for new programs. Frequently, a program is planned, such as a blood pressure screening, to meet an expressed community need. Then, it is continued for years without an evaluation of relevancy. The question should be asked routinely—is the program still needed? Clearly, evaluation is not necessary just for new programs but for all programs. A common constraint to beginning a new program is inadequate staff or budget. A remedy to that constraint can be a relevancy evaluation of existing programs. Staff and budgets from a program that is no longer needed can be redirected to the new program.

Progress

Are program activities following the intended plan? Are appropriate staff and materials available in the right quantity and at the right time to implement the program activities? Are expected numbers of individuals participating in the scheduled program activities? Do the inputs and outputs meet some predetermined plan? Answers to these questions measure the progress of the program and are part of process or formative evaluation.

Cost Efficiency

What are the costs of a program? What are its benefits? Are program benefits sufficient for the costs incurred? Cost-efficiency evaluation measures the relationship between the results (benefits) of a program and the costs of presenting the program (such as staff salary and materials). Cost efficiency evaluates whether the results of a program could have been obtained less expensively through another approach. Cost-benefit analysis requires skills beyond the scope of this text, but references abound, particularly in economics and management literature.

Effectiveness (Impact)

Were program objectives met? Were the participants satisfied with the program? What behaviour changed as a result of the program? Were program providers satisfied with the activities and client involvement? Effectiveness focuses on formative evaluation as well as the immediate, short-term results.

Outcome

What are the long-term implications of the program? As a result of the program, what changes in quality of life or health can be expected in 6 months or 6 years? Effectiveness measures the immediate results, whereas outcome evaluation measures whether the program activities changed the initial reason for the program. The fundamental question is this: Did the program meet its goal? (Was health improved?)

Evaluation Strategies

Program "...evaluation can be defined as the consistent, ongoing collection and analysis of information for use in making decisions" (W. K. Kellogg Foundation, 1998, p 14). As such, the choice of approach or method to collect the information is an important decision in itself and needs to be agreed on by all involved from the beginning. Realize that there is no one best approach to evaluation, but whichever approach is chosen needs to "fit" the questions you wish to answer.

Selected Methods of Data Collection

Four key points need to be considered as you decide which method to use:

1. What resources are available for the evaluation tasks?
2. Is the method sensitive to the respondents/participants of the program?

3. How credible will your evaluation be as a result of this method?
4. What is the importance of the data to be collected? To the overall program? To participants? (W. K. Kellogg Foundation, 1998)

Consider, too, that there are several frameworks or paradigms that may inform your choices. A summary of five such paradigms is included in Table 13-2.

Taking the key points and paradigms into consideration, let's review the various methods of data collection: case study, surveys, experimental design, process monitoring, and cost-benefit and cost-effectiveness analyses.

Case Study

A case study looks inside a program to determine its adequacy to meet stated needs. The case-study method provides insight into an entire program and, unlike many forms of evaluation, can be started at any time during the program. The data collected during a case study include observation of program activity, reports prepared by the program, unstructured conversations with program personnel, statistical summaries of program activities, structured or unstructured interview data, and information collected through questionnaires. Subjective data and objective data can both be collected. Subjective data include information collected primarily through observations of participants or program staff. Objective data are collected from organization or program documents or structured questionnaires and interviews. The distinction between subjective and objective is not readily perceptible. All questionnaires, regardless of how carefully written, have a subjective component, and, likewise, "objective" records or documents are all written by people and, therefore, introduce a subjective factor. It is optimum to have a mix of both objective and subjective data.

OBSERVATION

Observation is one method of collecting data for a case study. Observation can be participatory or nonparticipatory. The participant observer assumes a working role in the agency or organization and collects data about the program while working within the group. The nonparticipant observer remains an "outsider," does not assume a working role within the agency, and reviews and examines the program for designated periods.

The *types* of observations that are made are determined by the questions that have been asked about the program. For example, if the question is one of rel-

TABLE 13-2 ◆ PARADIGMS FOR EVALUATION

	Natural Science Research Model	Interpretivism/ Constructivism	Feminist Methods	Participatory Evaluation	Theory-Based
Roots	Western "science"; European, white, male	Anthropology	Feminist research, power analysis	Education, community organization, public health, anthropology	Application in comprehensive community programs
Key points	Control of variables	Study through ongoing and in-depth contact with those involved	Women, girls, and minorities historically left out; conventional methods are seriously flawed	Create a more egalitarian process, make process more relevant to all, democratizing	Every social program is based on a theory—the key to understanding what is important is through identifying the theory
Approach	Hypothetico-deductive methodology, statistics	In-depth observations, interviewing	Contextual, inclusive, experiential, involved, socially relevant	Practical, useful, empowering	Developing a program logic model—or picture—to describe what works
Purpose	To explain what happened and show causal relationships between outcomes and "treatments"	To understand the targets of the program and the program's meaning to them	To include the feminine voice in all aspects of evaluation, being open to all voices	Actively engage all in process, capacity building	Revealing what works in comprehensive, community-based programs

From W. K. Kellogg Foundation. (1998). *Evaluation handbook.* Battle Creek, MI: Author; Minkler, M. (Ed.). (1997). *Community organizing and community building for health.* New Brunswick, NJ: Rutgers University Press.

evancy, the observer would concentrate on the "who, what, why, and when" of the program. Who is using the services? Record the demographics of age, ethnicity, geographic location, educational level, and employment status. What services are the participants receiving? (For example, what services are offered in the well-child clinic? Immunizations? Physicals? Health teaching? Screening? How often are the services offered, and what are the ages of the children who use the services?) Why is the population using the offered services? (Availability? Affordability? No other options?) Lastly, when are the services accessed? (Do people come at appointed times or only when they are ill? Or do people tend to cluster at opening and closing times?)

Some data can be collected from agency records; other information can be collected by informal conversations with the participants—both the professional health care providers and the clients. When interviewing, always have a checklist of topics you want to consider, arranged in a logical sequence, along with the who, what, why, and when questions. Unstructured interviews in the form of informal conversations afford the opportunity to explore with the participants their perceptions of the program. The results of unstructured interviews provide specific areas from which a "structured" interview can be developed. Recall from Chapter 11 that an interviewer conducts the interview, whereas a questionnaire is self-administered. Observations and interviews share the criticisms of selective perception and interactiveness.

1. *Selective perception* is the natural tendency of everyone to consciously classify into categories the behaviours or statements of others. These categories have been established by our cultural values, learning, and life experiences. To a certain extent, this process is desirable because it limits the number of observations that need conscious consideration and permits the rapid and effective handling of information. For example, if it were observed that a client waited 1 hour for a scheduled appointment, most people, based on the common orientation to time, would classify that observation as a negative aspect of the clinic's functioning.

   Herein lies the major problem of selective perception. Statements and behaviours are classified according to the selective perception of the observer, which may be completely different from the selective perception of the client or provider. The most dangerous effect of selective perception in program evaluation is when the observer has a *preconception* that a program will be successful or unsuccessful. This can produce a self-fulfilling prophecy because the biased observer may unconsciously record only data that support the preconceived belief. Both selective perception and self-fulfilling prophecy are sources of subjective data. Perhaps the most important point is that you should be aware of the problem of selective perception and share your observation and interview data with a mixed group of clients and providers. Ask the group for categorization and summation implications.

2. *Interactiveness* is an additional event to be aware of during all observations. When an observer, whether participant or nonparticipant, observes and records program activities, the person's presence affects and shapes the activities observed. Productivity may increase because staff members are aware of being observed or because they are concerned about client satisfaction or dissatisfaction. All evaluation strategies can have an interactive component, but perhaps the interactive consideration is strongest in case studies because of the presence of an observer.

Two additional techniques of the case-study method are nominal group and Delphi technique. (References to both techniques and examples of their application are presented at the end of this chapter in the Suggested Readings.) Both techniques are based on the belief that the individuals in a program are the most knowledgeable sources on its relevancy.

NOMINAL GROUP

The nominal group technique uses a structured group meeting, during which all individuals are given a judgmental task, such as to list the functions of the program, problems of the program, or needed changes in the program. Each member is asked to write a response on paper and to not discuss it with other people. At the end of 5 to 10 minutes, all members present their ideas, and each idea is recorded (without discussion) so everyone can see all the suggestions. Once all ideas have been presented, a discussion is begun, during which ideas are clarified and evaluated. After the discussion, a vote is held to determine the order in which the group wants to address different areas. The nominal group technique allows all individuals to present their ideas before the entire group. Involving the entire group both decreases selective perception and promotes individual cooperation with the group's decisions because people believe they have been involved in the decision-making process.

DELPHI TECHNIQUE

The Delphi technique tends to be used in large survey studies but is also useful as a case-study method. It involves a series of questionnaires and feedback reports to a designated panel of respondents. An initial questionnaire is distributed by mail to a preselected group (this could be all staff members, a group of clients, or program administrators). Independently, respondents express their thoughts through the questionnaire and return it. Based on the responses of the group, a feedback report and a revised version of the questionnaire are sent to the respondents. Using the feedback information, the respondents evaluate their first answers and complete the questionnaire again. The process continues for a predetermined number of feedback rounds.

USEFULNESS OF THE CASE-STUDY APPROACH TO EVALUATION

The case-study method of program evaluation can help answer questions of *relevance*. Questioning clients and health care providers helps explore perceptions of how well the program is meeting its defined goals as well as ascertaining problem areas and possible solutions. The case-study method would not point to any one solution but rather would offer several possible choices.

Questions of *progress* can also be addressed through the case-study method. The extent to which a program is meeting predetermined standards of service indicates progress. Because the case study provides an examination of the program, much can be learned if program activities are already in place.

Cost efficiency of the program is difficult to evaluate using a case-study method. First, to evaluate if the program could have been offered more economically, a comparable program must exist, and second, the case-study method is designed to look at only one program. The method is not formatted to look at two programs and compare them. However, judgments can be made as to the operating efficiency of the program. These must be based on the experience and knowledge of the evaluator and cannot be based on comparisons with other operating programs.

Effectiveness determines if the program has produced what it intended to produce immediately after the program, as opposed to outcome, which measures long-term consequences. Although the case-study method may determine aspects of effectiveness, such as whether the aims of the program have been met in the short run, it is very difficult to measure long-term consequences unless the case-study method is conducted over a long period that allows a longitudinal or retrospective view of the program.

Surveys

A survey is a method of collecting information and can be used to collect evaluation information. Surveys are usually completed by self-administered questionnaires (the process used in DT5 to determine residents' perceptions of community health challenges) or by personal interviews. Surveys are formulated to describe (descriptive surveys) or to analyze relationships (analytic surveys). (Actually, most surveys can be used to both describe and to analyze.)

Surveys can be used to describe the need for a program, the actual operations of a program, or a program's effects. Along with the descriptive information, questions of analysis can be answered through a survey. For example, a survey could be used to describe the composition of the groups that attend crime prevention or weight reduction classes as well as to analyze the relationship between descriptive data of sex and weight reduction success.

Surveys are usually performed for *summative* (impact) evaluation. Did the program accomplish what it was proposed to do? Do clients perceive the program as successful? Program personnel? If the program was considered successful, what parts were most helpful? Least helpful? What should be changed? Left unchanged? The questions asked by the survey are determined by the initial list of questions about program evaluation.

Like the case-study method, the answers on surveys come from the perceptions, values, and belief systems of the respondents. The response given to questions of program usefulness by the team that planned and implemented the program may be very different from the answers of the participants. Awareness of perception bias can direct evaluation efforts to consider the perceptions of all people (providers, clients, and management) involved in program implementation.

Surveys that are used to measure program evaluation must be concerned with the reliability and validity of the information collected. *Reliability* deals with the repeatability, or reproducibility, of the data (i.e., if the same questions were asked of the same people 1 week later, would the same responses be recorded?). *Validity* is the correctness of the information. If questions are written to evaluate knowledge, and the answers of the respondents reflect behaviours, then the questions are not valid because they do not measure what they claim to measure.

USEFULNESS OF SURVEYS TO EVALUATION

Surveys can be very valuable to answer questions of *relevance*, or the need for proposed or existing programs, especially if the perceptions of clients, providers, and management are solicited. In like fashion, *progress* can be measured. People critiquing surveys as an evaluation strategy may be concerned with the subjectivity of the survey—indeed, individual perception affects every response to every question. However, most decisions are based on subjective judgments, not objective reality. The important concern is to understand whose subjective impression is being used as a basis for judgment; it is imperative for community health workers to ensure that clients' perceptions are represented alongside those of health care providers and management.

Cost efficiency, effectiveness, and *outcome* are difficult to measure by using a survey. Although a survey can measure the perceived efficiency of the program or the acceptability of ideas on alternative ways of operating to make the program more cost efficient, these perceptions are formed only in the context of the existing program. There is no other comparison program against which recorded perceptions can be measured. A survey can provide information on the characteristics of program activities that are perceived by the respondents to have caused changes in their health status, but these impressions are reported in the absence of any comparison group. A comparison group is especially important with regard to effectiveness and impact because it is impossible to tell if an alternative program (or no program at all) might have been more or less effective in accomplishing the same objectives.

 TAKE NOTE

You may be wondering—if a comparison group is so important and if perceptions cloud the evaluation with subjective impressions, then why use surveys at all? Two pluses exist in surveys: a great deal of information for program evaluation can be obtained, especially about the activities of the program from the perception of several groups; and important evaluation data can be inferred if the instrument (questionnaire or interview schedule) is reliable and valid.

Experimental Design

Completed correctly, an experimental study can provide an answer to the crucial questions: Did the program make a difference? Are health behaviours, knowledge, and attitudes changed as a result of the program activities? Is the community healthier because of the programs offered by the Inner City Health Promotion Council? However, the problem with experimental studies in program evaluation is that they require selective implementation, meaning that people who participate are selected through a process such as random assignment to a control group and an experimental group. For many ethical, political, and community health reasons, selective implementation is difficult to complete and is sometimes impossible. Despite these problems, the experimental study remains one of the better methods to evaluate summative effects (outcomes) of a program and the only way to produce quantified information on whether the program made a difference.

✎ TAKE NOTE

Reviewing the steps of the research process at this point may be of help to you in understanding the examples to follow. Indeed, each issue—such as a theoretical framework, sampling, reliability, and validity—must be addressed if an experimental design is proposed for evaluation.

The following designs are the most feasible and appropriate to health care settings. Apply the research process to each design.

PRETEST–POSTTEST ONE-GROUP DESIGN

The pretest–posttest design applied to one group is illustrated in Table 13-3. Two observations are made, the first at Time 1 and the second at Time 2. The observation can be the prevalence of a health state (e.g., the percentage of adults in the downtown that exercise regularly, brush their teeth three times daily, or drink alcohol [beer, wine, liquor] more than five times a week; the teenage pregnancy rate; number of reported cases of domestic abuse, etc.), knowledge scores, or other important facts in the community. Between Time 1 and Time 2, an "experiment" is introduced. The experiment may be a planned program aimed at a target group, such as teen sexuality classes, or an intervention with a community-wide focus, like a crime prevention program. The evaluation of the program is measured by considering the difference between the health state at Time 1 and the health state after the program at Time 2.

If the experiment in Table 13-3 was teen sexuality classes for 10th-grade girls at Hampton High School, Time 1 was a teen pregnancy rate of 5/100, and Time 2 (1 year later) was a teen pregnancy rate of 3/100 among the girls taking the classes, then would you agree that the teen sexuality program was responsible for the decrease in teenage pregnancies? What other information do you need to know to

---

TABLE 13-3 ◆ PRETEST–POSTTEST ONE-GROUP DESIGN

	Time 1		Time 2
Experimental group	Observation 1	Experiment	Observation 2

decide? Are there other factors that could account for the decrease in the teen pregnancy rate? Perhaps family-planning programs have been focused on teenagers, or maybe local churches and social service agencies have sponsored teen sexuality programs. Teen access and use of contraceptive methods may have increased, or laws regarding teen access to contraceptive methods may have changed. None of these factors can be eliminated on the grounds of not being associated with the decrease in the teen pregnancy rate. To eliminate other possible explanations for program effectiveness, a control group must be added.

PRETEST–POSTTEST TWO-GROUP DESIGN

A pretest–posttest with a control group design is illustrated in Table 13-4. The design has both an experimental group and a control group. At Time 1, an observation is made of both the experimental and control groups. Between Time 1 and Time 2, an experiment is introduced with the experimental group. At Time 2, second observations are made on both the experimental and control groups. Program evaluation is the difference between Observations 1 and 2 for the experimental group when compared to the comparison (control) group (which has been selected to be as similar as possible to the experimental group). Will the pretest–posttest with a control group design eliminate the effect of outside factors that occurred simultaneously with the experiment and that might account for the change between Observation 1 and Observation 2, the very problem that plagued the pretest–posttest one-group design? The answer is yes, if the experimental and control groups are similar.

To explain, let's return to the idea of a teen sexuality class for 10th-grade students at Hampton High School. If a group of 10th-grade students, similar in social, economic, and geographic characteristics, were randomly selected and then randomly assigned to the experimental or control group, then it could be assumed that any other factors that influenced the experimental group would also affect the control group. However, frequently the decision is made that all students must be given the same program, thereby eliminating a comparison group. At the Health Promotion Council, when the information was received that all 10th graders must be given a teen sexuality program that had been proposed by the school nurse as a response to an increasing number of teen preg-

TABLE 13-4 ◆ PRETEST–POSTTEST TWO-GROUP DESIGN

	Time 1		Time 2
Experimental group	Observation 1	Experiment	Observation 2
Control group	Observation 1		Observation 2

nancies, the suggestion was made that perhaps another high school could be used as a control group. How would you respond to that suggestion? Perhaps another high school class of 10th graders could be used, if the students were similar in social, economic, and geographic characteristics to the students at Hampton High (an unlikely situation).

Another possibility mentioned by the Health Promotion Council was to offer the program in one school year to one half of the Hampton High 10th graders (using the other half as a control) and then in the following year to offer the program to the remaining students. This method would ensure that all students would be given the program but would also allow for an experimental pretest–posttest design for evaluation.

A third method that was suggested to ensure an experimental design was to give the control group sexuality education and give the experimental group sexuality education plus assertiveness training. The assertiveness training would differentiate the groups and allow an experimental design. All the suggestions were discussed with school officials, and it was decided to offer a traditional sex education class to half the 10th-grade students (the control group); the remaining students (the experimental group) would get the traditional sex education material but would also receive classes on assertiveness training and values clarification. This design will not allow for evaluation of traditional sex education classes versus no information, but it will provide all students with the health information (an ethical compromise) and allow for evaluation of a traditional program on sexuality versus that traditional program plus assertiveness and values clarification information (an approach to reduce teenage pregnancies that is supported in the literature).

✎ TAKE NOTE

Notice that the decision to offer information on assertiveness and values clarification as part of teen sexuality classes was based on documentation from the literature. Hampton High School is not the first school to offer health promotion programs. Many schools and communities have assessed the status and perceived needs of their publics and have followed up by planning and implementing programs that have been evaluated, and have reported their findings and results in the literature. One contribution that the community health team can make is to do a literature review about the ways in which other communities have addressed and evaluated similar programs, review and synthesize the results of these programs, and present this information to the community to use when making choices and decisions.

USEFULNESS OF THE EXPERIMENTAL DESIGN TO EVALUATION

An experimental design can yield data on whether a program has produced the desired *outcomes* when compared to the absence of such a program or, alternatively, whether one program strategy has produced better results with regard to the desired outcomes than some other strategy. However, the experimental design is not useful for evaluation of program progress or program cost efficiency.

Monitoring (Process)

Monitoring measures the difference between the program plan and what has actually happened. Monitoring focuses on the sequence of activities of the program, specifically, how the program is to be implemented (the activities), by whom (the personnel and other resources), and when (the timing of activities). Monitoring is usually done with a chart, and, although there are several different styles of charts, all arrange activities in a sequence and specify the time allotted to complete each task. In Chapter 11, Figure 11-2 illustrated one form of calendar chart for planning purposes. Figure 13-1 provides another example of a calendar chart that illustrates the sequencing of events in a program.

MONITORING CHARTS

To construct a monitoring chart for your program plan, information is needed on the inputs (resources necessary to carry out the program such as personnel, equipment, and finances), the process (the program activities, their sequencing, and timing) and outputs (the expected results of the program, including immediate and long-term health effects). It is helpful to make a list of inputs, processes, and outputs.

✎ TAKE NOTE

You have already recorded this information as part of your program plan. Refer to Chapter 11 and note that resources, program activities, and objectives were listed in the logic model. Resources are the same as inputs; program activities correspond to processes; and objectives designate expected outputs or outcomes. You may have also made calendar charts of the detailed processes for each program component as detailed in Chapter 11. So all that remains is to plot implementation information (i.e., what *actually* happened) onto the existing calendar chart for monitoring purposes—to see if activities happened on time, by the people who were assigned, and what effects (if any) the context had on the schedule.

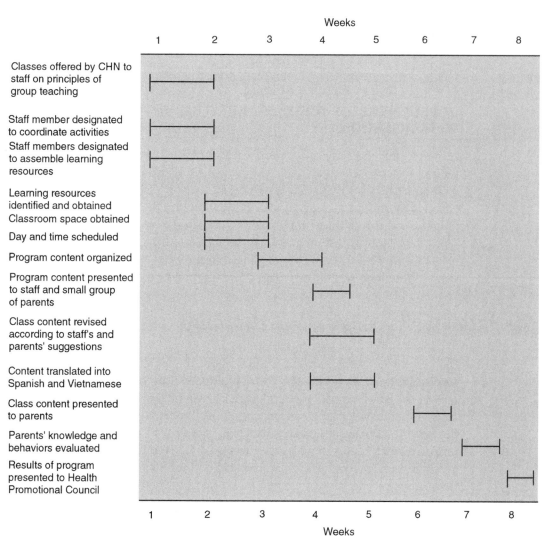

Figure 13-1 ◆ Sequence of events for program: Common health problems of children.

It is difficult to decide on the amount of time that will be needed to complete any task. After assessing the organizational structure and management methods of the agency, you determined the approximate amounts of time that would be needed to complete the activities of the program. Do not be surprised if you made errors in your estimates. With experience, you will begin to be more accurate in gauging time requirements for specific activities. Evaluation data will be valuable to future estimates. The Suggested Readings list at the end of this chapter includes references to several other types of monitoring charts, including the Gantt, Program Evaluation and Review Technique (PERT), and Critical Path Method (CPM). These provide a slightly different variation of the basic time-sequencing, activities-monitoring charts that appear in Figures 11-2 and 13-1.

USEFULNESS OF PROCESS MONITORING TO EVALUATION

A monitoring chart measures progress and can be used to evaluate whether a program is on schedule and within budget. Perhaps no other evaluation method is as perfectly suited to *process* evaluation as the monitoring chart. In addition, monitoring can provide information on the *cost efficiency* of the program by measuring the average cost of the resources required per client served. The *effectiveness* of the program can be measured by monitoring if the chart records outputs achieved. Monitoring charts cannot determine program relevance or the long-term impact of a program, however.

Cost-Benefit and Cost-Effectiveness Analyses

Much has been written and discussed about the escalating cost of health care services and on ways that cost can be reduced. The turmoil over health care reform in Canadian provinces and the intense debate regarding the pros and cons of various alternative approaches to health care delivery are testimony to the need to contain cost and yet increase access and maintain quality. Every program has a dollar price both in terms of the resources needed to offer the program (e.g., personnel and equipment) and the dollar benefits to be gained from improved health (e.g., increased worker productivity).

Two of the most common methods of analyzing the economic costs and benefits of a program are cost-benefit analysis (CBA) and cost-effectiveness analysis (CEA). Both CBA and CEA are formal analytic techniques that list all costs (direct and indirect) and consequences (negative and positive) of a particular program. The distinction between CBA and CEA is based on the value that is placed on the consequences of a program. In CBA, consequences or benefits of a program are valued in dollar terms; this makes it possible to compare different projects because all measurement is made in dollars. Therefore, the worth of a project can be judged by asking if dollar benefits exceed dollar costs and, if so, by how much. In contrast, CEA does not place a dollar value on either the consequences or the costs of a project. Another outcome is used for programs whose benefits or costs are difficult to measure. (For example, how could a dollar value be placed on each suicide prevented by a primary prevention program to decrease teenage suicide?) Therefore, CEA, unlike CBA, does not determine if total benefits exceed total costs.

However, CEA can be used to compare programs with similar goals and objectives. (For example, two different primary prevention approaches to decrease the incidence of teenage suicide share the same benefits, so only costs need be compared—a CEA.) A CEA can also be used if the costs of alternative programs are the same or if only a given amount of money exists and the objective is to select the program with the greatest benefits (not measured in dollar terms). The decision is obvious—select the program that produces the most effectiveness; that is, the most benefits per dollar spent or the least cost for each unit (individual, family, or community) benefited.

The choice between CBA and CEA depends on the type of questions and programs considered. Neither technique is superior to the other. Both techniques can be used in planning for future programs or as an evaluation strategy of present or past programs. The actual procedures for completing a CBA or CEA are beyond the scope of this book; however, several references that include the procedural steps are listed in the Suggested Readings list. Obviously, both CBA and CEA are strategies for measuring program cost efficiency and do not address the issues of relevancy, progress, effectiveness, or impact.

Summary

Several methods of evaluation have been presented and discussed. No one method will evaluate components of relevancy, progress, cost efficiency, effectiveness, and outcome equally well. It is important to be knowledgeable about different methods of program evaluation and to discuss the benefits and limitations of each with the community as the program is being planned and before program implementation occurs. Table 13-5 presents a summary table of appropriate evaluation methods for program components. Once evaluation methods

TABLE 13-5 ◆ EXAMINATION OF THE APPROPRIATENESS OF DIFFERENT EVALUATION METHODS FOR PROGRAM COMPONENTS

Components	Method			
	Case Study	Survey	Experimental	Monitoring
Relevancy	Yes	Yes	No	No
Progress	Yes	Yes	No	Yes
Cost efficiency	No	No	Yes	Yes
Cost effectiveness	Some	No	Yes	Some
Impact	No	No	Yes	No

are selected, then the methods (case study, experimental design, or process monitoring) become part of the program plan.

You may be wondering which evaluation methods were used to evaluate health promotion programs in downtown Calgary. A variety of strategies were used. To evaluate the relevancy of the crime prevention program, nominal group meetings were scheduled, and both human service providers (e.g., police service, public health, social services, community outreach agencies) and residents of the community attended. In addition, the utilization rates and demographics of the participants in the various crime prevention activities were assessed, as were the participants' perceptions of the value of the information. Crime reports and arrest and conviction data are being logged to determine if crime rates reveal a downward trend over time for the neighbourhoods in the program.

For the "Nobody's Perfect" program in Connaught, program progress was evaluated with monitoring charts; the effectiveness and impact of the program on individuals were evaluated with knowledge, attitude, and behavioural intent surveys (e.g., questionnaires) given to participants before the program began, immediately after the program ended, and at predetermined follow-up times (6 weeks and 3 months). As well, satisfaction was measured to make decisions about program adaptations that could be made before the next session was planned.

In both instances, costs were calculated, both real and in-kind, to determine the ongoing budget that would be needed to sustain the programs and perhaps expand to other communities as needs warranted. To assess impact, further data are required to measure and interpret the consequences (benefit and effectiveness) of the programs on the communities involved and the health of families and individuals residing there.

When providing a final report of your evaluation to the community, you will inevitably be asked to make recommendations for future action. This must be done with caution, and in consultation with the key stakeholders in community action—politicians, funders, informal leaders, local businesses, and the residents themselves. To help prevent people from taking offence, refer to community diagnoses and problems from a *positive* or *wellness* perspective, acknowledge the limitations as well as the strengths of the data collection processes, and defer to the wisdom of those who live in the community when suggesting future interventions.

One approach many evaluators find useful is to do a SWOT (strengths, weaknesses, opportunities, threats) analysis and use this to frame recommendations. For instance, the fact that residents were willing to bear the costs of leaving outdoor lights on all night (strength) could be used to overcome the darkness in the back alleys (weakness) that allowed drug deals and prostitution to occur. The risk of parental stress and consequent child abuse in a community with a high number of single-parent families (threat) was balanced by the opportunity for the community to come together to create healthy environments for child development and family support—school providing space for a parenting program, students volunteering for child care, and service agencies and businesses in the area supporting the initiative in many ways. Recommendations can take community strengths and opportunities into account when making recommendations for action against perceived weaknesses and threats.

You are ready now for program implementation and the reinitiation of the community process, namely, assessment of the program's effects. As you implement the planned program, data will be added to the community assessment profile, which will demand addition, deletion, and revision of the community diagnoses and the associated program plans and interventions. Let's take a final look at the community-as-partner model (see Fig. 8-2) and ask: Will the planned programs assist the community to attain, regain, maintain, and promote health? Strengthen the community's ability to resist stressors? Enhance the community's competence and self-reliance?

✎ TAKE NOTE

It is fitting that the final chapter of this section on the application of the community process in practice ends with questions. Community practice is the constant questioning, prodding, probing, and pondering of the health status of a population. Although individual and family health status are always important, the uniqueness of our field is the application of multidisciplinary professional practice techniques to the health and well being of a community. Each community is unique and special. There is no other community quite like the one in which you are practising!

References

Dignan, M. B., & Carr, P. A. (1992). *Program planning for health education and promotion* (2nd ed.). Philadelphia: Lea & Febiger.

Fetterman, D. M., Kaftarian, S. J., & Wandersman, A. (Eds.). (1996). *Empowerment evaluation: Knowledge and tools for self-assessment and accountability.* Thousand Oaks, CA: Sage.

Green, L.,W., & Lewis, F. M. (1986). *Measurement and evaluation in health education and health promotion.* Palo Alto, CA: Mayfield.

Minkler, M. (Ed.). (1997). *Community organizing and community building for health.* New Brunswick, NJ: Rutgers University Press.

Porteous, N. L., Sheldrick, B. J., & Stewart, P. J. (1997). *Program evaluation tool kit: A blueprint for public health management.* Ottawa: Public Health Research, Education and

Development Program, Ottawa-Carleton Health Department. Order form available on www.uottawa.ca/academic/med/epid/sld003.htm.

W. K. Kellogg Foundation. (1998). *Evaluation handbook*. Battle Creek, MI: Author.

Suggested Readings

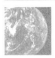

Allen, J. (1993). Impact of the cholesterol education program for nurses: A pilot program evaluation. *Cardiovascular Nursing, 29*(1), 1–5.

Birch, S. (1990). The relative cost effectiveness of water fluoridation across communities: Analysis of variations according to underlying caries levels. *Community Dental Health, 7*(1), 3–10.

Ervin, N. (2002). *Advanced community health nursing practice*. Upper Saddle River, NJ: Prentice Hall.

Finnegan, J. R., Murray, D. M., Kurth, C., & McCarthy, P. (1989). Measuring and tracking education program implementation: The Minnesota Heart Health Program experience. *Health Education Quarterly, 16*(1), 77–90.

Helvie, C. O. (1998). *Advanced practice nursing in the community*. Thousand Oaks, CA: Sage.

Horne, T. E. (1995). *Making a difference: Program evaluation for health promotion*. Edmonton: WellQuest Consulting. Available from tamhorne@web.net.

Kohler, C. L., Dolce, J. J., Manzella, B. A., Higgins, D., & Brooks, C. M. (1993). Use of focus group methodology to develop an asthma self-management program useful for community-based medical practices. *Health Education Quarterly, 20*(3), 421–429.

Nas, T. F. (1996). *Cost-benefit analysis: Theory and application*. Thousand Oaks, CA: Sage.

O'Brien, K. (1993). Using focus groups to develop health surveys: An example from research on social relationships and AIDS-preventive behavior. *Health Education Quarterly, 20*(3), 361–372.

Rossi, P. H., Freeman, H. E., & Lipsey, M. W. (1998*). Evaluation: A systematic approach* (6th ed.). Thousand Oaks, CA: Sage.

Smith, C. M. (2000). Evaluation of nursing care with communities. In C. M. Smith & F. A. Maurer (Eds.), *Community health nursing: Theory and practice* (pp. 407–423). Philadelphia: Saunders.

Thompson, J. C. (1992). Program evaluation within a health promotion framework. *Canadian Journal of Public Health, 83*(suppl 1), S67-S71.

Tonglet, R., Sorogane, M., Lembo, M., WaMukalay, M., Dramaix, M., & Hennart, P. (1993). Evaluation of immunization coverage at local level. *World Health Forum, 14*(3), 275–281.

Wheeler, F. C., Lackland, D. T., Mace, M. L., Reddick, A., Hogelin, G., & Remington, P. L. (1991). Evaluating South Carolina's community cardiovascular disease prevention project. *Public Health Reports, 106*(5), 536–543.

Internet Resources

http://www.heartfoundation.com.au/sepa/contents.html

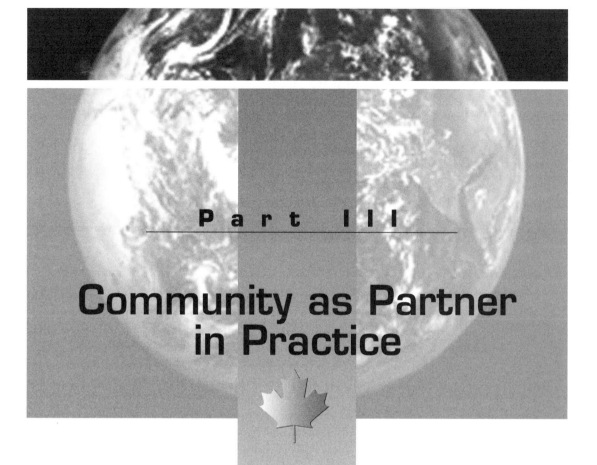

P a r t   I I I

Community as Partner
in Practice

This section is intended to serve two purposes: to offer an opportunity to share success stories and provide educators and students with case stories to study. Each author has presented a different story—of one community issue, with one target population, in one particular setting. The stories have been written with the community-as-partner model in mind, but different components of the process have been emphasized. These stories can be used to apply the model components. For instance, you can ask of each:

♦ What data represent the *community core?* Embedded within the stories are the social, economic, and demographic data relevant to the population of interest.
♦ What is the *normal line of defence?* Health status data are also contained within each story.
♦ What *stressors* are acting on the population and what *lines of resistance* are preventing them from invading the community core?
♦ What *flexible lines of defence* have been erected to preserve the integrity of the core when stressors have affected the health of the community?

Additionally, you can observe, vicariously, the processes undertaken in each of the stories. In each instance, assessment and analysis information is presented. Can you suggest community diagnoses from this information? Can you present them as problem statements and as positive statements? If you were involved in this project, how would you have presented diagnostic statements to the community or to funding agencies?

As you read about the interventions, are you able to discern the logic models inherent in the approach and activities? Are the indicators and evaluation processes coherent?

Critical reflection is an important component of learning. Reflection demands that we use various lenses to critique what we hear, see, and read. Using lenses of population health promotion (Chap. 1) and epidemiology and demography (Chap. 2), the authors have presented narratives of community practice that represent advocacy and ethical practice (Chap. 5) based on principles of public participation, partnerships, and accountability through evaluation.

This section is enriched by the addition of several chapters that have been generously contributed by authors in the fourth edition of the original publication by Elizabeth (Bets) Anderson and Judith McFarlane. These chapters reflect community practice in a variety of other settings and with other populations, written not as case studies but as information vehicles that overview a specific population group or setting, present salient issues regarding health/determinants of health, suggest opportunities for multidisciplinary population health promotion, and refer the reader to sites and references in the Canadian domain for further information.

There are many additional settings and population groups of interest to the Canadian community health worker. This section presents a small number of contributions for the reader to consider. I hope it will inspire you to do three things: inspire you to try new strategies in your community practice, share your stories (successes and challenges) with others, and be inspired to contribute to the next edition of this Canadian publication.

14

Community Profile:
Exemplar Health District

OBJECTIVES

After studying this chapter, you should be able to:

◆ Appreciate how large amounts of community assessment data can be displayed

◆ Understand how summary statements and inferences can be incorporated into text

◆ Recognize the utility of local, regional, and national data for comparison purposes

Introduction

This is a fictional case example that makes use of data available from various sources: Statistics Canada, Health Canada, Human Resources Development Canada, and others. No citations are given because the data have been adapted for presentation in this example and no provincial or local identifiers are used.

The current environment for the health professional, community board, citizen, and elected official in deciding health policy and expenditures is a challenging one. The cost of health care in the Province has been rising more rapidly than income and the cost of living. Public policy, at both the national and provincial levels, is clearly aimed at managing the debt and deficit.

These and other forces, such as reconceptualization of health from sickness care to wellness and health, the interest in coordinated local/regional decision-making, a more knowledgeable consumer, and so forth are causing health districts to initiate processes that will assess and improve the health of its citizens. One component of the process is the gathering of information on the health of residents. The purpose of this report is to gather data as it pertains to the health of residents in the geographic area of the Exemplar Health District (EHD).

The first issue that arises is, "What is an appropriate definition of health?" Increasingly, the trend is to a broader definition such as the one noted herein: health is a state of physical, mental, emotional, social, and spiritual well-being.

In deciding on the measures one might use to describe the health of a region and the categories is which data should be grouped, a review of similar studies and of health indicator literature was undertaken. The framework chosen for this project is a simple one with four categories of which only the first three are covered in this report:

◆ Demographic profile: a description of the population of the Health District, including data on birth rates, age, family characteristics, and so forth
◆ Determinants of health: socioeconomic, environmental, and lifestyle indicators such as measures of income, employment, social supports, and alcohol consumption
◆ Health status indicators: objective and subjective measures of well-being such as causes of death, dental health, communicable diseases, and mental health
◆ Health care system: descriptors of the health system, policies, use and cost, for example, inventory of health care facilities, medical services offered, actual services provided, patient days, and cost effectiveness

Where possible we have sought to obtain 10-year data and compare the information for the Health District geographic area with data for the Province. As might be expected, the desired information was not always available. Sometimes there was a problem in obtaining data for this length of time for the geographic area of the EHD, or the most recent data from the 2001 Canada Census was not published. This is not an unusual situation with which community workers must contend; census surveys are undertaken in different years and on different cycles for municipal, federal, or other purposes. Then there is a time lag between the collection of information and its publication. During this time the data are entered and statisticians prepare it for release, ensuring the accuracy of the data, the appropriateness of the display methods, and the relevance of the interpretations of the data.

Demographic Data

Population

The population in the EHD geographic area has decreased from 29,305 in 1991 to 27,525 in 2001. The Health District contributed 1.3% of the Province's total population in 1991 but decreased to 1.08% in 2001. The population growth is detailed in Figure 14-1; you will notice that the bars go below zero, indicating net population loss in Exemplar. Comparatively, the Province had a net population gain.

Age Distribution

In comparison to the Province, the Health District area's population has a much higher concentration of seniors (Fig. 14-2). However, the percentage of people in the Health District geographic area over 65 years of age has declined over the last 10 years from approximately 24% to 19% of the total population.

Birth and Death Rates

Because of the preponderance of seniors, the death rate in the Health District area has been higher than the provincial average. The death rate in the Health District geographic area has been increasing over the 10-year period (1991–2001), while the rate in the Province is remaining fairly constant.

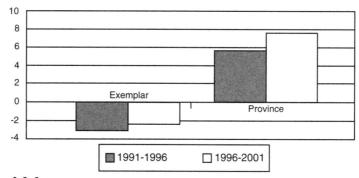

Figure 14-1 ◆ Population growth for the Exemplar Health District geographical area and Province, 1991–1996 and 1996–2001.

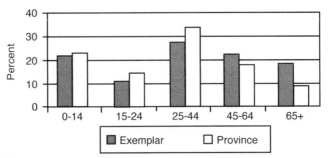

Figure 14-2 ◆ Population distribution by age category for the Exemplar Health District geographical area and Province, 2001.

The birth rate per thousand population has been correspondingly lower in EHD than in the Province. In 2001, the birth rate per thousand population was 13.70 in the Health District and 16.64 in the Province. However, women in the Health District geographic area are giving birth at the same rates as women in other regions of the Province. In 2001, there were approximately 54 babies born per thousand girls/women aged 10 to 49 in both the Province and the EHD geographic area.

Occupational Distribution

Generally, in 1996, approximately half of the EHD geographic area work force is employed in farming or processing occupations compared to about 30% in the Province (Fig. 14-3). The number of persons employed in the professional/managerial type occupations increased from 1991 to 1996 (the most current

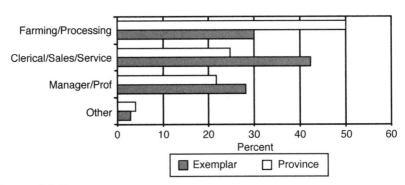

Figure 14-3 ◆ Occupational distribution for the Exemplar Health District geographical area and Province, 1996.

information available). There are more women than men in the clerical/sales/service professions in both the Province and the Health District geographic area, although there are more people in those professions in the Exemplar area than in the Province.

Single-Parent Families

The number of single-parent families in the EHD geographic area as a percentage of all families is lower than in the Province: 7.65% for the Health District in 2001 compared to 12.4% for the Province. Female-led single-parent families represent approximately 75% of all single-parent families in the EHD geographic area as compared to 82% for the Province.

Young Age and Old Age Dependency Ratios

A dependency ratio is the expression of the number of persons belonging to a certain age category of the population who are dependent on the "working population" (persons 15–64 years of age).

The young age dependency ratio (YADR) is those aged 0 to 14 expressed as a percent of those aged 15 to 64. In the EHD geographic area the YADR was 39.4 in 1991 and declined to 38.5 in 2001. In the Province, the YADR was 35.3 in 1991 and 35.1 in 2001. That is, there is .35 of a child for each adult (15–64), in 1991. The YADR in the EHD geographic area is only moderately higher.

The old age dependency ratio (OADR) is those aged 65+ expressed as a percentage of those aged 15 to 64. The OADR for the EHD geographic area in 1991 was 25 and rose to 28.8 in 1996 and to 32.4 in 2001. The Province OADR in 1991 was 10.7, 11.9 in 1996, and 13.5 in 2001. This means that the working population in the Health District geographic area "supports" about 2.5 times more seniors than the number supported by 15- to 64-year-olds in the Province as a whole.

Living Status of Persons 65 and Older

The biggest difference between the living status of those persons 65 and older in the EHD geographic area and the Province is the number of nonfamily persons living alone. As illustrated in Figure 14-4, 32% of those persons 65 and older in the Health District are living alone compared to 29% in the Province.

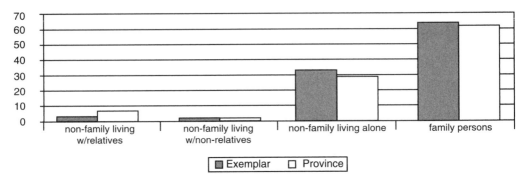

Figure 14-4 ◆ Living status of persons 65+ as a percentage of total persons 65+ for the Exemplar Health District geographical area and the Province, 2001.

This suggests that more seniors are living without family or companion support in the Health District area than in the Province.

Health Determinants

Income

The EHD geographic area had the lowest average private household income of all the Health Districts in the Province as of 1996. The average private household income for provincial Health Districts in 1996 was $36,800 in contrast to $28,784 in Exemplar.

The median income per tax filer in 1996 was lower in Exemplar ($14,943) than in both the Province ($19,900) and Canada ($19,200), as illustrated in Figure 14-5.

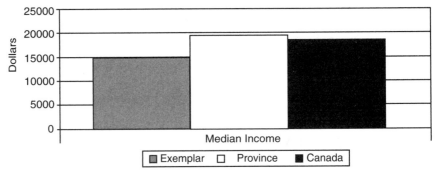

Figure 14-5 ◆ Median income in dollars for the Exemplar Health District geographical area, the Province, and Canada, 1996.

Levels of Education

In the EHD geographic area in 1991, 25.8% of the population 15 years of age and over had less than grade 9 education (12.7% for the Province) and 9.1% had university education (18.4% for the Province). These figures are illustrated graphically in Figure 14-6.

The percentage of people with some university education increased from 8.1% in 1991 to 11% in 1996. The percentage of people with less than a grade 9 education declined from 25.8% in 1991 to 22% in 1996, a change that is possibly related to a reduction in the number of older, less educated citizens. The proportion of people with more than a grade 9 education but no university education also increased slightly from 65.1% in 1991 to 67.1% in 1996.

Labour Force

The EHD experiences a higher unemployment rate than the Province or the nation, with similar participation and employment rates as the national average. However, in comparison to the Province, these rates are somewhat depressed.

The *unemployment rate* is the percentage of the labour force that actively seeks work but is unable to find work at a given time. Discouraged workers—persons who are not seeking work because they believe the prospects of finding it are extremely poor—are not counted as unemployed or as part of the labour force.

$$\text{Unemployment rate} = \frac{\text{Number of unemployed people}}{\text{Number of people in the labour force}} \times 100$$

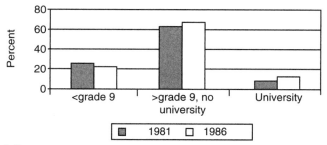

Figure 14-6 ◆ Levels of education for the Exemplar Health District geographical area, 1991 and 1996.

The number of persons unemployed is not the same thing as the number of people receiving employment insurance (EI, formerly unemployment insurance) benefits, because not all unemployed people are eligible for those benefits and some people receiving EI benefits for things like maternity leave and fishing benefits may not be considered unemployed.

The labour force *participation rate* is a measure of the extent of an economy's working-age population that is economically active; it provides an indication of the relative size of the supply of labour available for the production of goods and services. The labour force participation rate is calculated by expressing the number of persons in the labour force as a percentage of the working-age population. The labour force is the sum of the number of persons employed and the number unemployed. The working-age population is the population above age 15.

The employment rate—also called the employment-to-population ratio—is the percentage of working-age people who have jobs. For example, in 2001, there were 24.6 million Canadians of working age (aged 15 years and over). Of those, 15.1 million were employed full-time or part-time. The employment rate was therefore 61.2%.

The *employment rate* denominator is the source population, not the labour force. The source population includes all working-age people not in the military or institutions, but the labour force includes only those persons who either have a job or are looking for one. In 2001, the latter number was 16 million people. Whereas the source population grows fairly steadily from one year to the next, the labour force tends to fluctuate as persons become encouraged or discouraged by prevailing economic conditions. The employment rate shows a country's ability to put its population to work and thereby generate income for its citizens. Countries with higher employment rates are likely to have higher standards of living, other things being equal. As you can see from Table 14-1, Exemplar's unemployment rate is nearly double that of the Province, and higher than the national rate.

TABLE 14-1 ◆ UNEMPLOYMENT, PARTICIPATION, AND EMPLOYMENT RATES PERCENT FOR EHD, THE PROVINCE, AND CANADA, 2001

	EHD	Province	Canada
Unemployment rate	8.0	4.6	7.2
Participation rate	66.3	72.3	66.0
Employment rate	61.0	69.0	61.2

At present the number of active EI claimants in the Province is 130,000 people, a number typical of the last several years. The two largest cities each have about 40,000 to 50,000 claimants with the remainder scattered throughout other regions of the Province.

In both the Exemplar sample area and the nearest large city region, approximately 67% of all claimants are men and 33% are women. By age, in both the Exemplar sample area and the nearest large city region, about 20% are in the 15- to 24-year age category. About 58% are in the 25- to 44-year age category and 22% are in the 45 and older category. The average length of time on EI is currently 10 to 12 weeks.

Female claimants are concentrated in the clerical, service, and health areas, whereas male claimants are most likely to be in the construction trades, transportation, and resource operations. The unemployment rate by age and sex for the province indicates that unemployment for men is higher than for women. Table 14-2 compares the rate of EI claimants in Exemplar with that of the Province in several employment categories.

TABLE 14–2 ◆ PERCENT OF REGULAR* ACTIVE CLAIMANTS BY OCCUPATION IN EHD, GEOGRAPHIC AREA AND PROVINCE, VARIOUS DATES, 2001

Title	EHD	Province
Managerial and professional	2.6	4.7
Natural sciences, English and math	2.1	3.4
Social sciences	1.8	1.2
Religion	—	—
Teaching and related	0.3	2.0
Medicine and health	4.2	1.8
Artistic, literary, and performing arts	0.3	0.8
Sport and recreation	0.3	0.4
Clerical	15.1	15.7
Sales	5.7	6.3
Service	5.6	11.1
Farming and related	2.6	2.3
Fishing, hunting, and trapping	—	—
Forestry and logging	—	0.4
Mining, oil, and gas	3.7	2.4
Processing	2.1	2.0
Machining and related	3.7	3.5
Production fabric, assembly, and repair	4.4	6.3
Construction trades	32.8	25.4
Transport equipment operation	6.3	5.5
Material handling	3.5	1.5
Other crafts and equipment operating	0.8	0.7
Occupations not elsewhere classified	1.6	2.1
ALL OCCUPATIONS	100.3	99.9

*Excludes claimants on maternity or sick leave or receiving other special benefits.

Social Allowance

Social Allowance (SA) benefits are to be used for shelter, food, clothing, and household goods. The SA program encourages independence and encourages the individual's responsibility to work toward self-sufficiency.

The SA caseload in the Province increased substantially throughout the 1990s and reached historically high rates in early 1993. There is an average 1.8 people per case. The caseload for the Exemplar Regional Office of Social Services has again shown growth in the 3 years from 1998 to 2001, as is shown in Table 14-3. There is some difficulty in interpreting these data because the social services regions are not contiguous with the health regions.

TAKE NOTE

This is a situation that often arises in community assessment; for instance, data may be available for electoral wards, but not by neighbourhood, which may include parts of several wards.

Those receiving assistance through the SA program are placed into one of five categories: the Aged (60+), Lone Parent, Physical Illness or Disability,

TABLE 14-3 ◆ SOCIAL ALLOWANCE CASES EXEMPLAR (REGION 3) REGIONAL OFFICE* BY MONTH, FY† 1997–1999			
	1997–1998	**1998–1999**	**1999–2001**
April	331	351	452
May	307	353	419
June	318	352	421
July	300	351	427
August	301	349	437
September	307	367	456
October	320	375	466
November	327	396	486
December	334	415	500
January	357	449	529
February	360	474	504
March	326	458	513
Yearly Average	324	391	468

*Approximately equals the EHD excluding an estimated 750 people in Township 4 that are covered by the Region 2 Office of Social Services.

†Fiscal year runs from April of one year to March 31 of the next year. For example, the 1997 fiscal year runs from April 1997 to March 31, 1998.

Mental Illness or Disability, and Employable. This breakdown is graphically illustrated in Figure 14-7.

Child Protection Cases

The number of child protection cases in the Province as of March 31, 2001 was 8000, whereas the number of cases being administered on that date by the Exemplar Regional Office of Social Services was 88.

Over the last decade there have been changes to the legislation as well as to the methods by which the child protection caseload is determined. The most significant legislative change was the introduction of a new Child Welfare Act. One of the aspects of the new law was the view that the families of origin are generally best able to provide the child the warmth and stability it requires. This led to a drop in the number of cases in this period.

Further, the transfer of 3500 Disabled Children's Service Agreements from the Child Protection Services caseload in 1996 further reduced the size of the Child Protection Services caseload. Hence, as of March 31, 1997, the number of Child Protection cases stood at 7684, down from 11,263 the previous year. The data prior to 1995 are not comparable to that of following years because of the changes in legislation and also because of the reorganization of health, children's, and social service regions in the Province. Table 14-4 details the number of children in protection by the legal authority that governs them.

For the first 4 years of the period (1995–2001) being covered, the Exemplar area had less than 1% of all child protection cases in the Province. However, during the last 3 years the Exemplar area has exceeded the 1% rate and hence rose above the provincial average based on population. (With the provincial population growing and the Exemplar population declining, the rate of cases

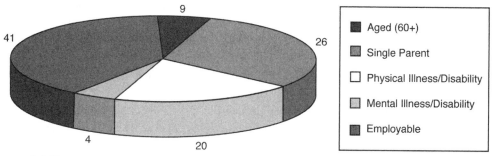

Figure 14-7 ◆ Active cases for social allowance program for the Exemplar regional office as of March 31, 2001.

TABLE 14-4 ◆ PROVINCIAL CHILD WELFARE CHILD PROTECTION CASES BY LEGAL AUTHORITY, EXEMPLAR REGIONAL OFFICE,* CASES ACTIVE AS OF MARCH 31, 1995–2001

	1995	1996	1997	1998	1999	2000	2001
Custody agreement	6	3	4	13	6	1	3
Support agreement	27	14	22	23	45	28	35
Apprehension	0	0	4	0	0	0	0
Permanent guardianship order	31	20	21	17	16	17	18
Supervision	0	0	3	4	0	0	3
Temporary guardianship order	5	6	5	7	8	4	5
Extend custody to 3 yr	—	—	—	—	0	0	0
Extend care past age 18	—	—	—	—	0	3	3
Interim custody order	—	—	—	—	0	1	2
Other	6	2	1	2	0	4	2
No legal authority in effect	1	0	4	1	0	28	17
TOTAL	55	45	64	67	75	86	88
Province total	7584	7712	8247	7855	7520	7109	7998
Exemplar Office as % of Province	0.9	0.6	0.8	0.9	1.0	1.2	1.1

*Approximately equals the EHD excluding an estimated 750 people in Township 4 covered by the Region 2 Office of Social Services.

in the Exemplar area is somewhat greater than these percentages would suggest).

Over the 6-year period, the number of provincial cases varied by as much as 9% from the base of 1995, with the number of cases in 2001 being about 4% higher than 1995. The number of cases in the Exemplar Regional Office declined by 32% between 1995 and 1996 but has been climbing every year since and presently stands at 33% higher than the number of cases in 1995.

Alcohol Sales

Excessive use of alcoholic beverages can be detrimental to the heart, primarily by increasing blood pressure, raising serum cholesterol levels, and increasing the ability to gain weight and fat. Excessive consumption is also closely linked to cirrhosis of the liver, poisoning, falls, domestic abuse, violence, psychosis, vehicle collisions, and problems in the workplace.

The preferred indicator relating to alcohol would be one based on consumption of ounces of alcohol. The published data by the Provincial Alcohol Office uses very large regions and the EHD geographic area is combined within a larger rural-urban region. An alternative indicator using sales data of 11 liquor stores within the EHD geographic area was chosen; these data are presented in Table 14-5.

Alcohol sales per capita within the EHD geographic area appear to be three quarters the level of sales in the Province. Sales per capita in these 11 stores

TABLE 14-5 ◆ ALCOHOL SALES IN DOLLARS, BY STORES IN EHD GEOGRAPHIC AREA, 1996–2001

	1996	1997	1998	1999	2000	2001
Area sales	8,367,038	8,523,988	8,525,213	8,690,137	8,436,464	8,514,585
EHD sales/capita	297.07	304.37	306.27	313.89	306.50	Not available
Province sales	942,061,103	994,895,681	1,003,436,423	1,044,804,522	1,019,915,078	1,004,989,345
Province sales/capita	395.76	410.60	413.07	423.03	400.67	392.97

increased between 1996 and 2001, peaking in 1999 at $314/capita. A similar trend is noted for the Province with a peak of $423/capita that year.

As noted, the data presented above relate to sales. When converted into quantity, there has been a steady decline in consumption in the Province during the 1990s (there was a slight increase in beer consumption in the 1990s). The consumption pattern in Canada has been similar to that experienced in the Province.

Alcohol consumption is quite strongly correlated to age and sex with high consumption by young in their late teens and twenties. With the EHD area consisting of a generally older population, lower sales per capita would be expected. More specific information is needed to confirm the extent to which patterns of consumption are of concern. Finally, notwithstanding that recent research notes that moderate alcohol consumption can provide a degree of protection against coronary heart disease, the impact on overall mortality is not clear. However, as a local physician noted, alcohol consumption ought not to be promoted if it involves "trading a couple of months of extra life in a nursing home, in the case of an older person who benefited from alcohol consumption, for decades of lost life in the case of a 20-year-old who dies on the road." Such minor health benefits cannot be compared with the tremendous social costs of alcohol use by young people and those who are addicted.

Health Status

No report on the health status of a community would be complete without a discussion of physical indicators of health. The following discussion summarizes the physical indicator findings presented in the main report. The physical indicators presented here include the leading causes of death; injury deaths and hospitalization; potential years of life lost (PYLL); the incidence of low-birth-weight births; congenital anomalies; teenage pregnancy; communicable diseases; sexually transmitted diseases (STDs); and dental health.

Causes of Death

Table 14-6 gives the actual frequencies of the seven leading causes of death in the EHD geographic area between 1991 and 2000. Diseases of the heart and cancer claimed more lives than any other cause. This was true for both the EHD geographic area and for the Province overall throughout the entire time period. In the EHD geographic area and in the Province, suicide was the least frequent major cause of death.

From 1995 to 2000, the annual number of suicides in the EHD geographic area fluctuated between 2 and 10. In 4 of the 5 remaining years during this time period, the number of suicides was four or fewer. However, in 2000, the number of suicides in the EHD area increased to 10 (7 men and 3 women). The predominance of male suicides over female suicides was consistent for every year from 1995 to 2000. The suicide rate in the EHD geographic area did not differ significantly from the provincial suicide rate during the 5-year period from 1995 to 2000.

The number of deaths from accidents and adverse effects in the EHD geographic area showed no apparent trend. On the other hand, the number of accidental deaths in the Province as a whole decreased between 1995 and 2000, although there are considerable fluctuations from year to year.

In comparison with provincial data, the rate of death from heart disease increased slightly more in the Province as a whole than it did in the EHD geographic area between 1995 and 2000 (32% and 26%, respectively).

Table 14-7 presents the rates per 100,000 of the seven leading causes of death in the EHD geographic area and in the Province in 1996 and 2001.

Generally the rates of death from the seven major causes were higher in the EHD geographic area than the corresponding provincial rates. However, it should be kept in mind that in both 1996 and 2001, the EHD geographic area

TABLE 14-6 ◆ INCIDENCE OF SEVEN LEADING CAUSES OF DEATH IN EHD GEOGRAPHIC AREA, 1995–2000

	1995	1996	1997	1998	1999	2000
Diseases of the heart	98	89	103	96	105	100
Malignant neoplasm (cancer)	73	73	73	70	84	89
Cerebrovascular disease (strokes)	18	22	22	23	21	34
Accidents/adverse effects	14	15	19	19	16	19
Chronic obstructive lung disease	4	10	12	7	14	18
Pneumonia/influenza	6	12	13	9	16	11
Suicide	2	4	3	4	4	10
Other	47	38	50	69	55	63
TOTAL	262	263	295	297	315	344

TABLE 14-7 ◆ MORTALITY RATES PER 100,000 OF THE SEVEN LEADING CAUSES OF DEATH IN EHD GEOGRAPHIC AREA AND PROVINCE, 1996 AND 2001

	1996		2001	
	EHD	Province	EHD	Province
Diseases of the heart	310	157	382	149
Malignant neoplasms (cancer)	240	135	305	145
Cerebrovascular disease (strokes)	71	44	76	41
Accidents/adverse effects	64	43	76	41
Chronic obstructive lung disease	18	21	51	23
Pneumonia/influenza	35	20	58	22
Suicide	18	18	14	18
Other	208	124	200	128
TOTAL	964	562	1144	559

had more than twice as many persons over the age of 65 as the provincial average. Elderly persons tend to die from all causes at higher rates than the general population and this can inflate the overall death rates. The specific trends and differences between the EHD geographic area and the Province are described below.

The overall death rate in the EHD geographic area rose between 1996 and 2001. Of the specific causes of death, chronic obstructive lung disease had the sharpest jump. In the EHD geographic area the rate of death from cancer and pneumonia/influenza also increased substantially. The rate of death from heart disease also rose but the rate of death from other (miscellaneous) causes dropped between 1996 and 2001.

Injury Deaths and Hospitalization

A more detailed examination of injury deaths indicates that in the 6-year period 1995–2000, there were three times as many male as female fatalities from injuries. Figure 14-8 notes the three most significant causes of injury death for the EHD geographic area and the Province.

The number of persons hospitalized due to injuries increased from 572 in 1999 to 653 in 2000. The average length of stay remained constant at 8 days. Falls and motor vehicle crashes were the two leading causes of hospitalization due to injuries. The rate of hospitalization due to motor vehicle crashes was, as with deaths from motor vehicle crashes, significantly higher than the provincial rate.

Motor vehicle crash data obtained from Provincial Transportation indicates that four of five of motor vehicle crashes in the EHD area resulted only in property damage.

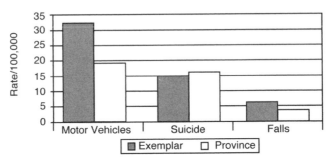

Figure 14-8 ◆ Injury death rate for the Exemplar Health District area and Province, 1995–2000.

Potential Years of Life Lost

The number of potential years of life lost, or PYLL, is a measure of premature death. It is based on the assumption that all people have the potential to live up to an average life expectancy of 75 years of age. Table 14-8 compares the total number of PYLL in both the EHD area and in the Province in 2000 broken down by the leading causes of death.

When considering these data, it is useful to keep in mind that the population of the EHD area represents approximately 1% of the total population of the Province. Using this rough estimation, it is clear that the number of PYLL in the EHD area in 2000 was higher than 1% of the provincial figure for all of the leading causes of death, with the exception of pneumonia/influenza and miscellaneous causes. In these two cases, the figure for the Health District area was slightly less than 1% of the provincial rate.

Also note that when ranking causes of death in the EHD geographic area with PYLL, accidents move from fourth to second and suicide from seventh to fourth.

TABLE 14-8 ◆ TOTAL NUMBER OF POTENTIAL YEARS OF LIFE LOST IN EHD GEOGRAPHIC AREA AND PROVINCE, 2000

	EHD	Province	EHD (% of Province)
Cancer (malignant neoplasms)	473	35,688	1.3
Ischemic diseases of the heart	294	17,128	1.7
Strokes (cerebrovascular disease)	66	3818	1.7
Chronic obstructive lung disease	40	1854	2.2
Suicide	237	16,764	1.4
Pneumonia/influenza	13	1531	0.8
Accidents	313	24,882	1.3
Other	635	72,310	0.9
TOTAL	2081	173,975	1.2

The PYLL for men in the EHD in 2000 exceeded the PYLL for women for ischemic heart disease, suicide, and accidents. On the other hand, women exceeded men in the total number of PYLL for strokes, chronic obstructive lung disease, and miscellaneous causes of death during 2000.

Low-Birth-Weight Babies

In the EHD area, the number of low-birth-weight babies born from 1991 to 2002 fluctuated between a high of 29 in 1991 and a low of 13 in 2002. The rates also fluctuated throughout this time period between approximately 3 and 7 low-birth-weight babies per 100 live births.

During the same time period, the number of low-birth-weight babies in the Province varied between 2699 and 2286. However, the rate of low-birth-weight babies per 100 live births in the Province remained fairly constant throughout this time period at approximately 5.7. The data for the EHD and the Province are located in Figure 14-9.

Congenital Anomalies

Figure 14-10 presents the rate of congenital anomalies per 1000 births in both the EHD geographic area and in the Province between 1990 and 2000. Through the entire time period, the rate of congenital anomalies in the EHD geographic area was lower than the provincial rate. The rate for the EHD geographic area fluctuated between a low of 12.6 in 1993 and a high of 42.7 in 1999. Between 1990 and 2000, the Health District area rate rose by a net 3.2%. In comparison, the provincial rate fluctuated between 35.9 congenital anomalies

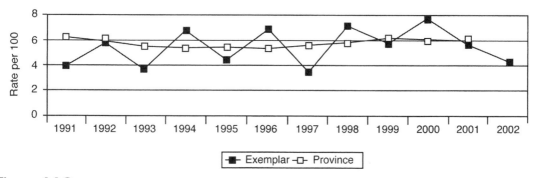

Figure 14-9 ◆ Rate of babies born weighing less than 2500 grams per 100 live births, Exemplar Health District and Province, 1991–2002.

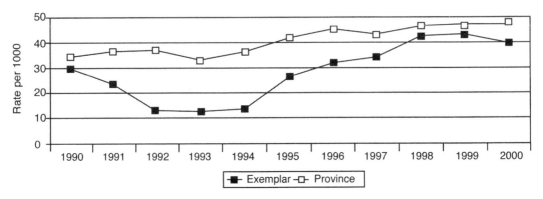

Figure 14-10 ◆ Rate of congenital anomalies per 1000 births, Exemplar Health District geographical area and Province, 1990–2000.

per 1000 births in 1990 and 47.8 in 2000, and increased by 33% during the same time period.

Adolescent Pregnancy

Table 14-9 shows the number of live births to all girls under the age of 19 in the EHD area and in the Province. In the EHD geographic area there was a total of 48 live births to girls 19 years and under in 1991. By 1998, the number of live births had dropped to 21, less than half of the 1991 figure. Although the total number of live births to girls aged 19 years and under also dropped in the Province during the same time period, the drop was less dramatic.

TABLE 14-9 ◆ TOTAL NUMBER OF LIVE BIRTHS TO GIRLS AGED 19 YEARS AND UNDER IN EHD GEOGRAPHIC AREA AND PROVINCE, 1991–2001

Year	EHD	Province
1991	48	4255
1992	27	4188
1993	26	4515
1994	25	3303
1995	23	3120
1996	23	3155
1997	22	3064
1998	21	3032
1999	37	3189
2000	25	3339
2001	16	3477

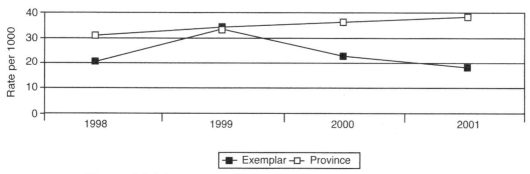

Figure 14-11 ◆ Live birth rates per 1000 females aged 15–19 years, Exemplar Health District geographical area and Province, 1998–2001.

In Figure 14-11 the rates of live births per 1000 girls aged 15 to 19 years in the EHD geographic area and in the Province during the years from 1998 to 2001 are shown. In the EHD geographic area, the rate of live births per 1000 girls aged 16 to 19 years decreased 47% between 1991 and 1997 (from 45.1 in 1991 to 23.9 in 1997). This trend continued during 1998 through 2001, with a further 9% drop in the rate of live births per 1000 girls between the ages of 15 and 19 occurring during this time period.

The provincial live birth rate for girls aged 16 to 19 years also decreased between 1991 and 1997 (−14%). However, between 1998 and 2001, there was a 22% increase in the number of live births to girls aged 15 to 19 years in the Province.

In Table 14-10 the percentage of teen mothers in both the EHD geographic area and in the Province in 1991 and 2001 who were not married at the time of their child's birth is illustrated. The proportion of single teen mothers more than doubled in the EHD geographic area during this time period (from 40% to 94%). In the Province, the trend was similar but not quite as pronounced (a rise from 53% to 84%).

The acquisition of a sexually transmitted disease (STD) is a health risk of sexual activity. Table 14-11 gives the number of reportable STDs among young

TABLE 14–10 ◆ PROPORTION OF ADOLESCENT WOMEN UNMARRIED AT TIME OF BIRTH IN EHD GEOGRAPHIC AREA AND PROVINCE, 1991 AND 2001

	1991	2001
EHD	40%	94%
Province	53%	84%

TABLE 14-11 ◆ NUMBER OF REPORTED STDS AMONG GIRLS AGED 15–19 IN EHD GEOGRAPHIC AREA AND PROVINCE, 1998–2000			
	1998	**1999**	**2000**
EHD	18	11	7
Province	2708	2896	2676

women aged 15 to 19 years in the EHD geographic area and in the Province from 1998 to 2000. In 2000, there were 7 reported cases of STDs in the EHD geographic area among young women aged 15 to 19 years, resulting in a rate of 6.84/1000. By comparison, the provincial rate was 30.3 in 2000.

Communicable Diseases

Tables 14-12 and 14-13 give the rates per 100,000 of vaccine-preventable and enteric communicable diseases in both the EHD geographic area and in the Province in 1996 and 2002. Enteric communicable diseases are infections that occur within the digestive tract or intestines.

An outbreak of pertussis (whooping cough), which began in 1999, is undoubtedly responsible for the large jump in the rates of pertussis in both the EHD geographic area and the Province between 1996 and 2001.

The number of diagnosed cases of measles in both the EHD geographic area and the Province dropped considerably between 1996 and 2001, with the rates also showing corresponding decreases.

There were no reported cases of either tetanus or poliomyelitis in the EHD geographic area between 1996 and 2002.

TABLE 14-12 ◆ RATE PER 100,000 OF SELECTED VACCINE-PREVENTABLE COMMUNICABLE DISEASES IN EHD GEOGRAPHIC AREA AND PROVINCE, 1996 AND 2001				
	1996		**2001**	
	EHD	Province	EHD	Province
Diphtheria	—	—	—	—
Mumps	14.1	9.8	3.6	3.7
Rubella	45.9	48.9	14.5	2.4
Haemophilus influenza b	3.5	6.1	3.6	1.9
Pertussis	7.1	7.8	32.7	42.0
Tetanus	—	—	—	0.1
Poliomyelitis	—	—	—	—
Measles	74.1	34.3	—	0.3

TABLE 14-13 ◆ RATE PER 100,000 OF ENTERIC DISEASES IN EHD GEOGRAPHIC AREA AND PROVINCE, 1996 AND 2001

	1996		2001	
	EHD	Province	EHD	Province
Giardiasis	70.6	68.0	21.8	61.2
Salmonella	21.2	32.0	18.2	35.8
Shigellosis	45.9	36.8	29.1	40.8
Campylobacter	7.1	7.6	14.5	7.8
Escherichia coli	—	6.2	—	4.1

The number of diagnosed cases of giardiasis in the EHD geographic area fluctuated somewhat but showed an overall downward trend, from 20 cases in 1996 to 6 in 2001.

The rate of campylobacter infection in the EHD geographic area more than doubled between 1996 and 2001 (two diagnosed cases in 1996 and four in 2001). Similarly, the yearly number of cases of salmonella in the EHD geographic area peaked at 23 (1998). In comparison to the Province as a whole, the rates of salmonella infection in the EHD geographic area were lower than the provincial figures in both 1996 and 2001.

There were no diagnosed cases of *Escherichia coli* in the EHD geographic area in either 1996 or 2001; however, there was one reported case in 1997 and another three in 1999.

Sexually Transmitted Diseases

Table 14-14 shows the rates per 100,000 of the three most common STDs (gonorrhea, NGU/MPC and chlamydia) for the EHD geographic area and for the Province in 2001. The EHD geographic area had substantially lower rates of all

TABLE 14-14 ◆ INCIDENCE RATES PER 100,000 OF SELECTED STDS IN EHD GEOGRAPHIC AREA AND PROVINCE, 2001

	EHD	**PROVINCE**
	Rate	Rate
Gonorrhea	7.3	54.7
NGU/MPC	18.2	133.0
Chlamydia	72.7	272.5

MPC, mucopurulent cervicitis.
NGU, nongonococcal urethritis.

three STDs than the provincial average. In the EHD geographic area the rate per 100,000 of chlamydia, the most frequently occurring STD, was approximately one quarter of the provincial rate in 2001 (72.7 and 272.5, respectively). The rates of gonorrhea and NGU/MPC in the EHD geographic area in 2001 were close to one seventh of the provincial figures. The positive diagnosis of a STD is a highly sensitive and confidential matter; thus, the following data need to be interpreted in light of the possibility that the number of reported cases may be less than the actual number of cases, particularly because infections such as chlamydia often exhibit few symptoms.

Dental Health

Figure 14-12 shows the average number of decayed, missing, and filled teeth (DMF) among school-aged children in the EHD geographic area between 1992–1993 and 2001–2002. During this time period, the average number of DMF teeth decreased by almost half (47%).

Observations and Recommendations

Frameworks and Understanding Health

It is clear that our concept of health is becoming broader. This is evident in both the reflections of local citizens and professionals. In a recent report of residents of five communities in the Province that were exploring concepts of

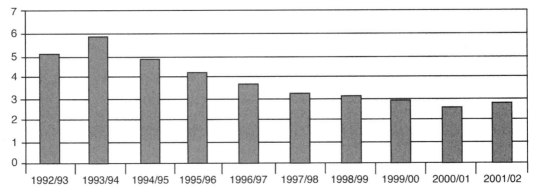

Figure 14-12 ◆ Average number of decayed, missing, or filled teeth among school-aged children, Exemplar Health District geographical area, 1992/93 to 2001/2002.

health, health issues, and making health information available in the community it was noted that rather than seeing health as something to work toward (i.e., dedication to a rigid regime) focus group participants tended to favour a balance of activities and interests, where enjoyment was the goal. The societal framework, the focus groups suggested, should be one that allows for individual differences in needs, tastes, capabilities, personal histories, and lifestyles.

A senior researcher in mental health of the Provincial Health Ministry has been examining data on mental illness and social problems and concluded physical health, mental vulnerability, social problems, and social structure are interconnected and interdependent. Further, although we still need to know more about the way in which these connections operate and how to deal with them, the evidence of their existence is clear enough to warrant, and in fact demand, a change in direction.

As our understanding of health and wellness grows and broadens, we will undoubtedly revise the frameworks used for data collection in similar health indicator studies so as to more clearly draw conclusions and develop useful strategies for improving the population's health.

Data

The limited availability of certain useful data, such as the lack of information about a condition in the desired geographic region, for enough years to discern possible trends, and so on, is generally acknowledged. Although the provincial Health Ministry has organized a committee to look at health indicator information, it is suggested that much more energy and attention need to be given to this area.

There is concern that the provincial government decisions to reduce expenditures will inhibit the availability of data on a timely basis. The regional office of Statistics Canada is a source for some data, but cost and turnaround time need to be factored into the data collection process if different breakdowns of data are needed.

Data Interpretation

Statistical information by itself would not normally be the sole basis for decision-making in a Health District or community. For example, low income has been closely correlated with poor health. Hence, one might conclude that because average income is high, good health should be expected. However, additional exploration might point to continuing concerns, for example, although the average family income in Canada rose during the 1990s there was also an increasing disparity between those with lowest income and those in the uppermost income categories.

With respect to "hard" data, one needs to be open to interpretations other than those initially considered. Qualitative data and measures that reflect health-promoting processes must also be given serious consideration in analysis of complex situations.

Additional Measures

Future health indicator studies should consider including data on:

♦ Prescription and over-the-counter drugs
♦ Mental health
♦ Spiritual health

Decision-Making Structure

In the development of comprehensive community health plan the community infrastructure and decision-making process must be considered. That is, health in the first instance is individual—it is based on each person's physical, mental, emotional, and spiritual condition. However, one could be in a healthy caring society or in a sick society; in one that promotes health and wellness of all or one that limits access or freedoms unnecessarily; or in one which ensures that legislation and decision processes reflect current issues and needs or one that neglects to change laws no longer current.

Regional Health Indicators

The core list of health indicators is presented in Table 14-15, within the Statistics Canada and Canadian Institute of Health Information (CIHI) indicators framework. The indicators included in this list (in italics) are available at the health region level and represent a subset of this core list of indicators. Subsequent releases will add indicators and time series as these data are developed at the regional level, and new health data are collected.

TABLE 14-15 ◆ HEALTH STATUS

Well-Being	Health Conditions	Human Function	Deaths
Self-rated health Self-rated 'excellent' health for two consecutive survey cycles Self-esteem Mastery	*Low birth weight* Overweight Arthritis Diabetes Asthma High blood pressure Cancer incidence Chronic pain Depression *Injury hospitalizations* Food and waterborne diseases	Functional health Disability days Activity limitation	*Infant mortality* *Perinatal deaths* *Life expectancy* *Total mortality* *Circulatory deaths* *Cancer deaths* *Respiratory deaths* *Suicide* *Unintentional injury deaths* *AIDS deaths* *Potential years of* *life lost*

Nonmedical Determinants of Health

Health Behaviours	Living and Working Conditions	Personal Resources	Environmental Factors
Smoking rate Youth smoking rate Smoking initiation (average age) Quitting smoking Regular heavy drinking Physical activity Breastfeeding	*High school and post-* *secondary graduation* *Unemployment rate* *Long-term and youth* *unemployment* *Low income rate* *Children in low-income families* *Average personal income* Income inequality *Housing affordability* Crime rate and youth crime rate Decision-latitude at work	School readiness Social support Life stress	

Health System Performance

Acceptability	Accessibility	Appropriateness	Competence
	Influenza immunization, 65+ Screening mammography, women age 50-69 Pap smears, age 18-69 Childhood immunizations	*Vaginal birth after caesarean* Breast-conserving surgery *Caesarean sections*	

Continuity	Effectiveness	Efficiency	Safety
	Pertussis Measles Tuberculosis HIV Chlamydia *Pneumonia and influenza* *hospitalizations* Deaths due to medically treatable diseases *Ambulatory care sensitive* *conditions*	Surgical day case rates *May not require* *hospitalization* *% alternate level of* *care days* *Expected compared to* *actual stay*	Hip fractures

(continued)

TABLE 14-15 ◆ HEALTH STATUS (*Continued*)

Community and Health System Characteristics

Population count	Coronary artery bypass grafting rates
Percent population over 65 yr of age	Hip replacement
Percent 'urban' population	Knee replacement
Percent Aboriginal population	Hysterectomy
Percent immigrant population	Myringotomy
Teen pregnancy/teen births	
Expenditures per capita	
Doctors (GP/FP and specialists)	
Nurses per capita	

Summary

In this chapter, the report of the EHD was presented to illustrate how an assessment and analysis of a geopolitical district might be consolidated in a form that could be taken to decision-makers for planning purposes. In the real world, this report would include a series of community diagnoses with recommendations for action. However, the report stops short to allow you, the reader, to take it further. You can contemplate the data, drawing on what you view as salient to generate community diagnoses, both risk related and wellness oriented, and postulate hypotheses for action. From this, an intervention plan, logic model, and evaluation guides can be created and used as templates to guide action. As you become familiar with the process by using this chapter as a case study, you will develop skills that are transferable to the community practice setting.

Internet Resources

http://secure.cihi.ca/indicators/en/tables.shtml
http://www.statcan.ca/english/freepub/82-221-XIE/free.htm
http://www.cich.ca/resource.htm
http://library.usask.ca/data/health/
http://www.canadian-health-network.ca/customtools/homee.html
http://www.utoronto.ca/chp/chp/consort/working.htm
http://www.ainc-inac.gc.ca/gs/soci_e.html
http://www.camh.net/research/research_ar2001/pop_life_course_studies.html
http://rhrg.brandonu.ca/
http://www.sustreport.org/issues/sust_comm2.html
http://www.sustainable.doe.gov/measuring/meother.shtml
http://www.ccsa.ca/stats.htm
http://www.cewh-cesf.ca/
http://www.spheru.ca/
http://www1.oecd.org

15

Okotoks, Our Healthy Home

LORI L. ANDERSON

OBJECTIVES

After studying this chapter, you should be able to:

◆ Understand the principles of the Healthy Communities movement
◆ Describe how support from key stakeholders can be generated for a community program
◆ Describe how health planners involve citizens in the program and its projects

Introduction

Positive health is believed to be achieved, at least in part, by the ability of individuals to be able to predict, control, and participate in the environment in which they live. The process of creating a healthy community provides people and organizations with the opportunity to do just this. This is the story of a healthy community process within rural Alberta that has positively contributed to both the health of the community and the way in which the community (Okotoks, Alberta) and the health authority (Headwaters Health Authority) work together to influence community health and well-being. Most importantly, it is about a group of dedicated community members who sincerely wanted to make a difference to the health of their community.

Background and Context

The Ottawa Charter (1986) emphasizes the importance of communities owning and controlling their own endeavours and futures. The Healthy Cities movement, known also as the Healthy Communities movement, was jointly developed by the World Health Organization (European Chapter) and Canadians Hancock and Duhl (1988) as a vehicle for achieving "Health for All" through primary health care (PHC), by applying the principles of health promotion as articulated in the Alma Ata Declaration (World Health Organization [WHO], 1978).

The WHO Healthy Communities project is a long-term international development project that is committed to a comprehensive approach to health and seeks to involve both the grassroots and policymakers at the national and local levels in the health agenda. The Healthy Communities concept has taken hold internationally and has grown rapidly since its inception as it responds to present and future concerns about health and pays attention to both outcomes and processes (Baum, 1993). The Healthy Communities movement encourages the formation of multisectoral partnerships among local government, businesses, nongovernment and community agencies, and individual community members. These partnerships draw on the existing resource base in the community to identify and prioritize local health-related needs and issues and plan, implement, and evaluate methods and strategies designed to improve the health of the community at large.

The core guiding principles of the Healthy Communities movement are:

1. Local government commitment
2. Broad community involvement and participation
3. Development of healthy public policy
4. Intersectoral collaboration and involvement
5. Broad definition of health with emphasis on the determinants of health

This case story focuses on the inception and development of the Healthy Okotoks Coalition (HOC). The HOC was created in the spirit of health reform as a concrete way for health authorities to work with communities to enhance health status. This initiative was developed as a tangible and collaborative way to achieve the health authority's goal of "improving the health status of the population within the region by facilitating the creation of healthy communities" (Headwaters Health Authority [HHA], 1998).

The political climate in which the HOC exists is one in which the status quo is being challenged and new approaches such as PHC (with its emphasis on the principles of accessibility, public participation, intersectoral and interdisciplinary collaboration, appropriate technology, and increased health promotion) are gaining recognition. The current fiscally driven political will within Alberta for health care restructuring and reform is providing a rationalization and affirmation of the value and worth of health promotion and PHC initiatives such as the HOC. The realization that health is affected by determinants far broader than the formal health care delivery system is influencing the shift away from the illness focus of the medical model to a perspective in which health is a holistic comprehensive construct and the combined responsibility of government, communities, families, and individuals.

Getting Organized

A Seed Is Planted

The inspiration to embark on a Healthy Community process came while I was attending the Health Care Forum in San Francisco in the spring of 1996 with two other members of our health authority. The conference theme that year was "Creating Healthier Communities." The quality of the speakers and the wonderful examples from a variety of communities and cities made us realize that HHA needed to explore new ways in which to engage with communities to enhance health and well-being. At the conference, Flin Flon, Manitoba received international recognition and a Healthy City award for its coalition's work in positively influencing its community's health. Inspired, and motivated to do something different within our newly formed regional health authority, the three of us made a commitment to pursue a healthy community project within the HHA.

What is a healthy community? The Healthy Communities vision goes far beyond a traditional view of medical health. A healthy community, according to the Ontario Healthy Communities Coalition:

◆ Provides a clean, safe physical environment
◆ Meets the basic needs of all its residents
◆ Has residents that respect and support each other
◆ Involves the community in local government
◆ Promotes and celebrates its historical and cultural heritage

◆ Provides easily accessible health services
◆ Has a diverse, innovative economy
◆ Rests on a sustainable ecosystem

The Healthy Communities model is one by which a community determines its own issues, needs, and action plans in building a healthier community (www.opc.on.ca).

Every community will go about enacting a Healthy Community process in a different way. For some, it is a grassroots movement with members of the community acting as the initiating parties; in others governmental and nongovernmental organizations act as the catalyst. There has been criticism (Baum, 1993; Hancock, 1993) that the Healthy Cities/Communities movement is too enmeshed in bureaucracy and that it has become a tool to transfer the responsibility of health to communities, using the rhetoric of community control and empowerment to hide the real agenda of withdrawing health services or providing token support. If health authorities are sincere in their efforts to develop meaningful partnerships with communities, the leadership provided to implement and facilitate innovative approaches to enhance community health should be embraced with minimal scepticism and in the true spirit of collaboration and partnership. The HOC provides a good example of this. A vision of a healthy community has been articulated by Roulier and McGrath and is shown in Box 15-1.

A template for how a healthy community should be created would never be imposed in the Healthy Communities movement; thus, communities have the flexibility to identify and assess needs that are relevant and important to them, as well as to plan, implement, and in many cases, evaluate their own strategies to address the identified needs. Further, this allows communities to take into account the space, time, and environmental conditions singular to each community and provide the opportunity for capacity building within a community itself (Hodson, 1999).

BOX 15-1. WHAT IS A HEALTHY COMMUNITY?

Many proponents see healthy communities as something broader than an attempt to improve the physical health of communities. They see it as an attempt to improve the quality of life, share power among groups and individuals, develop social capital and rekindle a spirit of community democracy. (Roulier & McGrath, 1998)

The process of creating a healthy community relies on certain values and beliefs that include:

◆ Health is removed from the disease continuum and aligns itself more close-ly to the WHO (1946, 1986) definitions that consider health as a state of physical, mental, and social well-being, and a resource for everyday living that emphasizes social, physical, and personal capacities.
◆ It is accepted that communities have both strengths and problems, but communities are also believed to have the ability to solve these problems by drawing on their strengths and by realizing their potential.
◆ The process should encourage individuals to identify their own needs, set priorities, and take responsibility for their own well-being, while fostering a supportive, nurturing environment.
◆ The process is believed to accommodate the context in which it takes place and is based on participation by all those affected, directly and indirectly, at each stage of the process (British Columbia Ministry of Health, 1989).

Creating Excitement

An action plan was developed for implementation following extensive research into Healthy Community processes and connecting with individuals across Canada with valuable experience. The community of Okotoks was selected by the HHA planning group to determine if there was interest on the part of the town in pursuing a Healthy Community partnership. Okotoks is a rural com-munity with agricultural roots, 20 kilometres south of the city of Calgary. The majority of residents commute to the city for employment. Okotoks is one of Alberta's fastest growing communities with a population of 12,000 that is expected to double in the next 20 years.

✎ TAKE NOTE

• Timing is everything! Our project fit well with stated provincial and regional health objectives for safe communities and with the town's inter-est in environmental sustainability.
• Planting initial seeds of interest with key stakeholders determines the level of interest and enthusiasm for a project.
• People need clarity about the proposed partnership to establish realistic expectations.

Generating enthusiasm and energy around a concept is critical to successfully building the momentum required to launch a significant process such as we envisioned. I had an informal meeting with the mayor of Okotoks and the HHA chief executive officer (CEO), where the idea for a Healthy Community project in partnership with the town was proposed. The CEO explained that we still had to gain the support of the HHA board, but wanted to determine first if there was any mutual interest around the concept prior to pursuing it further. The mayor could see the potential in such an initiative, and felt that the Town of Okotoks would be interested in pursuing the discussion. Thus, a seed was planted. When we would formally present the idea to the Town Council, we were assured that some internal support and understanding was in place.

Seeking Partners

It was imperative that the HHA board support the vision and commit the resources required to initiate the process. The proposal was placed on the HHA board agenda and, with the CEO and board chairperson (who had both been at the Health Care Forum) voicing support, presenting the guiding principles and philosophy underpinning the Healthy Communities movement, providing some of the tangible results experienced by Flin Flon, and indicating initial interest on the part of a local community, the proposal was accepted and funded. The board was interested in establishing innovative ways to work with communities and keenly endorsed the idea. It was determined that Okotoks, given its focus on sustainability and safe environmental practices, would be the community with which to pursue a partnership.

✎ TAKE NOTE

- Selecting a pilot community on identified capacity, interest, and a solid history of collaboration increases potential for success.
- Providing examples of results and tangible outcomes from other projects balances the conceptual and concrete for stakeholders.
- Academic connections add credibility to the process.

The next step was to introduce the concept to the Okotoks Town Council; a formal presentation was made to the council at an open (public) meeting.

Council unanimously passed a resolution endorsing its support to engage in a Healthy Community project with the HHA. Council members were able to see a direct link between the proposed initiative and the town's considerable work and commitment toward the creation of a sustainable community.

At the time of this project, I was engaged in graduate studies through the University of Calgary, Faculty of Nursing. This project was identified as an excellent opportunity for a practicum focus and thus the university also became involved. My professor provided access to theory and literature around the Healthy Communities movement. An academic connection ensured theory and evidence-based practice and created linkages to related research and projects. Now three parties had declared their interest in pursuing the adventure.

Finding a Local Champion

Following the passage of the town's resolution, the Community Support Services (CSS) coordinator became involved in the project; her role is to work with volunteers, facilitate the collaboration of allied service agencies within the community, and promote citizen participation in the planning and delivery of programs and services. She sits on all the primary community committees and chairs the Interagency Group* and is one of those people who have their fingers on the pulse of the community, and tirelessly works behind the scenes attending to detail, doing follow-up tasks, and carrying on the networking necessary to launch and sustain this new initiative. She immediately embraced the Healthy Communities concept because it fit with her professional emphasis on community collaboration and integration and her own personal worldview and, with her skills in community development, we knew we had found our local champion!

✎ TAKE NOTE

Finding a local champion who understands the community and has passion for health promotion is key to successful advocacy and legitimization and is critical for generating enthusiasm and building project momentum.

---

*An Interagency Group is a semiformal meeting of community agencies with the purpose of coordinating efforts, sharing information, and making effective use of each agency's resources to reduce duplication, fill gaps, and ensure that community needs are addressed.

Engaging the Community

With the backing of the town, HHA, and the support of a member of the academic community, it was time to introduce the idea to the different community sectors and general public. We sent a notice to several stakeholder groups inviting them to participate in a Healthy Communities initiative (Box 15-2). To gain support from the formal and informal "legitimizers" within the community and health authority, a number of presentations and consultations were carried out. A town councillor and I (representing the founding partners) facilitated a discussion with the local Interagency Group. Most communities have a similar forum for members of the different human service sectors to meet, network, and collaboratively address community issues of relevance. This proved to be an excellent forum for building support and energy around our idea for a Healthy Communities project. The Interagency Group had recently undertaken a significant needs assessment for children and family services and was cautious in making a commitment to another process that appeared at the outset to be slightly daunting. We agreed that the assessment phase would build from existing knowledge rather than duplicate the extensive research available.

Introductory presentations were also made to the local public health unit, clergy group, and local physicians. Most groups were supportive and expressed interest in the project, essential for the legitimization and community-wide acceptance of the initiative, while expressing caution about the potential time commitment the process would require to be successful. The physician

---

BOX 15-2. THE INVITATION TO PARTICIPATE

The Town of Okotoks and Headwaters Health Authority are embarking on a Healthy Community process. This process will result in the creation of a healthier community building on existing strengths, which will be accomplished through collaborative partnerships. The process will work from a community development framework in which the community will identify their health needs. Creative initiatives to respond to these needs will be explored and implemented.

The active involvement and commitment of key individuals and groups is imperative to the success of this initiative. A meeting is planned to outline this project and to solicit the support and participation of the health community. This meeting is scheduled for Friday, December 12th at 11:30 in the Health Unit meeting room.

We anticipate your participation at this meeting and look forward to seeing you there. Please RSVP regarding your attendance, as lunch will be provided.

group, however, had difficulty with the overall concept of Healthy Communities and did not readily see the relationship between community collaboration and health. Although they did not express an interest in becoming actively involved in the project, neither did they exert resistance to the process nor suggest the initiative was a means for the Health Authority to shirk its responsibility for health care delivery.

✎ TAKE NOTE

- Carefully select the individuals to introduce the idea to the community; ensure they are well known and trusted and have a positive history within the community.
- Seek the involvement of local physicians; they play a leadership role within health care and the community and are in positions of perceived power and influence (Bracht, 1990).
- Not all parties will share your enthusiasm or interest; focus on those that do rather than expending energy on convincing others.
- Use creative approaches that provide an enthusiastic high-energy message that will engage and excite the audience.
- Meet and talk with groups and individuals at every opportunity—you never know where you will find supporters (and detractors).

To engage community members in the Healthy Community process it was essential to establish key community relationships. The initial success and general acceptance of the idea within the community could be attributed, to some degree, to the positive reputations of the individuals promoting the initiative, community familiarity with them, and the respect they enjoyed within the community of Okotoks.

Public Forum

After initial support was garnered from some key community groups and members, a town hall meeting was organized to present the idea to the community at large and to generate interest in forming a coalition that would move the process forward. A series of newspaper articles, posters, word of mouth, and information packages sent out broadly to all community groups and organizations announced the meeting. The public forum was held on an evening where it would not compete with other ongoing community functions, and a venue was selected for comfort and a positive atmosphere.

The planning committee gave special attention to the format of the meeting and selection of speakers. To present not only the concept, but also outline the potential outcomes of a Healthy Community initiative, a representative from the Healthy Flin Flon Coalition was invited to attend the meeting and share that town's experiences. Experts in the area of health promotion and healthy communities were also present and responded to some of the questions put forward by the public.

✎ TAKE NOTE

- Consider providing childcare so that young families are able to attend.
- Think about engaging volunteer drivers to provide transportation to increase access to the meeting by seniors, those with limited mobility, or people without vehicles.
- Arrange refreshments for participants; social opportunities relax people, making them more receptive to ideas.

More than 70 Okotoks residents attended the open forum. The format for the evening included the following:

◆ A presentation was given on the principles of PHC and the Healthy Community movement.

◆ A slide presentation by the Healthy Flin Flon Coalition shared examples of tangible outcomes (e.g., a partnership with the smelter to improve air quality, the development of an adult literacy program), photos, and anecdotes.

◆ A discussion of general interest from the community was facilitated by Dr. David Swann, local medical officer and a leader in the Alberta Healthy Communities movement, and audience questions were addressed.

◆ A sheet was circulated at the end of the meeting for individuals interested in signing up to develop a coalition to put the Healthy Community project into motion and more than 30 of the 70 people in attendance expressed an interest in becoming involved to turn the concept into reality!

Building a Coalition

Once HHA and the Town of Okotoks committed to the Healthy Okotoks process and the list of interested parties was obtained from the open forum, it became apparent that the formation of a coalition was indeed viable to take ownership for the project and move the process ahead. The founding partners felt that the coalition should be action oriented to stay true to the principles of the Healthy Community process. Those factors that might influence participation were discussed, and the Chavis (1985) perspective was selected to provide guidance to the initiative (Box 15-3.)

A coalition model was chosen because it utilizes linked community organizations and groups to tackle issues. Because coalitions tend to be fluid in nature, individuals and organizations are able to become more involved when a topic of interest and relevance to them is being addressed, and less active at other times (Bracht, 1990). Coalitions offer the networking opportunities, efficient use of resources, and collective strength in addressing community issues. Some possible disadvantages are the degree of commitment required from participants, the complexity of decision-making, and the risk of personal agendas.

An initial coalition meeting was held to which all the people who had expressed an interest were invited. Vision and mission statements were created. *"Okotoks, Our Healthy Home"* captured the vision. To the Coalition the word "home" represented ownership, responsibility, care, and the need to nurture. The mission statement stated: *"To facilitate and promote wellness through community partnerships."* One of the Coalition's first tasks was to develop some terms of reference and begin to form as a group. Coalition members made a decision to measure success by a focus on community assets and existing strengths, rather than by a focus on needs or deficits. The following objectives were outlined:

- ◆ To facilitate networking and collaboration with community
- ◆ To provide a means of identification and resolution of community health issues
- ◆ To facilitate and promote cooperation and commitment of partnerships
- ◆ To bring all sectors together to create a healthier community
- ◆ To learn and develop skills in community development and Healthy Communities processes
- ◆ To demonstrate some quick successes

BOX 15-3. WHAT INFLUENCES PARTICIPATION?

Active participation does not seem to be related to demographic characteristics of members; rather, member satisfaction, commitment, expectations about outcomes, and a sense of citizen duty appear to be more influential. (Chavis et al., 1985)

◆ To not get caught up in bureaucratic process
◆ To make a difference to the health of the community
◆ To have fun!

An asset map was developed and it was apparent that one of the strengths of the newly formed Healthy Okotoks Coalition (HOC) was the number and variety of "hats" worn in the community by its members.

Celebrating Success

The HOC has now been in operation for 6 years and has gone through the normal ups and downs that most groups experience. There have been periods of intense planning and action and other times when smaller ongoing projects have sustained the group. The HOC has become well known and respected within Okotoks and is often called on to facilitate processes requiring community collaboration and partnership. There are currently more than 50 declared members of the HOC with a core group of 10 to 15 who meet twice a month. Many of the initiatives with which the HOC has become involved are a direct result of a member being at another meeting and suggesting that the HOC may have a role to play in the issue being discussed. Butterfoss, Goodman, and Wandersman (1993) state that one of the defining characteristics of a coalition is that members act not only on behalf of the organization they represent, but also advocate on behalf of the coalition itself.

The terms of reference and Healthy Community principles are reviewed annually to ensure that the coalition is staying on target. Goals and objectives are developed as community health issues are identified. Some of the successes, as identified by members, the HOC has achieved are:

◆ Creating a fun and light-hearted culture that does not interfere with progress but adds to the emotional climate and contributes to a sense of unity
◆ Strong Coalition membership that represents many community sectors
◆ Submitting a community transportation review report with recommendations to the Town Council and other key stakeholders
◆ Creating a community garden with 30 plots in partnership with the local gardening club
◆ Being the local advisory committee for a new Community Health Centre that will contain a healing garden on its grounds as suggested by the HOC

◆ Disseminating knowledge by presenting the HOC experience at provincial and national conferences, and by providing support to other communities engaged in Healthy Community projects

◆ Participating in a variety of health-related partnerships (e.g., a helmet safety initiative with the Rotary Club and Community Health Council; FAS/FAE Council in partnership with a First Nations community to increase awareness and reduce incidence; and with Habitat for Humanity to create affordable housing)

◆ Partnering with the Town of Okotoks on environmental issues (e.g., responsible pesticide use, autumn and spring community clean up, holiday tree recycling and chipping, and projects exploring sustainability of the Healthy Community process)

◆ Building youth capacity (e.g., youth forum, training youth facilitators, survey of Okotoks youth, and assistance to develop a presentation to the Town Council regarding its curfew policy)

◆ Enacting tobacco reduction strategies (e.g., advocacy for smoke-free public policy, recognition of local businesses that are nonsmoking, community education sessions)

◆ Developing visibility initiatives (e.g., HOC logo that was developed as a donation by a local graphic artist, nonprofit charitable status, grant support, HOC web page)

◆ Ongoing involvement of local government and the health authority for political, legislative, and administrative support and legitimacy

For more information and photos, go to the Internet site: http://www.foothillsbiz.com/communities.htm.

Meeting Challenges

The HOC evaluates its effectiveness on a regular basis and debriefs following major initiatives. The challenges faced have evolved as the Coalition has matured and grown with the community. In the formative stage of the HOC tensions existed as personal agendas became apparent and "storming" of group process played out (Dimock, 1994). By establishing in the "forming" stage clear terms of reference as well as processes for conflict resolution and decision-making "norming," most challenges were addressed in an honest and open manner.

We did not conduct a formal community health needs assessment because the Coalition felt there were adequate, recent, and relevant data already available. An ongoing challenge for the Coalition is to ensure that any projects with which it becomes involved are not reactive to personal interests, political influence, or opportunities, but are genuine efforts to address the determinants of health and offer potential benefits to all residents. Box 15-4 summarized what we learned from the process.

The core group of the Coalition has remained somewhat static with new members joining based on the particular initiatives in which the HOC is engaged. Because of familiarity, the group battles "group think" by ongoing recruitment to ensure diversity of ideas, experience, and beliefs.

At the beginning of the project, it was an ongoing challenge to get administrative support. Without the dedication of the CSS coordinator the sustainability of the HOC would have been in jeopardy; she took and distributed meeting notes and did the necessary follow-up, reminding people of the commitments they made. At present, the town and the health authority jointly provide administrative support by circulating minutes electronically and by mail to those without computers. Although the two key partners provide support, the HOC does not have a dedicated budget, allowing the HOC members to develop capacity in generating funds. Members attended a training session on proposal writing, and the Coalition became so proficient at obtaining grants that it ends most years with a budget surplus!

Sustainability and Conclusion

Hodson (1999) investigated the sustainability of the HOC and the process of creating a healthy community by using qualitative research methods to gather and analyze data from in-depth interviews and observation of HOC meetings. Study findings suggested that the process is dependent on both the framework and functional aspects of a coalition. The framework includes a coalition's purpose and the criteria and characteristics of membership. This framework sets the conditions for a coalition to function and influence factors that ultimately affect the health of the community. A coalition's functional processes include

---

BOX 15-4. WHAT WE LEARNED

- Celebrate results and successes of the Coalition and its members.
- Use shared leadership models; step back to encourage leaders to emerge.
- Create a fun, lively environment.
- Invest in learning opportunities to build group capacity.
- Involve the local media.

BOX 15-5. ADVICE TO OTHERS

- Health professionals/organizations should act as a catalyst for projects not as controllers or dominators.
- Develop annual work plans based on identified need and create measurable indicators for evaluation.
- Establish detailed action plans with assigned responsibilities.
- Strike a balance between process and action, realizing the value of meeting the needs of those members motivated by action and those requiring adequate planning and process time.
- Be patient with process and chaos—order will emerge; develop flexible processes that do not impose a restrictive structure.

---

needs identification, decision-making, action, mobilization, and evaluation. Resources, as well as political and human factors (e.g., capacity, energy), sustain a coalition as an organization and its activities. Others considering a Healthy Communities project have asked for our counsel; our advice is located in Box 15-5.

The HOC is heading into its seventh year. The Coalition remains committed to making a difference to its community's health. The Coalition acknowledges that members must not become complacent and must consider whether it is staying true to the principles of the Healthy Community movement and to PHC. With its foundation of enthusiasm and dedication, the HOC hopes to continue to evolve and become increasingly more effective at working together to achieve its vision: "Okotoks, Our Healthy Home."

References

Baum, F. E. (1993). Healthy Cities and change: Social movement or bureaucratic tool? *Health Promotion International, 8,* 31–40.

Bracht, N. (Ed.) *Health promotion at the community level.* Newbury Park, CA: Sage.

British Columbia Ministry of Health. (1989). *Healthy communities: The process. A guide for volunteers, community leaders, elected officials and health professionals who want to build healthy communities.* Victoria, BC: British Columbia Ministry of Health.

Butterfoss, F. D., Goodman, R. M., & Wandersman, A. (1993). Community coalitions for prevention and health promotion. *Health Education Research, 8,* 315–330.

Dimock, H. & Devine, I. (1994). *Making workgroups effective* (3rd ed.). Concord, ON: Captus Press.

Hancock, T. (1993). The evolution, impact and significance of the healthy cities/healthy communities movement. *Journal of Public Health Policy,* November, 5–18.

Hancock, T., & Duhl, L. (1986). *Healthy cities: Promoting health in the urban context. Healthy Cities Paper #1.* Copenhagen, Denmark: WHO Europe.

Headwaters Health Authority. (1998). *Strategic planning: The products and the process.* Internal planning document. High River, AB: Author.

Hodson, B. A. (1999). *The process of creating a healthy community in rural Alberta.* Faculty Graduate Studies and Research, Centre for Health Promotion Studies. Unpublished Master of Science Thesis, University of Alberta, Edmonton.

Roulier, M., & McGrath, M. (1998). Healthy Communities: The movement. *Partnership Perspectives*, Spring.

World Health Organization. (1946). *Constitution.* New York: Author.

World Health Organization. (1986). *Ottawa Charter for Health Promotion. First International Health Promotion Conference.* Ottawa: Author.

World Health Organization. (1978). Declaration of Alma Ata. International Conference on Primary Health Care, Alma Ata, USSR, Sept. 6–12, 1978. www.who/int/hpr/archive/docs/almaata.html.

Suggested Readings

Chalmers, K. I., & Bramadat, I. J. (1996). Community development: Theoretical and practical issues for community health nursing in Canada. *Journal of Advanced Nursing, 24,* 719–726.

Dehar, M., Casswell, S., & Duignan, P. (1993). Formative and process evaluation of health promotion and disease prevention programs. *Evaluation Review, 17,* 204–220.

Flynn, B. C. (1992). Healthy cities: A model of community change. *Family and Community Health, 15,* 13–23.

Hancock, T. (1995). Creating healthy communities: The role of the health care organizations. *Canadian Health Care Management*, November, 133–135.

Hayes, M. V., & Willms, S. M. (1990). Healthy community indicators: The perils of the search and the paucity of the find. *Health Promotion International, 5,* 161–166.

Kickbush, I. (1989). *Good planets are hard to find, WHO healthy cities papers #5.* Copenhagen, Denmark: World Health Organization.

Labonté, R. (1993). *Issues in health promotion series. #3 Health promotion and empowerment: Practice frameworks.* Toronto: Centre for Health Promotion, University of Toronto and ParticipACTION.

McGraw, S. A., McKinlay, S. M., McClements, L., Lasater, T. M., Assaf, A., & Carlton, R. A. (1989). Methods in program evaluation: The process evaluation system of the Pawtucket Heart Health Program. *Evaluation Review, 13,* 459–483.

Nuñez, A., Colomer, C., Peiro, R., & Alvarz-Dardet, C. (1994). The Valencian community healthy cities network: Assessment of the implementation process. *Health Promotion International, 9,* 189–198.

Pearson, T. A., Bales, V. S., Blair, L., Emmanuel, S. C., Farquhar, J. W., Low, L. P., MacGregor, L. J., MacLean, D. R., O'Connor, B., Pardell, H., & Petrasovits, A. (1998). The Singapore declaration: Forging the will for heart health in the next millennium. *CVD Prevention, 1,* 182–199.

Poland, B. D. (1996). Knowledge development and evaluation in, of, and for, Healthy Community initiatives. Part II: Potential content foci. *Health Promotion International, 11,* 341–349.

Internet Resources

Directory of Canadian Healthy Community networks: **www.ulaval.ca/fsi/oms/p2En.html**

16

School as Community: Springhill School Summer Camp Project

LYNN CORCORAN

OBJECTIVES

After studying this chapter, you should be able to:

◆ Describe the use of the community-as-partner process to plan a population-focused program

◆ Understand how a multidisciplinary and interagency partnership functioned

◆ Describe how process evaluation was used to assess program success

Introduction

Springhill School is a high-needs, inner-city school, many of whose children are challenged by poverty, family violence, poor nutrition, and lack of social support for their families. Some families do not have enough to eat. Some families are led by single-parent mothers (who gave birth to their babies as teenagers) and experience difficulty with accessing education for themselves, finding meaningful work, or obtaining reliable, safe child care. Some families live in apartments where drinking parties, followed by fights, occur week after week. The consequences of these challenges are reflected in children's social skills, behaviour, and academic performance. Some children display aggressive behaviours and lash out verbally with profanities and physically by punching and kicking. Some children are extremely withdrawn and barely able to express their needs or feelings. Some children have poor problem-solving skills and low self-esteem. Some children perform well below academic standards for their grade level. What could be done to help the children from these families?

In 1991, a public health nurse, a mental health therapist, a special needs teacher, and a police officer working together at Springhill School gathered to discuss the possibility of providing a summer camp for a small group of children whose behaviour was beginning to reflect the influence of living in poverty, with family violence, with poor nutrition, and in social isolation.

Assessment: Discovering the Population, Uncovering the Needs

Teachers from kindergarten through grade 3 classes at Springhill School were asked to identify potential campers who met the following selection criteria:

◆ Child would benefit from social interaction
◆ Child exhibits "problem" behaviour (e.g., swearing, fighting, withdrawing)
◆ Child is at risk for neglect or abuse
◆ Child is experiencing reading delay

The initial list of potential campers was given to the special needs teacher and public health nurse. Based on her experience with the children in the school, at homes with their family, and in the clinic, the public health nurse was in a unique position to offer her observations of the children and their families in an effort to narrow the list. The assistant principal of Springhill School was consulted for final approval of the proposed candidates. Additional criteria for selection evolved, after consultation, to include:

◆ Children from single-parent families
◆ Families with more than one child eligible to attend camp
◆ Children with little parental supervision
◆ Children with little structure/activity during the summer

Once a final list of potential campers was determined and a priority order established, the special needs teacher telephoned the parents to inform them of the opportunity for their child to attend the Springhill School Summer Camp. When verbal affirmation of attendance was obtained, a letter describing the camp and a consent form were sent home with the children. The public health nurse facilitated this process by making a home visit to those families of potential campers who did not have a telephone. Like the special needs teacher, the public health nurse was able to describe the camp to the parents and invite their participation. If a family did not want to be involved with the camp, another child was selected from the list.

The campers included an equal number of boys and girls, aged 5 to 9. They came from single-parent, blended, and two-parent families from diverse cultural backgrounds.

Planning: Building Authentic Partnership

The camp was conceived and developed by the spring following the initial idea proposal the previous September. It took another full school year to complete the preparations for the first Springhill School Summer Camp.

Nine community agencies formed a consortium: Provincial Family and Social Services; Provincial Mental Health; City Board of Education; City Health Services; City Police Service; City Social Services; City Parks and Recreation; Springhill Community Association; and a local charitable organization. The logistics of getting people of these agencies together for a meeting was challenging. To create "buy in" for the summer camp project, several "levels" of people working for the same agency were invited to meetings. For example, the Springhill School police officer and his supervisor would attend the meeting as representatives of the City Police Service. Similarly, the Springhill School public health nurse and her district office manager attended meetings to represent City Health Services. Involving multiple levels of people within an agency was essential to:

◆ Maintaining awareness about the project
◆ Securing funding
◆ Sharing ideas and expertise
◆ Supporting communication within and among agencies

A planning committee was formed from the consortium; it included one person from all agencies except the Springhill Community Association, Provincial Family and Social Services, and the local charitable organization. These agencies opted out of the planning process but provided ongoing support in the areas of funding and support of the camp philosophy. With this support, the planning committee was able to go forward with the work of planning and organizing the Springhill School Summer Camp.

Camp Philosophy, Goal, and Objectives

Developing and agreeing on a philosophy, goal, and objectives was time consuming and frustrating, engaging and rewarding. This framework provided the foundation for the camp and was referred to when struggles occurred with decision-making in all phases (from assessment to evaluation) of the camp planning process.

The philosophy of the camp was that play and recreation provide a child with relationship requisites (i.e., attachment, trust, safety, positive self-image) that are the foundation of social skills. The overall goal was to develop and enhance the campers' social skills through play and recreation. Specific camp objectives were to:

- Create a safe and fun environment for the campers
- Increase campers' self-esteem
- Reduce campers' aggressive/withdrawn behaviour
- Increase campers' problem-solving skills
- Increase campers' competence in reading

Implementation: The Fun

Logistics

The camp operated Monday through Thursday from 9:30 AM to 3:30 PM for 4 weeks during July. Camp counsellors, hired specifically for this project, took the lead role in planning activities for the campers. Themes such as "Beach Day" and "Krazy Kite Day" were incorporated into the camp. The City Boys and Girls Club provided breakfast and mid-morning snacks; campers' parents supplied lunch. Most days were spent playing games and sports as well as doing arts and crafts. A reading area was created in the main camp room; it was stocked with books designed to address feelings and issues such as loss and separation. Stories were read to the campers almost every day; a volunteer came to camp several times to read one-on-one with some of the children. Off-site trips were taken to the public library, the fire station, the community swimming pool, an amusement park, and the city zoo. Special guests visited the camp, including a group of physically challenged people who spoke to the campers about their experiences with disability, a dog trainer and her dog who showed the campers their skills, and a local women's group who treated the campers to a hotdog lunch.

Staff

Camp staff and support persons represented six agencies: three camp counsellors (one position hired and funded by City Social Services, two positions hired and funded by City Parks and Recreation); a mental health therapist (Provincial Mental Health Services); a police officer (City Police Service); a public health nurse (City Health Services); along with a special needs teacher, a teen volunteer, and a school janitor provided by the City Board of Education. Some campers' parents also participated as volunteers.

Process

The children were expected to participate in the planned activities. When activities were in process, the children used social skills (e.g., listening, controlling impulses, and cooperation) that were necessary requisites for participation. These social skills were modeled by the camp leaders and positively reinforced by leaders' praise and encouragement.

When social skills were performed poorly by the children and replaced with negative behaviours (e.g., hitting, yelling, and withdrawing), the activity was stopped. Staff initiated a process where the "problem" was explored with the child involved; they took the child aside, helped the child identify the issue (with an emphasis on feelings of self and others), think about alternatives, choose the best alternative, act on this choice, and rejoin the activity. The skills and expertise of a full-time mental health therapist facilitated this process.

Evaluation: Examining Process and Outcome

Overall camp attendance was good. During the camp, children exhibited a wide range of behaviours and emotions: negative social behaviours such as aggression, hitting, kicking, biting, choking, spitting, swearing, and throwing objects; emotional responses such as whining, withdrawing, running away from activities, and fear; and positive social behaviours such as sharing with each other, including others in their play, showing concern for others, and resolving conflicts effectively.

There were several occasions when children were sent home because they were unable to exercise control over their behaviour. There were a few occasions where planned activities could not be completed due to the children's lack of cooperation. These incidents were managed by strategies such as modeling and time out. In some cases, activities were changed or feedback statements were made about the individual or group process. Off-site trips seemed to be an impetus for the group as a whole to exhibit challenging behaviours. Campers were permanently expelled from the public library on their second visit due to running around and too much loud talking. Campers received repeated feedback from swimming pool staff regarding inappropriate behaviour; they came close to being permanently expelled from the pool as well. The off-site trips to the fire station, the zoo, and an amusement park were successful. However, on the way to the amusement park, the bus driver pulled the bus over to the side of the road to warn the children that if the noise level continued unabated, he would turn around and go back to Springhill School.

Formal Evaluations

Campers

Campers completed a social skills checklist on a one-to-one basis with the mental health therapist on the first day of camp and approximately 2 months after the camp ended. The evaluation comprised 20 questions on self-esteem, social skill development, aggressive/withdrawn behaviours, and problem-solving skills. The children reported most improvement in self-esteem, with small improvement reported in aggressive/withdrawn behaviours and social skills. The children reported a slight decrease in problem-solving skills.

Parents

Parents were interviewed before and after the camp session, primarily by the mental health therapist, assisted by the public health nurse and special needs teacher. In June, prior to camp, they were asked to describe changes they would like to see occur with their child as a result of participation in this program. In

September, following camp, they were asked to describe any changes they noticed with their child. Additionally, parents were asked for comments and suggestions. Only half of the parents participated in the postcamp survey that was conducted by telephone; some families had moved and several families did not have a telephone. Further, resources did not allow the use of home visits and other extraordinary means to contact the parents. This experience is informative; frequent moves are often characteristic of families struggling with many challenges. In general, the parents who responded reported a high level of satisfaction with the camp. Some parents reported improvements in their child's behaviours. One parent reported that there was a negative change in her child's behaviour. She felt the other children had been a "bad influence" on her son because after the camp experience he began to use profane language at home.

Teachers

Kindergarten to grade 3 teachers completed brief surveys that were very general in nature before and after the camp. In June, they were asked to describe specific changes they would like to see with each child. In September, teachers reported on any changes they had noticed in the children after attending camp. Data were available on only eight children because some families had moved away and other children had different teachers in the new school year. Teachers reported improvements in five of the eight campers' social skills behaviour, for example, children playing better with classmates and cooperating better in classroom group activities.

Camp Counsellors

Camp counsellors completed a 4-page standard City Program Evaluation form consisting of 13 questions. In summary, the four camp counsellors:

◆ Suggested the camp was not long enough
◆ Reported they need additional information in how to deal with "problem behaviour" in children
◆ Agreed they had support from the planning group
◆ Agreed the camper-to-counsellor ratio was adequate
◆ Would return to work at camp, if asked
◆ Believed the counsellors were an extremely cohesive group

Planning Committee

Approximately 3 months following the camp, planning committee members from six community agencies met to discuss what was learned from the experience and future directions. Recommendations were made based on the results of the camp evaluations; these recommendations were implemented for the next summer's camp.

Analysis: What Worked and
Why It Worked: Authentic Partnership

The Springhill School Summer Camp began with the "seed" of an idea. Several factors were in place prior to embarking on the journey to the creation of the camp. The special needs teacher, public health nurse, police officer, and mental health therapist working at Springhill School cared deeply about the children and their families. Although their work at the school involved very different tasks, their work with the children was done with respect, sensitivity, and patience. Further, the teacher, nurse, police officer, and therapist had exemplary professional working relationships based on respect, trust, and flexibility for years before the camp. They had previously worked together on many smaller projects within the school. Panet-Raymond (1992) stated the "human factors" influencing partnerships include "open-mindedness, tolerance, patience, respect and sensitivity" (p. 163). I believe these human factors were present in the initial small group and served to foster a similar atmosphere at the levels of the planning committee and consortium.

Although there were time lines for the completion of tasks set by the planning group, there was a commitment to not pushing the process. Much planning occurred in the first year, even though a camp did not take place. It was decided that more groundwork needed to be done. The group remained committed to the camp, but they were not willing to rush to the implementation phase without consensus from all agencies, secure funding, and attention to fine details such as liability insurance for children at a school during the summer.

The development of a camp philosophy, overall goal, and specific objectives was absolutely key to the success of the Springhill School Summer Camp. This process is supported in the literature on partnerships (Kang, 1995; Labonte, 1993; Panet-Raymond, 1992; Scott & Thurston, 1997; Stewart, Banks, & Crosman, 1995). The camp philosophy guided the agencies as a consortium and was used frequently throughout the planning process to keep activities "on track." In the process of creating evaluations, the camp philosophy, overall goal, and objectives provided guidelines for measuring outcomes. With this in place, it was easy to analyze the evaluations and make recommendations. Several changes took place from the first to second camp, including the revision of camp goals, more orientation and training days for camp counsellors, and revised evaluation forms for children, parents, and teachers. This feedback loop enabled the planning committee to confidently act on information from the first camp and make the necessary adaptations for the next camp. We celebrated success; we learned from mistakes.

One of the strengths of the Springhill School Summer Camp was the equal distribution of power. Without a doubt, each person involved in the camp was invested within the context of his or her work life. The therapist was most interested in the mental health of the campers; the public health nurse was most concerned about children's health issues; the special needs teacher was most interested in improving the campers' academic performance; and the police officer was most concerned about the campers becoming good citizens. Somehow, these particular interests became secondary to what the group was hoping to accomplish together. As such, all professionals shared their skills and knowledge, and it was in this "letting go" of specific interests that power was shared equally among group members. The camp counsellors were very aware of what was going on with each camper because they were at the camp all day, every day, with the children; this knowledge was appreciated by the professional staff. The volunteers were honoured for their generosity, time, energy, and commitment. The planning group and consortium were appreciated for providing the counsellors with the structure and vision from which to operate the day-to-day activities. Shared power is critical to the formation and maintenance of partnership initiatives (Labonte, 1993).

Ongoing verbal and written communication kept all agencies informed, a very important action, because three agencies involved in the consortium were not involved in the planning group. Also, managers and supervisors were involved more at the level of the consortium and involved less in the planning group where the front-line staff had more to offer. Minutes of meetings and draft copies of forms and evaluations were circulated to all parties to keep all agencies informed. This attention to the "big picture" helped to sustain commitment from all parties in the consortium to support the camp and secure further partners and funding.

There were many decisions to be made over the course of assessing, planning, implementing, and evaluating the camp, such as what the optimal age range of campers might be, what action steps might take place when dealing with a child's inappropriate or unsafe behaviour during camp, and what questions might be posed in an evaluation interview with the campers' parents. With these decisions, the consortium, planning group, and camp staff experienced conflict. The foundations of trust and respect and regard for one another enabled individuals to stay engaged in the process of decision-making to reach consensus by actively listening and considering all points of view. Consensus building was viewed as a process of allowing everyone to be heard; it was not railroading, bulldozing, or co-opting others. Chinn (1995) stated that decisions reached by consensus are stronger than any decision made by an individual; consensus decisions embrace different perspectives and build unity around the group's purpose. As difficult as it was at times, those involved with the Springhill School Summer Camp used consensus to reach decisions and, in so doing, created stronger partnerships.

Summary

The Springhill School Summer Camp ran for two summers. Its end came in the context of massive provincial government cuts influencing restructuring of agencies and policy. The consortium and planning committee were not able to maintain partnerships in the face of significant political changes involving critical loss of funding and personnel resources. Despite this, for the two summers that it operated, Springhill School Summer Camp provided a safe place for children challenged by poverty, family violence, and poor nutrition to participate in fun activities while learning the social skills necessary to enjoy being part of a group.

References

Chinn, P. L. (1995). Cooperation and collectivity in action: Consensus. In *Peace and power: Building communities for the future* (4th ed., pp. 53–61). New York: National League for Nursing.

Kang, R. (1995). Building community capacity for health promotion: A challenge for public health nurses. *Public Health Nursing, 12*(5), 312–318.

Labonte, R. (1993). Community development and partnerships. *Canadian Journal of Public Health, 84*(4), 237–240.

Panet-Raymond, J. (1992). Partnership: Myth or reality? *Community Development Journal, 27*(2), 156–165.

Scott, C. M., & Thurston, W. E. (1997). A framework for the development of community health agency partnerships. *Canadian Journal of Public Health, 88*(6), 416–420.

Stewart, M. J., Banks, S., & Crossman, D. (1995). Health professionals' perceptions of partnership with self-help groups. *Canadian Journal of Public Health, 86*(5), 341–344.

17

Community Care for Perinatal Women Living With HIV

JEANNE M. SARGENT
ARDENE ROBINSON VOLLMAN

CHAPTER OUTLINE

Introduction
Assessment
Project Implementation
Summary

OBJECTIVES

After studying this chapter, you should be able to:

◆ Describe the health challenges faced by childbearing women living with HIV

◆ Describe the impact of the determinants of health on women living with HIV

◆ Note the planning issues involved in integrating services across levels of care (primary care, hospital care, and community care)

Introduction

Globally, the number of women living with HIV infection has been increasing steadily. By 2001, 16.4 million women were living with HIV and AIDS, accounting for 47% of the 34.7 million adults living with this infection (World Health Organization [WHO], 2000). According to the National

Institute of Allergy and Infectious Diseases (NIAID) of the U.S. National Institutes of Health (NIAID, 2001), women face the greatest risk of acquiring HIV infection from sexual intercourse due to substantial mucosal exposure to seminal fluids, high prevalence of nonconsensual sex, sex without condom use, and unknown high-risk behaviours of their partners (e.g., unprotected sex with others, particularly men, injection drug use, and needle-sharing).

Women suffer from the same complications of AIDS that affect men, but also experience sex-specific manifestations of disease (e.g., recurrent yeast infections, pelvic inflammatory disease). Similarly, women may experience different complications from antiretroviral therapy than men. Frequently women with HIV have trouble gaining access to care and carry the burden of caring for children and other family members who may also be infected with HIV. They often lack social support, which interferes with their ability to comply with treatment regimens (NIAID, 2001).

In Canada, the number of women diagnosed with HIV continues to increase. Although there has been an overall drop of 25% in the number of new HIV infections in Canada since 1995, the female infection rate has increased from 10% prior to 1995 to 25% in 2001 (Health Canada, 2001). The major reported modes of transmission in women with AIDS include injection drug use (36.8%) and heterosexual contact with an infected partner (50.0%, including 23.7% from contact with a partner from a country where AIDS is endemic, and 26.3% from contact with partners who are at risk from lifestyle choices). In 13.2% of cases, there is no identified risk (NIR) except heterosexual sex. Approximately 80% of total AIDS cases among Canadian women are in the childbearing age (15–44 years). Of pediatric cases the majority (84%) can be attributed to mother-to-child (vertical or perinatal) transmission (Health Canada, 2001).

Although pregnancy is not harmful to the health of a woman living with HIV/AIDS, there is a risk of vertical (perinatal) transmission to the infant; statistics vary, but estimates range from 8% to 25% of infants born to HIV-infected mothers will become infected. Transmission depends on a number of factors: the amount of virus in the blood (viral load), general health status, effect of antiretroviral drugs, other STD infections, unprotected vaginal intercourse with an HIV+ partner, and aspects of the labour and delivery experience. The baby is more at risk if the mother is seroconverting (i.e., in the first 3 months of infection) or if she has progressed to AIDS. The longer the time between rupture of membranes and delivery, the greater the risk of transmission. After birth, breastfeeding increases the possibility of transmission from mother to infant (Family Planning Australia [FPA Health], 2001).

In Canada, 121 infants were reported exposed perinatally to HIV, estimating that from 10 to 30 infants would have become infected. Of 119 follow-up reports, 5 were confirmed infected, 82 confirmed not infected, and 32 cases had not yet been confirmed by June 30, 2001. All babies carry their mother's HIV antibodies for the first 12 to 18 months of life, so they will initially test positive. More complex tests for the virus itself are done with infants to determine the presence of infection.

Assessment

In the Calgary Health Region the proportion of women newly infected with HIV in the year 2000 was 21% of the total cases diagnosed. Immigrant (44%) and First Nations' (33%) women are overrepresented relative to their proportion in the population. In 1999, the Southern Alberta Clinic provided treatment to more than 83 women living with HIV; of these, over 80% are of childbearing age (15–44 years). Since universal prenatal screening for HIV came into effect in 1998, approximately one pregnant woman is reported every 6 weeks to be HIV+ in Calgary. However, less than one third are diagnosed during prenatal screening; two thirds have had very late or no prenatal care where screening would be conducted. Not having a pregnant woman's HIV status on record can place health professionals at risk and also risks the health of the infant. In 1999, over 20% of infants born to HIV+ women were placed into foster or adopted care.

To identify and address concerns of women living with HIV in Calgary, stakeholders in reproductive health services, community agencies, and women living with HIV gathered informally to discuss action on the issue. In 1999, a focus group identified some of the major concerns expressed by women living with HIV as fear of death, people finding out, being ostracized, not having all the facts about their illness, and not knowing the impact of the diagnosis on the family. When asked about their experience with health care workers, focus group participants stated their major concerns were not being addressed; they found most health care professionals not up-to-date regarding HIV; and they needed to find information themselves so they could ask the proper questions. In talking about where they received support, the majority listed family, health care professionals at the HIV treatment clinic, voluntary AIDS organizations, and positive women's groups. The focus group participants expressed that there was a general lack of information about pregnancy, safer sex, and sexual health resources available specific to women.

In light of the findings from the focus group and the perceptions of stakeholders in the reproductive health field, an environmental scan was conducted. A review of HIV/AIDS resources revealed a paucity of information specific to women's reproductive health. Most information available was meant for a broader audience; there were no resources available for women with low literacy levels or in languages other than English and French. The scan also revealed a lack of coordination among organizations providing services to women living with HIV/AIDS, requiring women to go to different locations and agencies to receive the treatment, information, support, and resources they needed.

Project Implementation

A steering committee of concerned stakeholders in reproductive health was created and, in 1999, a proposal was submitted to the Alberta Health and Wellness Health Innovation Fund (HIF) to support an initiative that would address the issues identified. In response, a project was funded for 3 years to provide comprehensive, integrated reproductive and perinatal care for women living with HIV in the Calgary Health Region. The steering committee acknowledged that it would be a challenge to maintain privacy with a small target group. There is a danger of overresearching this population of women and care providers. Because of the vulnerability of the target group there will be, inevitably, many sensitive ethical issues to be addressed as the project unfolds.

The overall goal of the project is to reduce vertical transmission of HIV. Objectives of the project are:

◆ To understand the reproductive and perinatal needs of women living with HIV
◆ To provide service providers with current information about the reproductive and perinatal needs of women living with HIV
◆ To develop and initiate a coordinated community referral mechanism for women living with HIV
◆ To provide special services to women living with HIV
◆ To provide a coach-advocate to act as a bridge to the health care system, women living with HIV, and their community
◆ To identify and address gaps in service to women with HIV

The logic model for the project is shown in Table 17-1 and outlines the service and capacity building components, activities, processes, outcomes, and indicators of success.

A master's-prepared nurse was hired as project director. Accountability for the project rested with the steering committee; financial accountability was through the Communicable Disease Unit of the Calgary Health Region.

TABLE 17-1 ◆ PROJECT LOGIC MODEL

Project Goal   Reduce vertical transmission of HIV

Based on a prior needs assessment that increased understanding of the reproductive and perinatal needs of HIV+ women in Calgary through the use of focus group methods, literature review, and an environmental scan. It is intended to incorporate this knowledge into services developed and provided in this project.

Project components

1. Care Provision

	Training	Referral Services	Special Services
Processes	Curriculum developed Training sessions Agency training Use of modules	Referral process developed Protocols disseminated Protocol utilization Database developed Practice guidelines developed Guidelines disseminated	Development and utilization of: • Infant formula • Transportation assistance • Contraception materials • Counselling services • Respite
Outcomes	Increased knowledge Improved attitudes Trainee satisfaction	Protocols Practice guidelines Communication strategy Reports generated from database Satisfaction of users/clients	Utilization reports Client/caregiver satisfaction Gap analysis
Indicators	Pretests and posttests Interviews Survey	Descriptions Expert review Descriptive statistics Surveys/interviews	Descriptive statistics Vignettes Interviews/surveys

2. Empowerment and Self-Care/System Capacity

	Coach Advocate Service	Sustainability
Processes	Hiring coach-advocates Training of coaches Service provision	Project advisory committee Agency involvement In-kind contribution
Outcomes	Increased awareness Client utilization Client satisfaction Advocate satisfaction	Strategy for ongoing funding Statement of contributions Outreach workers, PHNs in place
Indicators	Employment statistics Descriptive statistics (Re: utilization) Interviews/surveys	Grant proposals submitted In-kind contributions detailed Staffing plans enacted

Services to Women Living With HIV

As a first step in the project, the project director initiated the process of hiring the coach-advocate, a social worker with extensive experience with Aboriginal and street-involved women. Concurrently, contacts were made to arrange for special services for women in the target group (e.g., transportation to appointments, free infant formula, respite care for other children, contraception advice and materials, and social support services). The coach-advocate and project director made home visits; accompanied women to medical appointments (e.g., HIV care, prenatal care, infant care, postnatal care); interfaced with literacy agencies, utility companies, landlords, food banks, and social services on behalf of the women in the project; and translated information received into lay language for them. En route to and from appointments the project staff would debrief with the women what they had been told; counsel them on actions needed; teach them about medications, formula preparation, and child care; and encourage them to ask questions of their health care providers. As women became more knowledgeable, they became more able to speak up with questions to providers, attend appointments on their own, and take care of their daily affairs and children. The vignette in Box 17-1 illustrates the experience of one woman.

The story contained in Box 17-1 is not the same for street-involved women who have substance use issues. In this case, the coach-advocate reaches out to them in shelters and at soup kitchens. They occasionally contact the project staff when they are in crisis. Most of these women have had their children apprehended, and one recently had a late-term stillbirth. These women live with violence every day and are difficult to locate and maintain contact with. Sometimes they move out of the region and are lost to follow-up.

The scope of coach-advocate services over 8 months for one client admitted to the program 5 months prior to the birth of her first child is illustrated in Box 17-2.

Coordination of Services

As project staff accompanied women in their quest for services, it became increasingly evident that the perception of fragmentation of services was accurate. The steering committee developed a flow sheet and protocol for referrals to make the experience more seamless for women. The committee was committed to improve coordination among agencies but needed to overcome the reticence of providers to share confidential information. To address this concern, project staff asked clients to consent to release of information among key providers. This consent was not open-ended; it stipulated who could be contacted on the client's behalf and what information could be released. In this way clients could control the degree to which agencies could share information about them. They could choose to use project staff as liaison or could receive advice regarding which agencies they could contact themselves for service, support, and counselling.

BOX 17-1. A WOMAN'S STORY

A woman, call her Jane, was admitted to the project at the time of the birth of her second child. Jane had had no prenatal care; she was an immigrant and not literate, and her husband did not take her to the doctor. Her oldest child was 2 at the time of admission; he is not HIV+.

The HIV status of Jane's husband is not known. He came to Canada before Jane, went to school, and is now "working" and is reportedly involved in substance use. He used to beat Jane and the children and kept Jane very isolated from people. Jane had no friends or relatives in Calgary. When the baby was only a few weeks old, he left Jane and the children and has had no further contact with them.

Immediately following the birth of Jane's daughter, the coach-advocate tried to provide assistance, but was rebuffed by the husband, who was still in the home. Initially, minimal services were accepted, in terms of formula and transportation to appointments. The coach-advocate tried to maintain contact, telephoning during the day when the husband was out, offering support and suggesting community resources. On one occasion, the coach-advocate made a follow-up contact and, finding the phone out of order, went to the home. There, she found Jane and the children in a cold apartment, no food, no clothing for the children or herself, and without utilities or telephone service. She had not received welfare cheques for 3 months, since her husband left, and she had been reporting to the coach-advocate "all was fine." It was not fine—she had trusted no one, told no one of her real situation, and was in desperate straits as a consequence.

The coach-advocate immediately contacted the social worker at the AIDS clinic and over the next few days, between the two of them, had the utilities and telephone reinstated to the apartment, found emergency funds for rent, connected Jane to community resources for clothing and childcare supplies, and arranged for a trip to the food bank.

Once stabilized, the coach-advocate took Jane to the bank to set up an account, to pay her bills, and had her enrolled in an English as a second language (ESL) class. The children were placed in subsidized day care that had a program in place to provide stimulation and language training.

Jane, however, was reticent to speak up in ESL class, felt embarrassed by her single-parent status, her lack of money, and her inability to read and write. The coach-advocate attended a class with her, spent a few hours weekly with Jane in her apartment teaching and demonstrating how to carry out the activities of daily life. Eventually, she captured Jane's trust. Then, little by little, the severe challenges of Jane's everyday life were revealed. She began to reach out, asking questions of her teachers at school, talking with classmates, and transferring that trust to others.

(continued)

BOX 17-1. A WOMAN'S STORY (*Continued*)

Now, after this intense period of intervention, the coach-advocate is in brief contact about once every 10 days. Jane's teachers report: "she has become a different person" and attribute this to the "bridge created by the project." Jane attends class regularly, is able to pay her bills, shop, and maintain her treatment regimen. As her English improves, she is more self-confident because she has become more able to take care of herself, her children, and her affairs.

Jane is attending medical appointments regularly for herself and the baby. She appreciates that the coach-advocate drives her to the appointments, stays with her and "rehashes what happened" with her on the way home. The coach-advocate puts instructions in plain language and draws pictures as necessary so that Jane can follow instructions.

The baby is healthy and both children are thriving. Jane hopes to be able to get a job soon, once her son is in school full time.

Training Care Providers

As the project gained visibility among community agencies, the need for training became more urgent. The intent of the project's training component is to develop, implement, and evaluate an effective, sustainable model of peer HIV education by training staff educators and staff nurses to provide on-the-job training to coworkers. The goal of training is to increase knowledge, reduce fear, and create positive attitudes among those who work with women living with HIV infection. A resource manual with seven modules was developed to support training efforts: basic facts about HIV/AIDS, hepatitis B and C; working with women living with HIV; HIV antibody testing; infection prevention and control; women, HIV, and pregnancy; women, HIV, sexual and reproductive health; and women, HIV, and substance use. The manual, which also contained teaching/learning resources, an extensive bibliography and pre/post tests, was developed by the project staff, reviewed and approved by the Steering Committee, and printed and disseminated to stakeholders by Planned Parenthood of Calgary. People selected to become peer trainers had knowledge of adult learning principles, teaching and presentation skills, interest in gaining knowledge about women and HIV, and were motivated to facilitate education and support to coworkers. Agencies involved in the project agreed to provide time for facilitators to attend the initial training sessions, and to create opportunities for peer-based learning on the job for remaining staff.

There is a definite need for effective and efficient means of continuing education; workshops continue to be the vehicle of choice because they are cost effective, reach large numbers, and provide an efficient means for information dis-

---

BOX 17-2. SERVICES PROVIDED TO ONE CLIENT OVER 8 MONTHS

Transportation: 33 hours

Accompaniment to high-risk prenatal clinic (6 visits)	15.5 hr
Accompaniment to ESL classes (2 classes)	3.0 hr
Accompaniment to medical centre for intravenous meds	5.0 hr
Accompaniment for baby care (children's hospital, pediatrician)	9.5 hr

Contacts for other purposes: 38 (approximately 60 hours)

Taxi chits	9
Phone consultations	15
Home visits by project staff	9
Formula deliveries	4
Family planning clinic visits	1

Services accessed by the client:

Southern Alberta Clinic
Interfaith food bank
Thrift store
Family physician
Obstetrician
Pediatrician
Infectious Diseases Children's Hospital
Public health nursing
Best Beginning Program
English as a second language
Immigrant women's aid
Social welfare
Respite care (Children's Cottage)

---

semination. The degree to which they are effective for attitudinal change is, however, unknown. In this project, knowledge acquisition was a large part of the desired outcome, but it is hoped that with knowledge, changes in attitudes about HIV care and toward HIV+ women and their infants would be also achieved. To measure these objectives in the short term is impossible; nevertheless, the details of the workshops were reviewed for the purposes of documenting the process, challenges, and solutions during the pilot-testing phase. Methods used to collect evaluation data included interviews with project staff, consultant, and manager; training manual review; and the analysis of manager and staff nurse before workshop questionnaires, pretests and posttests, and workshop evaluations.

Inputs into the training component were primarily the time of the educator (a half-time position), project coordinator, and the time contributions of managers and educators (meetings) and staff (training). The educator, new to the project and the substantive area of practice, underwent an abbreviated orientation period where she met key contacts, stakeholders, and the steering committee. Audiovisual, electronic and print resources were sought and reviewed; the manual was reviewed; expertise was sought from consultants (instructional design and evaluation); Powerpoint presentations were developed; instruments, notices, and forms were designed; and workshops were planned, scheduled and conducted. A teaching and learning module was outlined as suggested by the educator, but not completed due to project constraints for the first round of training. Because of the educator's knowledge of public health nurse (PHN) practice and the needs assessment carried out in support of the second round of workshops (with PHNs) she developed a Powerpoint presentation on adult education principles for the first workshop and accompanied this with supplemental handouts and readings on adult learning and the facilitation process.

Project staff underestimated the time that needed to be allocated to the training process in several ways: the manual was clinically focused and needed some revision to make it user-friendly for educational purposes (i.e., more interactive learning activities); resource review time was minimal, given the imperative to search nationally for resources; tools for learning needs assessment needed to be developed; and there was need to build rapport and market the training workshops to managers, staff educators, and nursing staff, as well as to establish roles and relationships for sustainability.

Training was carried out in a climate of restraint and budget cuts; nursing contractual obligations that require payment for all professional development activities, including preparatory reading; few HIV+ women were receiving nursing care at certain sites compared to HIV− obstetric cases; other competing demands for education; and demands on staff educators' time.

The training process was adapted by putting manuals on all regional obstetric nursing units in advance of the first workshops; project staff conducted the workshops with nursing staff; with future in-services to be conducted by site-specific staff educators and infectious diseases personnel. For the public health nurse facilitator workshops, participants were given manuals after the first workshop day and had an opportunity to review the modules, along with supplemental readings, in the interim before the second workshop day 2 weeks later. Workshop content was determined by the pre-surveys, questions submitted by attendees, and issues known by project staff to be concerns as expressed by client and advisory committee feedback.

The training process was carried out as designed only in the Public Health Service, although not fully honoured in terms of one facilitator per community district. Significant adaptations were made to accommodate the challenges and constraints of the hospital sites. Participants expressed a high level of satisfaction with the workshop; pretest and posttest scores indicated that knowledge was gained, but that attitudes remained fairly constant.

Sustainability

For this HIF Project a working definition of sustainability reads:

[T]he ability to improve institutional capacity in order to adopt a realistic and innovative strategy to provide quality comprehensive integrated reproductive and perinatal care to HIV positive women in the Calgary region with a view to effectively incorporating and utilizing the array of resources available, and expanding services to a wider population of HIV-infected women.

With this suggested definition in mind, the International Planned Parenthood Federation's framework for sustainability (February 2000) is germane. Its goal of sustainability is to create an efficient and entrepreneurial culture in which to develop human resources and management capacity.

Three key components and their respective strategies have been proposed for this HIF project, as illustrated in Table 17-2.

This project faces some complex sustainability questions, some fraught with organizational tensions:

◆ Will the Health Region incorporate this service as part of its regular programming?
◆ If yes, where will it be housed? Who will staff it? How much budget will be allocated?
◆ If not, from where will the ongoing funding come? What sorts of grant proposals and evidence will be required? Who will write these?
◆ If not, what will happen to these women and their children?

Summary

At the time of writing, this project has 6 months to completion. It is on track, on budget, and is meeting its interim objectives. The quality of services is exceptional; care providers and clients express a high level of satisfaction. The project meets the health needs of perinatal women infected with HIV and is innovatively and collaboratively addressing a gap in services to this population. No infants born to women enrolled in the project have acquired a vertically transmitted infection.

TABLE 17-2 ◆ COMPONENTS OF SUSTAINABILITY APPLIED TO THE PROJECT

Institutional Sustainability

Developing sound management practices	
• Conducting a needs assessment	Early in the project a needs assessment was conducted and findings incorporated into program planning.
• Using financial and evaluation data	The costs for taxi chits were very high in the early months of the program. Directions of evaluation have been guided by findings.
• Purchasing equipment and training staff	A car seat has been purchased to safely transport children. Respite workers and outreach staff have been trained in its use.
• Marketing and promoting the project	Key stakeholders are aware, but more primary care physicians need to be informed. October 2000—newsletter to physicians. Article in "Frontlines" 2001.
• Evaluating cost effectiveness	In progress. Services are being tracked so costs can be calculated. Cost effectiveness may not be possible with such small numbers of clients.
Strengthening leadership skills and investing in staff training	Obstetric nursing staff is being trained in the hospitals that deliver babies. Eight public health nurses from 8 of 12 offices are being trained as a trainer.
Building partnerships	Stakeholders represent the range of health providers for HIV⁺ women. No social service organizations are formal partners. Informal relationships in place with ESL, shelters, food bank, CIWA, Children's Cottage, and others
Investing in information systems	The population is too small to make a database cost effective; confidentiality is also an issue. A website has been suggested by a stakeholder, but staff nurse and PHN access to computers on the job is extremely limited.
Developing marketing and communication strategies	In progress

Sustainability of Quality Services

Expanding services	Not a part of the project at this time to extend the services to all HIV⁺ women—focus on those who are in the childbearing years. Expressed desire to expand services to include a wider catchment area (e.g., southern Alberta) to match partner mandates
Investing in service providers	Hiring coach advocate, and educator. Training. Shared case conferences with SAC
Evaluating quality	In progress—focus on satisfaction and process

Financial Sustainability

Developing financial management	
• Developing financial systems	CHR
• Identifying potential cost savings	Because taxi expenses were high, clients have been transported by project staff.
• Developing financial projections	Not yet
Resource mobilization	
• Designing a mobilization strategy	In the initial funding proposal; in-kind contributions tracked
• Developing proposals for additional resources	Not yet
• Sharing costs and capitalizing on economies of scale	SAC and CD unit with the project
Income generation	
• Exploring the sale of products	Training manual
• Creating private sector partnerships	Donations or supplies at cost (e.g., female condoms)

CIWA, Calgary Immigrant Women's Association; SAC, Southern Alberta Clinic; CD, communicable diseases.

References

Family Planning Australia. (2001, March 28). *Sex matters: Women and HIV fact sheet 5—pregnancy*. Sydney, NSW: Author.

Health Canada. (2001). *HIV/AIDS in Canada: Surveillance report to June 30, 2001*. Ottawa: Author.

International Planned Parenthood Federation. (2000). *Sustainability initiative*. Retrieved from website: www.ippf.org/initiatives/sustainability/2000feb/index.htm.

National Institute of Allergy and Infectious Diseases. (2001, May). *Fact sheet: HIV infection in women*. National Institutes of Health Bulletin. Washington, DC: Author.

World Health Organization. (2000, December). *UNAIDS/WHO AIDS epidemic update*. Geneva, Switzerland: Author.

Internet Resources

AIDS hotlines: **www.cdnaids.ca** and click "Community Contacts" for a hotline in your area

General information on AIDS: **www.aidsvancouver.bc.ca**

Health Canada Division of HIV Epidemiology: **www.womenfightaids.com/epistats.html**

Kidshelp Line: **www.kidshelp.sympatic.ca**

Motherisk HIV Healthline and Network: **www.motherisk.org**

Planned Parenthood Canada: **www.ppfc.ca**

18

TRAC: Community Mobilization for Healthy Public Policy

MARLIES VAN DIJK

OBJECTIVES

After studying this chapter, you should be able to:

◆ Understand the health effects of environmental tobacco smoke

◆ Appreciate the potential of electronic technologies in health initiatives

◆ Describe how the project mobilized the public to influence public policy

Introduction

This chapter chronicles a campaign initiated by a community group (Tobacco Reduction Action Coalition, "TRAC") that mobilized citizens with the intent to change a public policy. The public policy in this case was a municipal smoking bylaw for a large urban centre in Western Canada.

TRAC began 6 years prior to the launch of the bylaw mobilization campaign when a group of concerned citizens and agency representatives gathered to discuss the high consumption of tobacco in the region.

The agencies involved in TRAC consisted of both provincial and local organizations such as the Cancer Society, provincial Lung Association, Heart and Stroke Foundation, provincial Pharmacy Association, local postsecondary institutions, and the regional health authority (Health Region). In the early years they formed as a coalition (Box 18-1) and focused on developing operating guidelines and structure with a broad mandate to reduce tobacco use in the Health Region.

Some of TRAC's early projects included developing as a coalition (Box 18-2), creating a campaign to publicize and acknowledge smoke-free restaurants, providing education and doing health promotion projects with youth, increasing partnership building among health organizations, and producing improved tobacco cessation materials for the public. Its next step was to strengthen the existing municipal bylaw to advance toward the goal of a smoke-free city.

Assessing Public Support

A public consultation survey conducted by TRAC about smoking and smoking restrictions was a springboard for the bylaw campaign. The goal of the survey was to assess the opinions and beliefs of city residents about smoking, health, and smoking restrictions in public places. A total of 626 residents completed a telephone survey conducted by a random digit dial method. Results showed

---

BOX 18-1. WHAT IS A COALITION?

A coalition is an organization of concerned citizens that advocates for services, policies, and programs to accomplish specific goals. A coalition monitors, analyzes, and mobilizes community efforts. A local coalition may assume several roles:

- Monitoring existing programs, services and policies
- Providing information and advice to decision-making officials in the community
- Undertaking special projects or activities
- Providing public awareness and information with suggestions for how the community can address issues of interest
- Initiating policy ideas and programs

Adapted from Institute of Food and Agricultural Sciences. (1998). *How to create a coalition. The disaster handbook* (national ed.), section 20.7. University of Florida. IFAS publication DH 2007. Web: http://disaster.ifas.ufl.edu/chap20fr.htm.

BOX 18-2. FORMING A COALITION

Concerned citizens, as individuals or as representatives of existing groups, are encouraged to take the initiative to mobilize community coalitions. Starting the process requires the commitment of at least one organization or person ("champion") to do some preliminary work related to defining the issue, specifying the location for coordinated efforts, and making the initial selection of key people and groups to involve.

It is important that the group have broad representation from professional and community leaders. To form a representative group of people who are concerned about or affected by the issue, determine who is missing from the group, which population groups are most likely to be interested in the group's goals and issues, what motivation can be provided to get people to join the effort, and what steps need to be taken to achieve balanced participation.

Steps	Rationale
Call a meeting	Use advance publicity all meetings. Use existing networks (e.g., schools, churches, neighbourhood groups, businesses) and the media. At the meeting, encourage discussion of problems caused in your community by the issue. These problems can be documented through data available from your local officials, health departments, etc. Statistics on the number of people affected by the issue help to assess the scope of the problem.
Select a chairperson	A designated chairperson facilitates the operations of the coalition. That person should chair the meetings, delegate responsibility, and coordinate the group's community efforts. It is important to include professionals, but strong leadership should come from private citizens.
Define the mission	A mission statement states the coalition's overall purpose. It explains what the coalition is, why it exists, and what it does. Because the coalition is made up of many organizations and people, a mission statement can help provide an identity for the coalition and clarify its role. There should be a direct relationship among the coalition's mission statement, its definition of the issue, its goals and objectives, and the steps it will take to reach goals.
Set goals and objectives	Establish well-defined goals as well as methods for evaluating progress.
Sustain involvement	Emphasize creative efforts directed toward a solution; progress and success serve to encourage participation. Establish a timetable, set tasks, delegate responsibility, determine deadlines, and schedule work to achieve goals.

Adapted from Institute of Food and Agricultural Sciences. (1998). *How to create a coalition. The disaster handbook* (national ed.), section 20.7. University of Florida. IFAS publication DH 2007. Web: http://disaster.ifas.ufl.edu/chap20fr.htm.

that a large majority of respondents (88%) were in strong support of smoking restrictions to protect children from second-hand smoke. Although the economic impact of smoking restrictions is always a main concern for the business sector, 33% of respondents reported that they would go out more often if restaurants were smoke free. Because 16% said that they would go out less frequently, this means that a net 17% of respondents would go out more often if restaurants were smoke free. It was discouraging to learn that fewer than half (43%) the respondents were aware that second-hand smoke causes ear infections in children. Survey results clearly indicated that the majority of city residents polled support some form of smoking restriction, in particular, one that would protect children from second-hand smoke.

Influencing Decision-Makers

TRAC compiled the highlights of the survey in an easy-to-read document (http://www.crha-health.ab.ca/pophlth/tobacco/Winit2Web.pdf). A press conference was organized that resulted in wide distribution of the main survey findings to the local media. The document was also circulated widely to many stakeholders but was primarily used as a gateway to local politicians. Members of TRAC, accompanied by a ward constituent whenever possible, met with each elected City Council member over a period of several months to present the survey findings to them and initiate a dialogue about future steps in the policy process. It was a very encouraging meeting with the city's mayor that gave TRAC the impetus to launch a bylaw campaign.

Planning the Campaign

TRAC had a mere 2 months to plan and prepare to launch a campaign that avoided an upcoming municipal election. In anticipation of a campaign, TRAC had successfully secured support funding. The next step was to develop a campaign theme and slogan. To assist in slogan development, coalition members decided to conduct focus groups with citizens opposed to, or "on the fence" about, smoking restrictions. Most focus group participants were comfortable with the idea of protecting children from second-hand smoke, which corroborated the survey findings. On the other hand, participants believed that adults have the right and ability to decide if they want to be exposed to second-hand smoke. Box 18-3 provides an overview of the health issues around second-hand smoke.

BOX 18-3. SECOND-HAND SMOKE AT A GLANCE

Second-hand smoke, also called environmental tobacco smoke (ETS), is a combination of exhaled smoke and the smoke that comes from the end of a cigarette, cigar, or pipe. Scientists have identified more than 4000 chemicals in second-hand smoke, including nicotine, carbon monoxide, ammonia, formaldehyde, and arsenic. Fifty of these substances are known to cause cancer.

Did You Know?

- Tobacco smoke is the most harmful and widespread contaminant of indoor air. Canadians spend about 90% of their time indoors.
- Every year about 3500 otherwise healthy nonsmokers in Canada—people who breathe second-hand smoke at work, at home, and elsewhere—die from second-hand smoke-related diseases.
- Second-hand smoke has been linked to heart disease, various cancers, and numerous respiratory diseases.
- Children are particularly vulnerable to second-hand smoke because they breathe faster than adults, inhale more air proportionate to their body mass, and their lungs are still growing and developing. Unfortunately children are limited in their ability to remove themselves from second-hand smoke.
- Studies show that ventilation systems are not capable of removing all of the air pollutants generated by cigarette, cigar, or pipe smoke, resulting in much of second-hand smoke getting recirculated.
- For years the tobacco industry has argued that smoking is a personal choice made by smokers. But research has clearly shown that smoking also poses a real health threat to non-smokers.

Facts on Second-Hand Smoke

- It is estimated that 33% of Canadian children under the age of 12 are regularly exposed to second-hand smoke in their homes. In addition, children continue to be exposed to second-hand smoke in arenas, malls, restaurants, and other public places.
- The Royal College of Physicians report that children of smoking parents inhale the same amount of nicotine as if they themselves smoked 60 to 150 cigarettes a year.
- Babies exposed to second-hand smoke are at increased risk for sudden infant death syndrome, respiratory diseases, and middle ear infections.
- In Canada, second-hand smoke is responsible for approximately 400,000 episodes of childhood sickness each year.
- Children who breathe second-hand smoke are at a greater risk for wheezing, coughing, asthma, ear infections, tonsillitis, bronchitis, and pneumonia.
- One in five Canadians has a pre-existing heart, lung, or allergic condition that can be aggravated by any exposure to tobacco smoke.
- Over 300 nonsmokers die each year in Canada from lung cancer caused by tobacco smoke. And almost 10 times that number die from heart disease caused by second-hand smoke—about 3000 each year.
- A 1998 survey reported that 81% of Albertans agreed that second-hand smoke is a health concern; 87% agreed that smoke-free indoor air protects the health of nonsmokers; and 74% agreed that there should be more smoke-free public spaces such as restaurants, hotels, and sports facilities.

www.smokefreecalgary.com/glance.html

Given the high use (65%) of the Internet by residents of the city, TRAC also decided that it would use the Internet as the main mobilization tool. A 24-hour telephone line was activated for those people who did not have Internet access but wanted to share their thoughts or register with the campaign. The primary goal of the campaign was to direct individuals to an interactive mobilization website and telephone line. The secondary goal was to provide an educational message that would resonate with the majority of citizens. Because the survey findings had clearly indicated a lack of knowledge that second-hand smoke can cause childhood ear infections, after much deliberation, and considering the focus group results, the slogan of the campaign became "Second-hand smoke hurts your children"—supplemented with a message to direct people to the campaign website (www.smokefreecalgary.com). To maximize the funds available TRAC decided to enact the following strategies:

◆ Interactive website
◆ 24-hour phone line number displayed at all media and other venues
◆ Billboards throughout the city
◆ Posters inside city light rail transit (LRT) system
◆ Media and resource generation
◆ Ballot boxes at high walking-traffic areas (e.g., tradeshows, hospitals)
◆ Letter writing campaign (targeting politicians and editorial boards of local newspapers)
◆ Media advocacy

Implementing the Action Strategies

Several very committed volunteers assisted with the ballot box strategies. Each volunteer was responsible for maintaining certain ballot box locations. Other volunteers wrote letters to local politicians and local news editors. After 6 months the ballot boxes had elicited 2500 registered names. These names were entered into a database that was used to activate a Call Centre at various points in the campaign.

The website was integral to community mobilization. The primary purpose for the site was to register supporters and to have the ability to communicate with those supporters who indicated the wish for ongoing information. The site also offered information on key issues such as ventilation, economic impact, and a list of other jurisdictions that had enacted bylaws regarding smoke-free areas. The website also began to serve other functions; for example, as electoral candidates declared themselves, TRAC surveyed them to ascertain their level of support of, or opposition to, an improved smoking bylaw. These results were posted on the website and shared with all registrants prior to the election.

Registrants of the website were updated via e-mail whenever a significant event, such as a meeting with City Council or a public hearing, was scheduled. Updates were sent approximately every 3 weeks, and generally TRAC would encourage supporters to be politically active. The request for action would suggest supporters call, write or e-mail their elected City Council member or write letters to the editors of local newspapers. TRAC was very cautious about not exhausting its supporters with e-mails and requests. After the first 6 months of the campaign, the website had 5000 people registered, with 3500 people indicating they wished to receive ongoing communication via e-mail. The website registration process had an evaluation component that asked participants how they learned of the web address. Registrants identified the LRT posters and e-mails from friends as the most common sources of information about the website.

While the website and ballot box names were growing in number, TRAC was also attempting to engage as many others stakeholders as possible. Coalition members made presentations to local groups such as the Chamber of Commerce, the Downtown Business Association, Hotel and Restaurant Association, and newspaper editorial boards while also working to establish a closer relationship with City Hall administration. Cognizant that the ultimate decision would lie with City Council, TRAC met with each council member at least once. During these meetings allies were identified and became the "eyes and ears" of the City Council back rooms; these supportive members would provide TRAC with direction and advice.

Activating citizens via a combination of Call Centre, e-mail, and website updates during crucial points of the campaign proved to be effective. Council members were overwhelmed with e-mails and phone messages each time the smoking bylaw was placed on the agenda. City administration announced they had never received such a high volume of calls and letters on any other issue in history. Despite the flood of messages, council members preferred to discuss the calls they received from unsupportive restaurateurs or community associations. It became clear to TRAC that council members weighed such messages more heavily than calls from residents of the wards they represented. Nonetheless, the media picked up the issue and headlines in papers across the city kept the issue in the forefront; Figure 18-1 is a collage of the headlines that appeared.

Once the smoking bylaw was brought forward to City Council, it was immediately redirected to the Standing Policy Committee (SPC) of City Council. The SPC held several meetings before finally announcing a public hearing date. Unfortunately, time had lapsed into the pre-election stage and the public hearing date was scheduled 1 month in advance of the municipal election. The public hearing itself was being organized by City Hall administration who, like

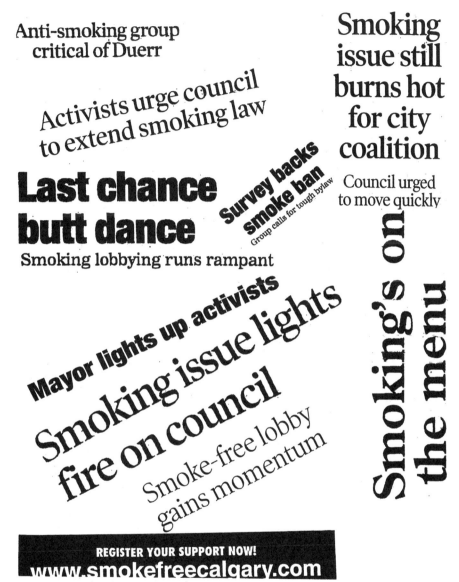

Anti-smoking group
critical of Duerr

Smoking
issue still
burns hot
for city
coalition

Activists urge council
to extend smoking law

Last chance
butt dance

Survey backs
smoke ban
Group calls for tough bylaw

Council urged
to move quickly

Smoking lobbying runs rampant

Mayor lights up activists

Smoking issue lights
fire on council

Smoke-free lobby
gains momentum

Smoking's on
the menu

REGISTER YOUR SUPPORT NOW!
www.smokefreecalgary.com

Figure 18-1 ◆ A collage of headlines.

TRAC, was aware of the potential drawbacks presented by the proximity of the election, such as Council delaying decision until a new Council was elected or voting to maintain the status quo. Nevertheless, TRAC recruited approximately 30 speakers to make presentations to the SPC, including experts from other Canadian urban centres with smoke-free legislation in place.

After the public hearing, and 2 weeks prior to the election, Council decided to amend the existing bylaw slightly to stipulate that children under 18 would no longer be allowed (as workers) to serve in, or be customers in, smoking areas as designated at the time. Council also appointed a committee of stakeholders and charged them to examine the issue further and to recommend to the incoming Council a revised bylaw 6 months after the election. City Council made a commitment (on which they did not vote, however) to make the city completely smoke free in the future, and further directed the stakeholder committee to provide input and direction to Council on the means to achieve this goal. TRAC was very disappointed initially with this outcome, but was encouraged when it learned that 150 restaurants became smoke free as a result of this small bylaw change. Several lessons were learned during this process; the pitfalls to avoid are listed in Box 18-4.

During a hiatus in the bylaw campaign during which the stakeholder committee deliberated, and recognizing the campaign had been active for almost a full year, TRAC decided to undertake an evaluation of the activities to date.

BOX 18-4. PITFALLS TO AVOID

- Neglecting to involve or at least advise key people in the community about the coalition
- Spending 6 months or more trying to define your purpose
- Starting a study or survey that takes a year and prevents other decisions or actions until completion
- Failing to reach a balance between process and task issues
- Developing wonderful plans, but neglecting to assign responsibility for carrying them out
- Neglecting to establish deadlines or at least target groups
- Failing to develop the ability to deal with hard issues such as group leadership and agency territoriality, local conservative or liberal attitudes
- Turning into a discussion group rather than an action group
- Failing to build in a process of self-evaluation
- Losing sight of the people the coalition should be assisting

Successful programs are based on community needs. Gaining support takes time, effort, and willingness to see all community segments as critical stakeholders.

Adapted from Institute of Food and Agricultural Sciences. (1998). *How to create a coalition. The disaster handbook* (national ed.), section 20.7. University of Florida. IFAS publication DH 2007. Web: http://disaster.ifas.ufl.edu/chap20fr.htm.

The evaluation process replicated the initial consultation survey with a few questions relating to the campaign added to the survey. A total of 729 individuals were interviewed using a random digit dial telephone survey. This time approximately 73% of respondents stated that they would like to see restaurants smoke free, a gain of 14% from the baseline survey. Like the first survey, 39% agreed that bars should also be smoke free. The following findings relate to the evaluation of the campaign itself:

◆ 94% were aware that there had been discussion about changing the smoking bylaw.
◆ 40% believe that the discussion over the past year influenced their opinion about smoking restrictions.
◆ 27% support smoking restrictions more than they did previously; 8% have not changed their opinion; and 4% are less supportive of smoking restrictions than they were previously.
◆ 42% have become more concerned about their exposure to second-hand smoke over the past year.
◆ 69% have become more concerned about children's exposure to second-hand smoke over the past year.

Summary

The results of the second survey confirmed to TRAC that the campaign had been a worthwhile venture. This campaign is a good example of how a community can influence policies so that residents can live healthier and happier lives. More people want smoking restrictions to protect people, particularly children, from second-hand smoke. More people are aware that second-hand smoke is harmful to adults and children. TRAC served as an effective conduit between the public and politicians by using mobilization tools such as an interactive website and a Call Centre to encourage political action. TRAC believes that the public dialogue that ensued as a result of the campaign is a solid foundation for changing attitudes to smoking, and will eventually result in modification of public policies that affect the health of all citizens.

References

Anderson, H. R., & Cook, D. G. (1997). Passive smoking and sudden infant death syndrome: Review of the epidemiological evidence. *Thorax 32,* 1003–1009.
Alberta Tobacco Reduction Alliance. (1999). *How Albertans view tobacco.* Calgary: ATRA
Calgary Regional Health Authority. (2001). A report on staff perceptions, attitudes and behaviours around CRHA's tobacco reduction policy. *Tobacco reduction policy newsletter:* http://www.crha-health.ab.ca/pophlth/tobacco/Winit2Web.pdf

Collishaw, N. E., Kirkbride, J., & Wigle, D. T. (1984). Tobacco smoke in the workplace: An occupational health hazard. *Canadian Medical Association Journal, 131*, 1199–1204.

DiFranza, J. R.,& Lew, R. A. (1996). Morbidity and mortality in children associated with the use of tobacco products by other people. *Pediatrics, 97*(4), 560–567.

Glantz S. A., & Parmley, W. W. (1991). Passive smoking and heart disease. *Epidemiology, Physiology and Biochemistry Circulation, 81*(1), 1–12.

Health Canada. (1998). *Passive smoking: Nowhere to hide*. Ottawa: Author.

Health Canada. (1999). Exposure to environmental tobacco smoke. *National Population Health Survey Highlights*, No. 1: Smoking Behaviour of Canadians (Cycle 2, 1996/97). Ottawa: Author.

Institute of Food and Agricultural Sciences. (1998). *How to create a coalition. The disaster handbook* (national ed.), section 20.7. University of Florida, IFAS publication DH 2007. Web: http://disaster.ifas.ufl.edu/chap20fr.htm.

National Clearinghouse on Tobacco and Health. (1997). *ETS & the tobacco industry*. Ottawa: Canadian Council for Tobacco Control. Located at www.ncth.ca.

National Institutes of Health. (1993). *Respiratory health effects of passive smoking: Lung cancer and other disorders*. Report of the U.S. Environmental Protection Agency. Washington, DC: U.S. Department of Health and Human Services.

Organization of Canadian Councils for Tobacco Control website: National clearinghouse for tobacco and health: www.ncth.ca.

Royal College of Physicians of London. (1992). Smoking and the young. *Summary of Report of a Working Party, 26*(4), 352–356.

TRAC website: www.smokefreecalgary.com

19

Promoting Healthy Partnerships With Refugees and Immigrants

CHARLES KEMP

OBJECTIVES

After studying this chapter, you should be able to:

◆ Differentiate between the terms *refugees* and *immigrants*
◆ Discuss the phases of health and adjustment for refugees and immigrants
◆ Describe health promotion strategies that focus at the individual/family and community levels

Introduction

Beginning in the 1970s and continuing into this century, the United States is experiencing the largest wave of immigration since the early 1900s. Refugees have come from Southeast Asia, Eastern Europe, Africa, and the Middle East; and immigrants (legal and illegal) have come from across the world, especially Latin America. Although some refugees and immigrants are at no population-specific risk for health problems, many are at very high risk for health problems in all spheres of being. To understand these populations, it is helpful to understand differences between refugees and immigrants.

◆ *Refugees* may be defined as people who are outside their own country and unwilling or unable to return because of persecution or a well-founded fear of persecution on account of race, religion, nationality, membership in a particular social group, or political opinion (Rasbridge, 1998).
◆ *Immigrants* are people who leave their homeland to seek economic or social benefit, and thus tend to be pulled to a new land by desire or need for benefit in contrast to refugees who are pushed from their homes.

Readers should understand that differences between refugees and immigrants may not be as clear-cut as presented above. For some immigrants, economic or social benefit may literally mean survival, whereas for others, the benefit may be a graduate degree or higher-paying job. For the purposes of this chapter, the focus is on refugee and immigrant communities that are at risk for acute and chronic health problems to a greater extent than the general population (i.e., those who live in poverty, have little education, and exhibit other characteristics of vulnerable populations in general).

Refugees and, to a large extent, immigrants go through a relatively predictable series of phases with respect to health and adjustment (Kemp, 1998; Rasbridge, 1998).

◆ The *acute phase* begins with arrival in the new country. Communicable diseases (e.g., tuberculosis, parasitism, and hepatitis B) are of particular concern to health officials. The new arrivals themselves may be more concerned about chronic symptomatic health problems. Mental health problems are seldom identified by either the new arrivals or by health officials.
◆ The *transition phase* is characterized by the emergence of secondary or hidden chronic health needs once the initial and more acute health needs are met. Diabetes, hypertension, and goiter are examples of health needs viewed as secondary by many refugees and immigrants. Mental health problems, notably chronic posttraumatic stress disorder (PTSD) and depression, also emerge.
◆ The *chronic phase* is the negative outcome of the refugee or immigrant experience. Long-term sequelae of hypertension, diabetes, and other chronic illnesses begin to emerge with concomitant morbidity and mortality. People with untreated mental illnesses drift into individual or even community (underprivileged enclave) seclusion, often including alcoholism or other

drug abuse. Family structure and roles deteriorate with marital breakup, family violence, and youth involvement in gangs common.

◆ The *resolution phase* is the positive outcome of the refugee or immigrant experience. When resolution occurs, individuals and families have access to health care and other essential resources. Physical, social, educational, mental, and spiritual needs are met to approximately the same extent they are met in other segments of the population. There is the essential characteristic of successful life: realistic hope for the future.

As with other theoretical or generalized stages applied to individuals, families, or populations, there are many exceptions or deviations from what is presented here. Nevertheless, these phases offer a structure to begin to understand refugees and immigrants and their health needs.

Strategies for Health Promotion: "Community Care"

"Community Care" had its roots in a community health nursing clinic in which students and faculty worked with Cambodian refugees in a large urban setting. Before beginning the health project, the class read Elizabeth Anderson's brilliant "A Call for Transformation" (1991), which discusses a district health model in which all people's health is addressed within the community. This would be a good time to stop, read, and discuss this short but very meaningful article. How does the article apply to the community you live in? Work in? Go to school in? Or plan to do your clinical experience in?

As part of "Community Care," students and faculty took responsibility for providing health care to a culturally diverse (primarily Asian refugee and Hispanic) inner city, low-income community with significant needs/problems. Rather than begin with a lengthy formal assessment process, students and faculty began working on one block of one street to assist people in the community to obtain health care and social services. Students went door to door, and every time a person was found with an unmet health or related need, the students stopped and, with the individual or family, figured out how to meet the need. In almost all cases, students later followed up on the solution.

Through the process of assisting people with the problems they believed were most pressing, students were able to develop a trusting and professional relationship with the community, identify needs and problems at all levels of care/prevention/promotion, and develop a meaningful understanding of available community services. Gradually, through this dynamic and continuing services-based community assessment, the program was expanded geographically from one block to more than 30 blocks and in terms of expanded individual, family, and community services as described below. Ultimately, the district health concept was realized.

District health is driven by individual, family, and community needs and encompasses individual- and family-oriented care such as outreach, primary care, case management, and home health care; and community-oriented care such as community assessment, disease prevention, and health promotion. Collaboration with a large number of providers and disciplines is necessary.

In addition to nursing students (from two universities), health promotion services are provided by seminary students, community health workers, lay health promoters, volunteers, and others. Services can be broadly classified as (1) individual- and family-oriented services and (2) community-oriented services. A differentiation of the two services follows.

Individual- and Family-Oriented Services

Individual- and family-oriented services include outreach, primary care, case management, and home health care. These services are focused primarily on care for people who are sick and are the means by which the program is able to move toward disease prevention and health promotion. Outreach, for example, is focused on individuals and families, but, without these personal contacts, health screening would never reach the most isolated people in the community.

Outreach

As noted earlier, outreach is implemented door to door through the apartments in the district. Although students carry flyers on the program in Spanish, English, Vietnamese, Khmer (Cambodian), and Laotian, they seldom just leave flyers on doors. Instead, students knock and, if anyone is home, inquire about health problems and check blood pressures, vaccination records, medications, and address other issues that arise in the course of the visit. Always, as much as is possible, students stop to solve problems wherever they are found.

Language is an issue in outreach and other program components. The primary languages spoken in this district (in descending order) are Spanish, English, Vietnamese, Khmer, and Laotian. Everyone involved in this work is acutely aware that there often are breakdowns in communication! Although there are now caseworker/translators with capabilities in Spanish, Vietnamese, Khmer, and Laotian working with the program, it is important to note that had services been delayed to wait for these capabilities, thousands of opportunities to serve this community would have been missed.

Primary Care and Case Management

When people are found with health or related problems, nursing students or other persons involved with the program help find appropriate resources, help clients access the services, follow up on the care given to be sure that clients understand treatments and medications, and, finally, provide further follow-up to determine if treatments were effective and if any new problems develop. Common individual problems encountered in the community include clients having difficulty obtaining and understanding:

◆ Primary care for hypertension, infections, and similar problems
◆ Prenatal care and family planning
◆ Specialty care for cancer, diabetes, and other chronic illnesses
◆ Preventive care, such as childhood immunizations, or early disease detection

Many health and social problems are handled in a student-operated clinic in the community. The clinic is held at a police storefront with a church health program providing internist services on Thursday mornings and the county hospital community-oriented primary care (COPC) clinic providing pediatrician services on Friday mornings. Clinic services include medical care, teaching, vaccinations, refugee screening, social work, pregnancy testing and counselling, and volunteer services. The program takes pride in the fact that medical services came to the nursing education program rather than the far more common case of nursing education programs attaching themselves to medical services.

When patients require care beyond the level of this clinic, students help obtain appointments. Students often accompany patients to appointments and thus provide essential advocacy and teaching services. In all cases, a goal of care is increasing patient independence so that, ultimately, the patient is registered with a provider such as the COPC clinic, knows how to make appointments, and is able to recognize the need to seek health care. This goal is not always reached. Access to care remains difficult for non-English or Spanish speakers, and current trends in health care have resulted in even public health providers demanding documentation that is impossible for some patients to provide.

Home Health Care

Home health care is provided independently of, or in cooperation with, home care agencies. Home care agencies have learned that, by cooperating with the program, the level of care exceeds that possible through funded sources. Some home care and hospice staff schedule visits on days when students are not available so coverage is doubled through cooperative care. In other cases, there is no coverage at all and students and faculty take on significant responsibilities for care.

For example, Mrs. C was a 58-year-old Cambodian woman who had undetected cervical cancer when students found her in door-to-door outreach. She had an 11-year-old son with Down syndrome, a 13-year-old daughter who provided most of Mrs. C's care, and a 15-year-old son who was sent to prison midway through the course of care. Students and faculty were instrumental in the cancer being diagnosed, played a critical role in getting the patient through two courses of treatment (surgery and radiation), and took responsibility for her home care after crises related to very severe complications of disease and treatment (septicemia, stroke, seizures, bowel obstruction, malnutrition, and dehydration). For 2 years, Mrs. C received at least three home visits each week. She agreed to hospice care about 2 months before dying. A faculty member was with her when she died at home.

Care is continuous between students across semesters. In summers, the clinic is operated by volunteers, faculty, and church health and COPC staff.

Community-Oriented Services

Community services currently under way include community assessment, immunizations taken into the community, women's health services, church health, and community development. These are not one-time projects! They are ongoing community care activities that, over time and with reinforcement and repetition, will change lives. Each is summarized below.

Community Assessment

Assessment of the community is services based. In other words, the community (problems, needs, strengths, and resources) is assessed primarily through the process of delivering services. Biostatistical data are also used, but to a lesser degree than direct experience in the community.

Vulnerable communities have been extensively studied here and elsewhere. For example, it is known that, nationally, Asian women underutilize cancer screening. Is it ethical, then, to take time to determine the degree to which Asian women in this community also do or do not underutilize cancer screening? Or, is the community better served by developing cancer screening programs and, through the process of screening, determining the degree of utilization or underutilization? The answer is obvious.

Immunizations

In going door to door in the community, students assess the immunization status of every child encountered. Immunizations are provided free every Wednesday by staff from a van from one of the nursing schools involved with the program and every Friday at the pediatric clinic by staff from the COPC clinic or county health department. Influenza immunizations for adults are provided by the COPC clinic and county health department at the community clinic site and at health fairs in the fall.

Women's Health

In addition to the already described outreach and assistance with family planning and prenatal care, each semester students plan and implement cancer screening events in which a portable mammogram unit is set up in the police storefront and women who otherwise would be highly unlikely to ever receive a mammogram come in for free screening. Along with mammograms, students teach breast self-examination one on one with the women, screen all participants (and others who come in the door) for other health problems (e.g., diabetes, hypertension, colon cancer, HIV infection), and provide follow-up care for all problems. Except for operating the mammogram unit and HIV testing, students are responsible for all aspects of the screening.

Here is the ethnic breakdown of the 240 women screened in eight mammogram events: African American, 10%; Anglo, 5.5%; Hispanic, 0%; Khmer (Cambodian), 21%; Laotian, 14%; Native American, less than 1%, and Vietnamese, 23%.

An example of how screening helps to identify other family health needs is the story of Sarath. Sarath was a 15-year-old Khmer girl in a dangerously abusive relationship with an older man. After initial failures in intervening, students, police, and a child welfare agency were finally able to help her move back to her mother in California. Students first made contact with her when she was helping translate for an older woman at one of the mammogram events.

Church and Lay Volunteers

One of the underutilized resources identified in this community work were the churches. On the basis of a community assessment, students made contact with a clergy member and obtained his agreement to work with students 1 day per week in a small church health effort. This effort quickly led to a relationship with a group of volunteer Hispanic (mostly Mexican) women, named the "CoMadres," at one of the elementary schools in the community. With the CoMadres, students developed a lay health promoter curriculum and provided training to the CoMadres. This curriculum may be viewed at www.baylor.edu/~Charles_Kemp/welcome.html. Students work with the CoMadres on a weekly basis and have held one cooperative health fair at the CoMadres' school.

Student work with the CoMadres and the clergy led to a close relationship with the previously discussed church health program. The Community Care program became an integral part of the church health efforts, and faculty from the two involved nursing schools were among the first church nurses. As noted earlier, the church health program provides an internist for the Thursday clinic and is chiefly responsible for the presence of lay health promoters at the clinic and in the community on Thursdays and Fridays.

Community Development

In all aspects of working in this community, whether with individuals or as part of community care, students affirm and strengthen the community's ability to grow and care for itself. Many referrals to people in need come from others with whom students have worked in the past and who have learned basic health measures from students. There is a growing corps of volunteers and a strong network of concerned individuals whom students helped equip to reach out and more effectively help their neighbours. Rather than depend solely on caseworker/translator services, relatives, neighbours, and friends often assist with translation, transportation, and other such services. Existing community groups are used to assist and promote health as much as possible.

The program recently outgrew the police facility that students call "home base." A small Vietnamese church in the heart of the community offered part of its facility for the clinic. People from the community and from churches outside the community are giving countless hours cleaning, remodeling, painting, and in other work to prepare the facility.

Challenges and Problems

Follow-up and evaluation are a constant challenge. Through the alliance with the church health program, the program is able to track "preventable admissions" (diabetes, asthma, etc.) to area hospitals from the district zip code. Data are encouraging, but direct cause and effect are difficult to show.

Compliance with treatment or health promotion is always an issue. Follow-up with patients with hypertension, diabetes, and other such diagnoses takes precedence over follow-up on compliance with health promotion measures such as breast self-exams after breast cancer screening. Efforts to utilize additional students to address the full spectrum of healthy behaviours are under way.

Summary

This program was designed and has evolved for the specific purpose of addressing the health care needs and problems of a community that, despite the relatively near presence of several health and social service providers, remained significantly underserved. The program is driven and defined by human needs. Through meeting the needs and priorities of the community, students and their partners in this work are able to gradually introduce services directed to health promotion and disease prevention and early detection. Rather than students coming into the health care system and working as students (whose work would be done whether the students were there or not), students in this program provide services that would not otherwise be provided.

References

Anderson, E. T. (1991). A call for transformation. *Public Health Nursing, 8*(1), 1.

Kemp, C. E. (1998). Mental health: Torture, PTSD, and grief. In C. E. Kemp and L. A. Rasbridge (Eds.), *Refugee health*. Online at www.baylor.edu/~Charles_Kemp/refugee_health.htm.

Rasbridge, L. A. (1998). Introduction: Background on refugees. In C. E. Kemp and L. A. Rasbridge (Eds.), *Refugee health*. Online at www.baylor.edu/~Charles_Kemp/refugee_health.htm.

Canadian Resources

Fowler, N. (1998). Providing primary health care to immigrants and refugees: The North Hamilton experience. *Canadian Medical Association Journal, 159,* 388(391.

Housing issues facing immigrants and refugees in Greater Toronto (article): **http://www.library.utoronto.ca/hnc/publish/issues.pdf.**

Listing of organizations that offer services to immigrants and refugees: **http://www.povnet.org/links/links_immigrants&refugees.htm.**

Metropolis Project: **http://canada.metropolis.net/.**

More than 250,000 new permanent residents in 2001 (press release): **http://www.cic.gc.ca/english/press/02/0211-pre.html.**

Ryerson University School of Journalism: Diversity Watch: **http://www.diversitywatch.ryerson.ca/backgrounds/immigrants.htm.**

Unfulfilled expectations, missed opportunities: Poverty among immigrants and refugees in British Columbia: **http://ftpd.maytree.com/resources_view.phtml?resid=185&catsid=23.**

20

Promoting Healthy Partnerships With Schools

NINA FREDLAND

OBJECTIVES

After studying this chapter, you should be able to:

◆ Design programs that are specific to the specialized school setting at the primary, secondary, and tertiary levels of prevention

◆ Implement programs that teach healthy behaviour to school-aged children, their parents, and school faculty and staff

◆ Involve the residents of the geographic community in which the school is located in program planning

◆ Utilize community resources specific to school-aged children and their parents

Introduction

Most health care providers would agree that a major goal for this, the 21st century, would be to create a nation of children who are optimally well so that they can lead long, happy, productive lives. How do we as nurses achieve this goal? This chapter focusses on strategies and partnerships within the community setting of the school. The school nurse or the community health nurse, depending on the community, is ideally situated to provide health care to school-aged children. Nurses with advanced preparation in child health, such as pediatric nurse practitioners and family nurse practitioners, are also well prepared to initiate partnerships with schools. An ideal model is one in which the school nurse or community health nurse collaborates with the advanced practice nurse. In this way, health promotion, disease prevention, and health maintenance are important components included within the delivery of health care. School-aged children are a captive audience, and their parents are closely connected to the school community. This makes the school community an ideal centre for health promotion activities for the entire family.

The health of our nation's children has been an area of concern for some time. Casual observations at any school note a high percentage of overweight children, youngsters easily fatigued while running around the playground, and children choosing nonnutritious snacks. Obviously, these children are at a disadvantage. Their health is compromised. One has only to observe adult role models to understand why children are making unhealthy choices. Therefore, health education approaches must be comprehensive and include the children as well as all groups of individuals involved in their care and nurturing. The school community encompasses:

◆ School-aged children and adolescents
◆ Parents and guardians
◆ School personnel (faculty, staff, and administrators)
◆ Neighbourhood residents, businesses, and service agencies

In addition to promoting the optimal health and preventing illness through the education of all members of the school community, school health programs must strive to identify and resolve existing health problems. Therefore, comprehensive school health programs should focus on delivering health services mandated by state laws and the individual school system as well as health education. Additionally, both internal and external environmental issues are critical areas of assessment and intervention for school nurses.

Delivering Health Services for Health Promotion

Each state mandates certain requirements to maintain the health of school-aged children. Programs for vision, hearing, and spinal screenings are required. Measurements of height, weight, and blood pressure are also usually part of these health services. Nutritional, dental, and developmental screening may also be required in the school setting. To find out about requirements in your state, contact your local state health department. The following list outlines some common state requirements.

> *Vision:* Screen all new students within 120 days of enrolment. Screen students in kindergarten, 1st, 3rd, 5th, 7th, and 9th grades by May of each school year.
> *Hearing:* Screen all new students within 120 days of enrolment. Screen students in kindergarten and grades 1, 3, 5, 7, and 9 by May of each school year.
> *Spinal:* Screen all students in grades 6 and 9.

Certification is required to perform vision and hearing screening. Certification training is available through state health departments or through individuals the state has designated with this authority. To find out how to receive certification training, contact your state health department. Certification for registered nurses is not usually required for spinal screening; yet, ancillary personnel or volunteer assistants are required to have attended an approved educational program. Therefore, it is important that student nurses be taught a thorough procedure for assessing spinal deformities as part of their health assessment curriculum.

Immunizations are required by state law to be current and on file before or on the first day of school. A school district can establish a short grace period, usually 30 days. Immunization requirements must be strictly supported by the school administration. Each state sets a standard for immunizations. A school district can increase the requirements but must include the minimum standard. For example, tuberculosis screening for school-aged children may not be required by state law; however, school districts can set a higher standard and require new students to have an approved skin test for tuberculosis screening within 1 year of initial enrollment. Furthermore, school districts can require school personnel to be tested biennially. The Centers for Disease Control and Prevention (CDC) is the best source for recommended immunization schedules for children and adults. The CDC website is www.cdc.gov. This would be a good time to familiarize yourself with this website and the current recommended immunization schedule for school-aged children.

In addition to mass screening programs, a nurse in the school setting identifies and monitors existing health problems, both acute and chronic, such as common respiratory infections and asthma. The school nurse is a referral agent and case manager and offers education within his or her scope of nursing practice.

Health Education for Health Promotion

Major issues affecting American children can be categorized under headings of nutrition, interpersonal violence, substance abuse, mental health issues, safety, sexuality; and environmental hazards, such as lead, asbestos, and air pollution. Health promotion strategies should focus on these important areas. Some topics from which you might select for health education programs are listed here. Some of these topics are more appropriate for children, parents, or teachers. As you are thinking of the topic, consider the audience you are targeting. For example, healthy food choices might be geared toward easy recipes that children can prepare. There are a number of cookbooks written with children in mind. My favourite is the American Heart Association's *Children's Help Your Heart Cookbook.* (To obtain this cookbook, contact your local chapter of the American Heart Association.) Eating disorders is a topic more suited for a parent session. The following health education list is not exhaustive. It is designed to promote your ideas. Consider how you might assess interest for any of the following programs.

Health Education Program Ideas

Nutrition
Healthy food choices
Healthy recipes for busy families
Healthy lunches children can prepare
Eating disorders (such as anorexia, bulimia, and compulsive eating)

Violence
Domestic violence—effects on children and sources of help for the whole family
Discipline versus child abuse

Anger management/impulse control
Gang behaviour
Date rape/acquaintance rape
Signs of child abuse/incest

Substance Use
Cigarettes and chewing tobacco
Underage drinking
Illicit drugs (marijuana, crack, cocaine, inhalants, speed, heroin, etc.)

Mental Health Issues
Self-esteem
Attention-deficit disorder/hyperactive disorder
Depression
Suicide

Personal Safety
"Latchkey" kids
Problem-solving/decision-making skills

Recreational Safety
Bicycles, in-line skates, sports
Vehicle safety (seat belts, booster seats, riding in open vehicles)
Water safety (swimming, boating, and skiing)

Sexuality
Personal hygiene
Teenage pregnancy
Teen parenting
Sexually transmitted diseases

Environmental
Internal (air, water, space)
External (pollution, noise)
Psychological (grade stress, parent–child discord, parent–teacher and
    teacher–teacher conflicts)
Societal influences
Changing family structure
Peer pressure
Media influences (video games, films, television)

Health Promotion Programs
for School-Aged Children

Programs for children and adolescents in the school setting must be age appropriate. Obviously, breast self-examination and testicular self-examination are not appropriate material for elementary school children. It is critical to assess the developmental and maturity level of the children before deciding on the educational content of a program or a strategy. Even if you think you know how to relate to a certain age group, each class is different. The youngsters may be a very young class for their grade level or they may be a very advanced group. The students may or may not be well socialized. Several may have attention-deficit disorder or exhibit hyperactivity.

Important information is gained from observing the student population before planning programs. Always visit the classroom and observe how the students and teacher interact. Classroom management skills are essential. It is difficult to successfully manage the classroom if the nurse's contact with the youngsters is only occasional. Relying on the regular classroom teacher for assistance works best. It is helpful to include key people, such as the teacher, counsellor, school nurse, and parents in the planning phase of all health programs. Outlining individual expectations of the teacher counsellor, school nurse, and parents will contribute to the overall success of the program. Another consideration is marketing your program. It may be the greatest idea; but, if no one comes or follows through, it is a waste of time and resources.

Use flyers, bulletin boards, and public address announcements to reach your audiences. Try various strategies to pique interest. For example, brightly colored signs and charts; guessing games; poster contests; door decorating competitions; age-appropriate, healthy food rewards (eg, juice bars, fruit) are a few suggestions. The following are examples of health promotion programs for school-aged children:

◆ Red Ribbon Week
◆ D.A.R.E. program
◆ Breast self-examination/testicular self-examination
◆ Muscle Mover Club or Triathlon or Walk-A-Thon/Swim
   to Bermuda
◆ Monthly health bulletin board
◆ Make a cookbook
◆ Pet responsibility

Red Ribbon Week

Red Ribbon Week occurs in October each year to celebrate being drug free. The Red Ribbon Campaign began in 1988 when the U.S. Congress established Red Ribbon Week. The goal was to increase the awareness of the dangers associated with the use of tobacco, alcohol, and other drugs. Since then, Red Ribbon Week has become the standard in many schools. The Internet has many examples of how different schools across the nation celebrate the week. An agenda for a week's program focusing on drug abuse prevention, which can be incorporated into the curriculum of an elementary school, follows. Each student recites a promise to stay away from drugs and wears a red ribbon for the week.

The community should be involved in the program along with the students in various ways. Parents can be invited to some programs. The parents' organization can be asked to decorate the school with red ribbons. Community leaders (e.g., church, civic, police) can judge contests. The police and fire departments can facilitate a parade route and provide security. Media coverage, such as local newspapers and radio and television stations, is an important strategy that schools should seek. (Often, worthwhile events are not covered by the media because media personnel have not been notified.) Older students and campus leaders can influence younger students by positive peer pressure, such as wearing their ribbons, participating in all activities, and having a major role in organizing and implementing the activities. This principal can be involved in this program.

It is very important to give clear messages to young people, particularly on the subject of drugs. The nurse should select speakers very carefully. Recovering drug abusers should not be used to speak to groups of students who are not users. It is also risky to choose high-profile role models, such as well-known sports or media individuals who may be positive nondrug users one day but in the news media at a later time for using drugs or violent behaviour. Consider asking the students to give 1-minute talks on why they are not going to use drugs. Have a poem or smart saying contest. Get the speech club involved.

D.A.R.E. Program

The D.A.R.E. (Drug Abuse Resistance Education) program is a substance abuse prevention program that originated with the Los Angeles Unified School District. The purpose is to teach students to resist peer pressure and say "no" to drugs. Decision-making is emphasized, and alternative ideas for dealing with problems are explored. D.A.R.E. is sponsored by the local community police department in which a specially trained police officer is assigned to the fifth grade class for a series of 17 weekly lessons. Other grade levels may be included in the educational process to a lesser degree than the targeted fifth grade. D.A.R.E. has also expanded to include high schools. The officer becomes an integral part of the classroom teaching team. This activity encourages positive relations between youth and law enforcement officers and provides children with accurate information about the hazards of drug use and useful strategies for staying drug free.

Muscle Mover Club or Triathlon or Walk-A-Thon

The Muscle Mover Club encourages physical activity by rewarding aerobic exercise, such as walking, running, swimming, and biking. Each child is given a badge and adds stickers for city blocks or track laps completed. Healthy competition can be encouraged by racing to a goal either individually or by a classroom. Another strategy is to include parent participation by having them sign off on triathlon or walk-a-thon mileage sheets. Encourage parents to do the activity with their child. A parent/teacher bulletin board recognizing athletic achievement, such as running a race or marathon, highlights adults leading healthy lifestyles. Children are very proud to have their parents and teachers value their achievements.

Health Promotion Programs for Parents

The following are ideas for healthy partnerships with parents:

◆ Parent information sessions
◆ Parent peer groups
◆ Late breakfast meetings; "second cup of coffee meeting"
◆ Grandparents day
◆ Breast cancer awareness
◆ Parents' nutrition committee
◆ Parent information sessions

The most difficult part of planning health promotion activities that include parents is timing. Most parents are employed and have very little flexibility in their work schedules. Breakfast meetings that are short and occur as children are brought to school may be well attended. Issues must be appealing to parents, and it is always a good idea to conduct a "needs assessment" before deciding on topics. In this way, you can include important health information as well as meet parental expectations. Below is an example of an agenda for a parent information session on nutrition. This was a program held in the evening. Marketing strategies include credit for parent volunteer service hours, a cooking demonstration with samples, and prizes, such as a 1-year subscription to a parenting magazine or a healthy fruit or vegetable basket. Always try to involve the community merchants in the donation of prizes. Perhaps the local grocery store will donate a fruit or vegetable basket or the hair salon will donate a free hair styling. The more involved community businesses are in school activities the better the community health nurse can promote the health of all citizens.

Healthy Habits, Healthy Kids! (An Evening for Parents)

Registration, sign up for door prizes, complete survey related to nutritional knowledge
Welcome and panel introductions
Healthy Habits, Healthy Kids overview
Effects of cholesterol, sugar, and salt on our daily diet
Making sense of food labels
Making good choices in the grocery store
Making choices in the restaurant
Making your family recipes healthy
Healthy heart discussion
Door prizes awarded

Parent Peer Groups

Establishing a parent peer group in which parents agree to certain rules of behaviour for the youngsters or teens, such as curfews and party rules, are helpful to parents and school personnel. Parents can agree not to allow drinking of alcohol, use of tobacco, or drugs at their house. Parents in the group can then feel comfortable when their children/teens are in the company of peers whose parents ascribe to the same rules. A consistent approach sets limits for youth while providing an atmosphere of positive peer pressure. Parents also feel comfortable consulting with each other and form a support system.

Grandparents Day

Grandparents Day is a day in which the school actively involves grandparents, many of whom may not have been in an educational setting for a long time. Activities of the day can include classroom visitation, a healthy lunch, and blood pressure screening. Seventh grade (or higher grade) students can be taught to measure blood pressure in science, physical education, biology, math, or health class. You can work with the respective teacher and conduct the practice sessions together. Youths take the elders' blood pressure under the supervision of a health professional such as yourself and volunteer nurse parents or other trained adult. This activity provides a service for the elderly guests as well as increases the awareness of the young students regarding the importance of preventing heart disease and monitoring blood pressure. If elevated blood pressures are noted, have a referral plan complete with name and phone numbers of clinics, the local health department, or private medical care providers that the person with an elevated blood pressure can be referred to. Also follow up on elevated blood pressure measures and offer every participant written information on elevated blood pressure and the association with poor health.

Mother–Daughter Programs

Cancer prevention programs for mothers and daughters can promote breast self-examination and mammography. Culturally appropriate programs can be designed to attract women of various ethnic backgrounds. For example, if it is not culturally acceptable to discuss breast matters in public meetings, perhaps you can involve the local worship centres or other culturally acceptable agencies where the information could be hosted. (The worship centre may also be able to provide a bilingual presenter for women not fluent in English.) Equally important is a cancer awareness for fathers and sons on testicular cancer and the correct technique for testicular self-examination. Perhaps mother–daughter talks can be scheduled at the same time with father–son talks. This can be fun for the whole family, regardless of age, and again involves the whole community. Girl Scout and Boy Scout troops or Future Farmers of America clubs might be interested in sponsoring a family awareness day because they are usually interested in hosting activities for the entire family.

Nutrition Awareness

If the school meal program is not healthy, form an ad hoc committee to study the problem. The committee should consist of parents, the community/school nurse, cafeteria personnel, representatives of the faculty and administration, and a dietitian, if available. (Hint: Seek consultation from parents. Frequently, a professional dietitian is among the parents.) Action steps would include:

1. Conduct a survey to assess parental interest and areas of concern. What would parents like to see happen? What are they willing to do to make change happen?
2. Conduct a survey to assess student opinion and food preferences.
3. Do a plate waste study to determine what children are actually eating (see below for how-to).
4. Form a committee, remembering to include the students.
5. Based on what you learned in steps 1, 2, and 3, identify other options to the present menu, such as hiring a nutritionist to study the present food service. You may also want to organize a committee to visit other schools to sample food, look at menus, and talk to those students about satisfaction.
6. Make recommendations to the school administration.
7. Make a presentation to the school board.
8. Pilot alternatives.

Plate Waste Study
1. Recruit parent volunteers, cafeteria staff, and teachers to help you.
2. Choose at least 2 days of the week to conduct the study.
3. Place volunteers next to the tray return and trash containers.
4. Record types and amount of food put into the trash.
5. Look into lunch bags for type of discarded, uneaten food.
6. Record all information (perhaps onto form with different food types).
7. You now have important information, such as nutritious food waste and the amount of soft drinks and candy consumed (from the wrappers).
8. Write a one-page report.
9. Give the report to parents, staff, and students.
10. Present the results to school administration along with suggestions to decrease food waste.

Health Promotion Strategies for the School

The following are additional ideas for health promotion strategies that can be used with groups such as teachers or staff in the school setting. Again, this list is not exhaustive but meant to generate ideas for viable strategies.

- ◆ Blood pressure screening on the same day each month
- ◆ Cancer awareness programs
- ◆ Stuffing payroll envelopes with health promotion material
- ◆ Healthy heart lunches, such as salad day once a week
- ◆ Referral and resource information
- ◆ Skin testing for tuberculosis

Health Promotion Strategies for the Community

- ◆ Involve elderly in school activities, such as reading programs, mentoring, and monitoring lunch hour
- ◆ Collaborate with the local civic association
- ◆ Establish a drug-free zone
- ◆ Have a community parade celebrating being drug free
- ◆ Establish a safe traffic pattern
- ◆ Contact radio and television stations and newspapers and ask them to report health promotion events
- ◆ Immunization programs
- ◆ School-based family clinics

Summary

This chapter has focused on health promotion strategies that can be implemented in the school setting to achieve the goal of optimum wellness for school-aged children. We have reviewed the components of health services, health education, and environmental issues. Suggestions regarding ways to incorporate groups associated with the school children, such as parents, teachers, staff, and the neighbouring community, in health promotion efforts have been outlined. Community resources specific to the school setting have been included in this chapter. Now, we hope you will have fun promoting healthy partnerships with schools.

Suggested Readings

Journals
Journal of School Health: Monthly journal, except for July/August
School Nurse: Health information publication; four issues per year
American Journal of School Nursing: Four issues per year

Books and Articles

American Heart Association. *American Heart Association kid's cookbook.* Atlanta, GA: Author. Healthful foods for ages 8 through 12. Available at local bookstores.

American Heart Association. (1993). *Children's help your heart Cookbook.* Atlanta, GA: Author. Low-cholesterol recipes that can be prepared by elementary and middle school children. No-cost item that can be ordered through the American Heart Association.

American Nurses Association. (1998). *Standards of clinical nursing practice* (2nd ed.). Kerneysville, WV: American Nurses Publishing.

Birch, D., & Hallock, B. (1998). School nurses' perceptions of parental involvement in school health. *Journal of School Nursing, 14*(3), 32–37.

Bryan, S. (1998). School nurses' perceptions of their interactions with nurse practitioners. *Journal of School Nursing, 14*(5), 17–23.

Cavendish, R., Lunney, M., Draynyak, B., & Richardson, K. (1999). National survey to identify the nursing interventions used in school settings. *Journal of School Nursing, 15*(2), 14–21.

Cowell, J., Warren, J., & Montgomery, A. (1999). Cardiovascular risk prevalence among diverse school-age children: Implications for schools. *Journal of School Nursing, 15*(2), 8–12.

Gaffrey, E., & Bergren, M. (1998). School health services and managed care: A unique partnership for child health. *Journal of School Nursing, 14*(4), 5–22.

Lunney, M., Cavendish, R., Luise, B., & Richardson, K. (1997). Relevance of NANDA and health promotion diagnoses to school nursing. *Journal of School Nursing, 13*(5), 16–22.

Newton, J., Adams, R., & Marcontel, M. (1997). *The new school health handbook* (3rd ed.). San Francisco: Jossey-Bass.

Pavelka, L., McCarthy, A., & Denehy, J. (1999). Nursing intervention used in school nursing practice. *Journal of School Nursing, 15*(1), 29–37.

Internet Resources

The following list contains websites that are of interest to those health care providers working in the school setting. It is important to note that Internet sites change rapidly and the information included below may not be the latest version. It is provided as a resource, and the reader is encouraged to recognize the need for periodic updating.

American Academy of Pediatrics: **www.aap.org**. An organization of primary care pediatricians includes information promoting health, safety, and well-being of children.

American Cancer Society: **www.cancer.org**. Not-for-profit voluntary health organization provides information to consumers related to the prevention of cancer.

American Diabetes Association: **www.diabetes.org**. Not-for-profit voluntary health organization provides information and resources related to diabetes.

American Heart Association: **www.americanheart.org**. Not-for-profit voluntary health organization provides information to consumers related to prevention and treatment of cardiovascular diseases. School site programs are highlighted, such as *Heart Treasure Chest, Getting to Know Your Heart, Heart Challenges, Hearty School Lunch, Heart at Work*.

American Lung Association: **www.lungusa.org**. Fights lung disease through community education, service, and research, particularly related to issues of tobacco use and asthma.

American School Health Association: **www.ashaweb.org**. Promotes the health of the nation's youth by advocating for comprehensive school health programs.

Centers for Disease Control and Prevention: **www.cdc.gov**. An agency of the Department of Health and Human Services, which promotes health by preventing or controlling disease, injury, and disability. Website includes data, statistics, and health information.

Children, Youth, and Families Education and Research Network: **www.cyfernet.mes .umn.edu**. Website includes resources for youth, parents, and professionals to promote healthy, safe individuals, families, and communities. Links with national, state, and international agencies, foundations, and associations.

Department of Health and Human Services, The Administration for Children and Families: www.acf.dhhs.gov.

National Assembly on School-Based Health Care: **www.nasbhc.org/**. Nonprofit private association promoting school-based interdisciplinary, accessible, quality primary and mental health care.

National Association of School Nurses, Inc.: **www.nasn.org**. Nonprofit specialty nursing organization. Website includes conference announcements and publications related to school nursing practice.

Partnership for School Health: **150.216.8.8/schealth/**. Website contains school health resources, information, and many links to health organizations and agencies.

School Nurse Forum: **www.schoolnurse.com/**. Accessible resource to link school nurses with current information and with each other through the web for the purpose of sharing ideas.

Sources for Canadian Information on School Health

Calgary Board of Education: **http://www.cbe.ab.ca/linknlearn/schoolhealth.htm**
Canadian Association for School Health: **http://www.schoolfile.com/CASH.htm**
City of Toronto Public Health: **http://www.city.toronto.on.ca/health/csh_index.htm**
Comprehensive school health: **http://www.hc-sc.gc.ca/hppb/children/english/**

Other Resources

D.A.R.E. (Drug Abuse Resistance Education). Contact your local police department

Guidelines/health manuals/continuing education programs for school nurses developed by local school districts

State associations for school nurses. Websites: access through state associations

State and local health department guidelines and laws

Volunteer agencies such as the American Heart Association, American Lung Association, American Cancer Society, and American Diabetes Association. Websites were given above.

21

Promoting Healthy Partnerships With Faith Communities

NINA FREDLAND

OBJECTIVES

After studying this chapter, you should be able to:

♦ Discuss the role of the community health nurse in promoting the health of faith communities

♦ Design and implement health promotion programs for faith communities

Introduction

In the face of the changing health care marketplace, congregations of worshipers are increasingly forming partnerships with nursing for health promotion programs. This movement of nursing in faith communities is based on the principles of holistic nursing that recognize the dynamic relationship of spirituality and health of mind and body throughout the life span (Solari-Twadell, 1999). Other influencing components are self-responsibility for health, increasing autonomous roles in nursing, and increasing lay ministry responsibilities in faith communities. *Congregational nursing* and *parish nursing* are descriptive terms found in the literature and apply equally to the concept of nursing in faith communities. For the purposes of this chapter, the term *faith communities* will be used. People of these communities will be addressed as *participants*.

Initiating Healthy Partnerships With Faith Communities

The roles of the nurse with faith communities are dictated as always by the needs of the people and include, but are not limited to, consultant, educator, counsellor, referral-agent, advocate, and facilitator (Westberg, 1999). Frequently, nurses with faith communities are licensed professional nurses, with varied educational backgrounds and areas of expertise, who share their nursing skills as a means to give something back to their community of spiritual support. However, in some settings, the nurses may be employed by the faith community. Frequently, the professional nurses donate their time and expertise as well as their own equipment (e.g., stethoscopes or sphygmomanometers). Some are advanced practice nurses in positions of clinical specialist in critical care, trauma, or ambulatory care, or are nurse practitioners with adult and family certification. Some are professional nurses in home health rehabilitation, nursing home, and acute care. Other volunteers are retired professional nurses. This is a rich group of nurses with varied experiences.

From the very beginning, nursing with faith communities has embodied the holistic approach to health care. This approach recognizes the dynamic relationship of all the needs (physical, psychological, spiritual emotional, social, and economic) to a person's health (Solari-Twadell, 1999). Nurses with faith communities are recognized members of the ministerial team. Home health care and invasive treatment procedures are usually not in this nursing practice; however, these procedures could be included should the faith community and the nurse so agree. Nursing with faith communities is not intended as a competitor to public or private health service organizations. Rather, a faith community-based program is simply another way to access the health care system. The holistic nursing approach is founded on the basic concepts of prevention, responsibility for one's own care, and partnership between individuals and providers (Schank, Weis, & Mateus, 1996).

If nursing with faith communities is based on a model such as the community nursing assessment, intervention, and evaluation model presented in Part II of this textbook, then the continuous growth and evaluation of programs are ensured. Assessments (monthly screenings), annual surveys, and analysis of the components of participants' needs tell us what intervention programs need to be implemented (e.g., healthy eating classes, exercise classes, walking clubs, or diabetes management instruction). These programs are implemented in a timely fashion that is most supportive of the participants. Evaluations of the programs led us to expand or to minimize programs depending on their effectiveness. Effectiveness is measured by the number of participants in the individual programs as well as individual goal accomplishment and overall satisfaction with the health outcomes (e.g., weight loss, increased feelings of fitness, decreased fatigue, better perceived control of stress with lowered blood pressure, and actual control and direction of one's lifestyle choices).

Here are some strategies for identifying faith community needs.

♦ Distribute an educational needs survey to various parish groups, such as the women's organization, the young mothers' support group, the elder group, the men's organization, and the non–English-speaking community.
♦ Attend meetings for the different groups.
♦ Form focus groups to discuss options to increase health or join an initiative already in progress, such as prayer groups or faith renewal focus groups.
♦ Provide a suggestion box.
♦ Form an ad hoc committee to study the health ministry and include key people such as clergy, lay ministers, school principal, social and health agency personnel, and so forth. Be sure that formal and informal leaders are included.
♦ Remember never to make decisions without input from the faith community.

The educational needs survey could be distributed at worship meetings to maximize the number of people reached. Of course, this should be available in all appropriate languages. It is helpful to have pencils available so surveys can be completed and collected at this time. After the information is gathered and synthesized, concerns and topics are prioritized. If an English version and non-English version are both used, respective priorities are noted.

Health Promotion Programs for Faith Communities

After assessing the faith community's educational preferences, the nurse plans intervention programs based on the results. Here is a listing of classes that may be of interest to members of a faith community.

♦ Exercise groups
♦ Nutrition classes

- CPR/choking awareness/first aid
- Positive parenting
- AIDS/HIV information sessions
- Planning for a healthy retirement
- Immunization program
- Health fair

If the community is interested in an exercise group, suggest a walking map. Walking maps are a self-directed exercise tool, which is popular particularly with the elderly. These maps have mileage-marked routes in each neighbourhood. Many members may be trying to begin an exercise program, but they do not know where to begin. Such maps can be helpful in starting and continuing a daily exercise program that contributes to the feeling of good health and, more importantly, can prevent or control high blood pressure. To construct a walking map, here is what you do:

- Design a 1-mile (or 1-km) map around the worship centre.
- Extend the map to include shopping malls, a recreational park, or neighbourhood school yards.
- Make sure the area is safe and accessible.
- Indicate $1/4$-mile (250-metre) markers, such as a retail store, a "no parking" sign, a mailbox, and so forth.
- Provide an opportunity for participants to learn how to do warm-up and cool-down exercises.
- Teach target heart rates and how to monitor pulses.
- Provide a mechanism for people to meet and become walking buddies, such as a kick-off party, convening at the worship centre, or meeting at the mall if it is nearby.
- Provide for ongoing encouragement and follow-up.

The Healthy Heart Club combines nutrition and education in a monthly gathering at lunchtime. This nursing action can be geared to adults, teens, or children. It is designed to teach the basics of eating a balanced diet, to provide tips on how to shop wisely for healthy food, and how to make good choices in restaurants. Here is a plan for Healthy Heart Club activities.

Healthy Heart Club Activities
- Gather in the faith community centre at a convenient time once a month.
- See if a faith community member who is a dietitian is available because it tends to attract people to the session.

◆ Identify content to be explored, such as healthy food recognition and preparation, economic purchases, eating out, and celebrating with healthy food choices.

◆ Include cooking demonstrations with healthy nonalcoholic drink or smoothie recipes that can be made in a blender and then sampled by participants.

◆ Recipe sharing that includes multicultural traditions is always popular for young and old alike.

◆ Offer tips on how to maintain favourite tastes in family recipes and still eat healthy, for example, substitution of 1% milk for whole milk, egg substitutes for eggs, or oil for lard.

◆ Field trips to ethnic restaurants and grocers can be scheduled.

This heart-healthy eating idea can be expanded to include children. Try starting a "Healthy Tots" or "Kid's Club" focusing on healthy food choices for healthy kids. How about serving chicken or tuna salad in an ice cream cone? Toss a banana, a peach (without the pit), some orange juice, and plain yogurt in a blender. Serve it over crushed ice. Challenge the children to come up with their own healthy, fruity concoction. Finally, celebrate with a heart-healthy party. Here is a healthy lifestyle program for youngsters that reinforces the notion that healthy choices can be incorporated into celebrations.

Pear and Apple Party Time Activity for Kids

◆ Pick a time when children are assembled. (Perhaps it is after the worship service.)

◆ Equipment you will need: pears, apples, toothpicks, little plates, napkins, a chalkboard (for tallying votes), cutting board, and knife.

◆ Have a variety of apples on hand (Red Delicious, Jonathan, McIntosh, Granny Smith, Golden Delicious).

◆ Have a variety of pears on hand (Anjou, Bosc, Comice).

◆ Cut the apples and pears into cubes.

◆ Have children taste each kind.

◆ Take a vote on what kind of apple and pear they liked most.

◆ Tally the votes on a scoreboard.

◆ Decorate the apple and pear with the most votes.

◆ Take a picture of everyone (and the pears and apples, of course).

◆ Celebrate and enjoy!

Cardiopulmonary resuscitation (CPR) training is another healthy lifestyle activity. This instruction is usually highly valued and can be an annual event.

Because CPR for community groups is an awareness session instead of a certification, it is less difficult. However, it still provides people with valuable information and skill should they be faced with a life-threatening situation. Attendees gain confidence in their ability to recognize warning signs and initiate lifesaving measures that perhaps can save loved ones. This training can include children over age 10 and teens as well.

If a faith community undertakes the project of a health fair, timing is important. One theory is that it should have its own special time of year. Another view is that it can coincide with an annual bazaar or fund-raiser. Personally, I always prefer as much fun as possible in everything I do. How about you? Because the community usually supports the annual fund-raiser, a captive audience is present. On the other hand, sometimes people would rather take health more seriously and not try to focus on fun and games and screening or health education activities at the same time. However, if immunizations are provided, sometimes this is an unpleasant association for children who set out for a fun time. Both situations can work with proper planning and marketing, depending on the commitment and support of the faith community. The following are steps to consider when setting up a health fair. This outline is not meant to be exhaustive but to provide ideas and some direction. Although the faith community is a church, synagogue, or temple, it is important to include the greater community in its health ministry. A health fair is a wonderful opportunity to open the boundaries of the faith community.

Organizing a Health Fair for a Faith Community

- Contact the clergy and lay council.
- Set the date (try to allow at least 6 to 8 weeks to arrange).
- Decide what health promotion areas to cover, depending on the audience (adults only, families, elders).
- Invite identified organizations to participate.
- Invite health care providers, health service vendors, and community resources from the geographic area.
- Solicit prizes from local merchants.
- Offer incentives for attendance, such as door prizes and coupons for free services (e.g., mammograms, heart scans).
- Collaborate with other professionals, such as a dental school, pharmacy school, or optometrist.
- Offer free immunizations.
- Have a women's health booth, a men's health booth, a teen booth, and a children's health booth.

◆ Include screening stations such as vision, hearing, blood glucose, blood pressure, lead, tuberculosis skin testing, depression, HIV testing, and counselling.

◆ Have a plan for referral and follow-up.

◆ It may be a good idea to have an HIV ministry booth providing information about HIV as well as providers from treatment centres.

◆ Have stations that focus on environmental health, including booths on mosquito control and water safety. People from rural areas can bring in water samples for testing.

◆ A home safety booth sponsored by the utility company or fire department can address ventilation, electrical hazards, and gas appliances.

◆ A crime watch booth sponsored by the police can address self-defense and home security.

◆ Set up computers for health risk appraisal programs.

◆ Assign booth areas considering flow pattern. Provide for privacy if breast self-examination is demonstrated or skin cancer checks are done.

◆ Invite the media.

◆ Include fun activities, such as craft booths for the children and adults.

Additional health promotion strategies for faith communities include:

◆ Blood pressure screening
◆ Glucose screening
◆ Vision and glaucoma
◆ Consultation and referral
◆ Bereavement program
◆ Weight management programs—how about "Weigh to go!" for a title?
◆ Smoking cessation programs
◆ Diabetes education classes
◆ Caregiver support groups
◆ Asthmatic support group
◆ Respite care programs

The nursing volunteers from the community ensure that the multicultural factor of the community can be mirrored in the nursing team. The problems of language are thereby mitigated by the volunteers who speak the same language as the attendees. Cultural practices that contribute to healthy lifestyle (e.g., Vietnamese and Chinese heavy use of vegetables in the diet) are emphasized at social and educational activities. Importance is placed on cultural recognition and adaptation of health-supporting behaviors.

Economic factors as well as cultural factors are essential concerns of problem identification and solution. The faith community is a microcosm of the larger economic pattern of the city. Services should be accessible to all members of the faith community as appropriate. The affluence of the community will affect the type of programs that can be implemented. It is an accepted fact that families that have more discretionary income are more able to engage in health promotion activities. This will have an impact on the overall health of the community. Economics also influences how members of the community obtain access to health services. The faith community may be the only consistent health care they receive.

Establishing a Lasting Partnership With Faith Communities

Now that background information and program strategies have been explored, let's focus on the essential elements of establishing a nursing partnership with a faith community. Here is one way to begin:

◆ Obtain support from clergy and administration.
◆ Identify a core of health professionals willing to participate. Ideally, they will be members of the faith community.
◆ Establish a marketing system.
◆ Find a college of nursing or a community college to assist you in developing the ministry.
◆ Identify sponsor support through parish members and neighbourhood establishments. (Local businesses are usually supportive because they recognize that their patrons are members of the faith community.)
◆ Acquire supplies, such as cotton swabs, rubber gloves, stethoscopes, blood pressure cuffs, glucose meters, and so forth, from various sources.
◆ Recruit additional volunteer health professionals to participate.
◆ Have a team meeting and plan nursing actions. Probably the first action would be to conduct a needs assessment. Be sure that it is conducted in languages that reflect the constituency.

It is acceptable to start small or to have volunteers who are only able to give a little time. The nature of the ministry is that it builds on itself as time and community needs dictate. A successful marketing strategy is critical to starting and maintaining an active program. Several approaches can be implemented. Depending on resources and community contacts, some may be more feasible than others. Local newspapers, radio and television spots, and civic association bulletins are possibilities. Posting on the church marquee or other community billboards is usually a very effective way of notifying the community of program activities. The most effective strategy is pulpit announcements during or immediately after regularly scheduled services. Surveys completed at this time usually yield excellent response. A nurse column in the faith community's bulletin announcing scheduled health-screening activities and health education programs can be a regular feature. Catchy names such as "Positively Healthy Choices," "Nurse's Notes," or "Here's to Healthy Choices" will focus attention on the health information, which should be published in all languages commonly spoken. Remember to partner with nearby or church-affiliated schools, community stores, and fast food restaurants. Ask to market the faith community "nursing news" and events in their flyers and newsletters and on their marquees.

Consulting with a community college or university school of nursing to assist with establishing the health promotion program really helps. Faculty members may be willing to assist with the writing of a needs assessment survey. Then, the church community can be assessed annually with a tool, an invaluable part of the process. Graduate student nurses can be lead players in the community assessment. They can work with lay members of the faith community and guide the actual assessment. This would be a tremendous asset to the nurse or nurses because most often they are volunteering and such needs assessments can be very time consuming. Reciprocally, the students would have an opportunity to participate in a valuable and realistic clinical experience. Another benefit to colleges is the opportunity for sharing research data.

Health care provider systems (hospitals, HMOs, PPOs) have come to realize the importance of collaborating with faith community health programs as a valuable model. Frequently, faith communities will sign agreements of support with health management systems such as hospitals, private clinics, or group medical practices. Depending on the type of agency, the sponsor provides continuing education for the volunteer nurses, screening services through a stationary or mobile health unit, and a speakers' bureau for health education programs (Gillis, 1993). This sponsor, who may be a local public health department, may also provide low-cost immunizations at health promotion activities (King, Lakin, & Striepe, 1993). Additionally, faith community nurses utilize the sponsor health care system, as well as other local health care providers, as referral options for faith community participants. Other types of nonhealth care sponsors include fast food restaurants, retail shops, businesses, colleges and universities, as well as civic and public service organizations (e.g., Lions Clubs, women's organizations, League of Women Voters). Frequently, national foundations, such as the March of Dimes, or local foundations may be receptive to being a sponsor, thus providing needed money for supplies, brochures, and other essential items. Because space on church property is limited, the program is totally portable. Many volunteers bring their own equipment (e.g., stethoscopes and sphygmomanometers). Representatives from drug companies and medical supply companies, who are members of the faith community, may supply the program with other needed equipment.

An example of how important this program is concerns a "healthy-feeling" parishioner who, because of his spouse's urging, had his blood pressure and glucose checked. The results were abnormal for age and gender. So, he was given the written test results, counselled, and referred to a health provider of his choice. A month later, the spouse reported that her husband was recuperating splendidly from coronary bypass surgery and learning to manage his newly diagnosed diabetes. Registered nurses, who are the diabetic management experts, and the nurse practitioners, with the support of the sponsor agent, can be the usual blood glucose screeners. Participants feel comforted and reassured when their screening data are within normal range. The participants who regulate their type 2 diabetes without monitoring at home, usually because of limited income, can use the screening program for self-management evaluation and further education.

Classes that are age or content specific are popular and well attended. A nurse with a background in men's health issues can speak to the men's club. A male nurse can make a particular contribution speaking to the group about testicular self-examination, prostate and colon cancer, and penile erection issues. Nurses have an opportunity to discuss domestic violence and abuse. Presentations focus on defining abusive situations, identifying community resources available to victims and perpetrators of abuse, and especially skills for relationships without violence. A special meeting of teens by way of youth groups should address the subject of dating violence.

Nurses support other ministries of the faith community by assisting with emergencies at services. They promote the health of Boy Scouts and Girl Scouts as well as Boys and Girls Clubs through education and immunization programs. Nurses team with men's and women's groups for monthly celebration activities. All events have health literature displays with generous amounts of health materials in all appropriate languages. Through these efforts, the nurses are recognized as a visible ministry of the faith community. The visibility contributes to the ongoing success of the partnership between the nurses and the faith community (Miles, 1997).

Summary

Nursing in faith communities is still in its early development phase. It has an enormous potential to grow and evolve into an enhanced health care delivery system. Nurses are singularly well equipped to use their multifaceted skills and their extensive body of knowledge to improve the health status of individuals, families, and communities in a changing health care arena. This nurse practice model is a relatively new and cost-effective way to help participants navigate the managed care environment. It is part of the solution to the problem of the ever-rising cost of health care. If programs such as this one can keep segments of society healthier through health promotion, disease prevention activities, and, in some cases, home care options, the quality of health care will be improved (Rydholm, 1997).

Through expansion of the nurse role, more services can be brought to the faith community. The sponsor agent relationship can facilitate the addition of services. Faith community nursing can be expanded to include well-child care, adult health, and minor acute care. This can be addressed by employing nurse practitioners, who will actually practise in a clinic in the faith community setting (Souther, 1997). Eventually, a community-wide needs assessment can be conducted to expand the annual faith community survey. Nursing students can assist with this activity. Analyzing databases to identify community assets as well as problems will provide information for the program.

One of the most important steps will be acquiring physical space for the nurse ministry to provide services. Clergy and administrative personnel who are supportive of the program and eager for it to advance will see this as a necessity. If renovation plans are under way, space for the nurse ministry should be incorporated. Although the program can be entirely mobile, it is more practical to have a designated space for storage and to render services. To maintain focus, ensure quality, and preserve the volunteer and multicultural components of the congregation, both long- and short-term goals are required. Identify a variety of health promotion strategies and health education needs to be addressed in the future. Then set realistic short-term goals that focus on the specific areas identified, such as enhancing the diabetic education, restructuring the weight management classes, or offering stress-reduction methods (e.g., aromatherapy, realistic relaxation techniques, caregiver support). Because members of the team are already often managing careers and professional commitments and family and personal responsibilities, limiting the focus at the beginning stage of development is the best strategy to ensure continued success of the program.

The practice model of nursing partnerships with faith communities described in this chapter is in evolution. Nurses need to be proactive in this area of continuous health care reform. We must participate in and help shape future decision making for health care delivery. This nurse ministry, whether a volunteer or reimbursed service, is a cost-effective enhancement of health care delivery systems. Nursing partnerships with faith communities are part of the solution.

References

Gillis, V. (1993). Sponsorship networks. *Health Progress, 4*, 34–41.

King, J., Lakin, J., & Striepe, J. (1993). Coalition building between public health nurses and parish nurses. *Journal of Nursing Administration, 23*(2), 27–31.

Miles, L. (1997). Getting started: Parish nursing in a rural community. *Journal of Christian Nursing, 14*(1), 22–24.

Rydholm, L. (1997). Patient-focused care in parish nursing. *Holistic Nursing Practice, 4*, 47–60.

Schank, M., Weis, D., & Mateus, R. (1996). Parish nursing: Ministry of healing. *Geriatric Nursing, 17*(1), 11–13.

Solari-Twadell, P. (1999). The emerging practice of parish nursing. In P. Solari-Twadell & M. McDermott (Eds.), *Parish nursing: Promoting whole person health within faith communities* (pp. 3–24). Thousand Oaks, CA: Sage.

Souther, B. (1997). Congregational nurse practitioner: An idea whose time has come. *Journal of Christian Nursing, 14*(1), 32-34.

Weis, D., Mateus, R., & Schank, M. (1997). Health care delivery in faith communities: The parish nurse model. *Public Health Nursing, 14*(6), 368–372.

Westberg, G. (1999). A personal historical perspective of whole person health and the congregation. In P. Solari-Twadell & M. McDermott (Eds.), *Parish nursing: Promoting whole person health within faith communities* (pp. 35–41). Thousand Oaks, CA: Sage.

Suggested Readings

Journal of Christian Nursing, published by the Nurses Christian Fellowship, Box 7895, Madison, WI 53707. Inquire about reprints of parish nursing articles and the availability of photocopies of selected articles.

Parish Nurse, a quarterly newsletter for practicing parish nurses. Issued by LCMS Health Ministries, The Lutheran Church—Missouri Synod.

Internet Resources

International Network for Interfaith Health Practices: **www.interaccess.com/ihpnet**. Includes practice models and resource links.

Parish nursing: **www.csbsju.edu/library/internet/parish.html**. Ecumenical perspective on health care ministry including Internet resources for parish nursing.

Canadian Resources

Clark, M. B., & Olson J. K. (in press). *Nursing within a faith community: Promoting health in times of transition.* Thousand Oaks, CA: Sage.

Solari-Twadell, P. A., & McDermott, M. A. (Eds.). (1999). *Parish nursing: Promoting whole person health within faith communities.* Thousand Oaks, CA: Sage. Two chapters of particular note to Canadian congregations are "The Canadian Experience" and "Perspectives on a Suburban Parish Nurse Practice."

Canadian Association of Parish Nursing Ministry: **http://www.capnm.ca/**.

Catholic Women's League: **http://www.cwl.ab.ca/EDCresolutions.html**.

United Church of Canada: **http://www.united-church.ca/exchange/1999/spring9901.shtm**.

22

Promoting Healthy Partnerships With Rural Populations

MARY WAINWRIGHT

OBJECTIVES

After studying this chapter, you should be able to:

◆ Discuss geographic and social factors that affect the health status of rural populations

◆ Describe health promotion issues that relate to rural populations

◆ Design and implement a health promotion project with a rural population

Introduction

What image comes to mind when you think of rural? Do you think of a farm at the end of a long dirt road where a large family is eating supper together? A place where neighbours know and care about each other? A place with close relationships and less hectic lifestyles? Most people have a favourable image of a rural lifestyle. Just like rural living, nursing in rural settings can be rewarding and challenging. In this chapter, we describe some general characteristics of rural populations and discuss strategies for developing healthy partnerships with rural populations.

Although most people recognize rural when they see it, defining the term has been a persistent unsolved problem. No operational definition of a rural area precisely differentiates rural from urban populations. A common distinction, especially for federal programs, is metropolitan areas and nonmetropolitan areas. These are designations made by the U.S. Office of Management and Budget (OMB) based on the integration of counties with big cities having a population of 50,000 or more (Baer, Johnson-Webb, & Gesler, 1997). Obviously, a small rural town isolated in a county designated as a metropolitan area would be lost in the OMB definition. A more common definition of rural population is people living in a sparsely populated place usually somewhat distant from a large city. Rural has a difficult-to-quantify feeling of close ties and strong community identity. It is not necessary to adopt a single definition for the purposes of this discussion. However, nurses should be familiar with the OMB designation of metropolitan and nonmetropolitan areas.

Engelken (1997) articulates the concept that rural is a tangible asset. However, not all attributes of rural populations fit with an idyllic image. The negative features of rural life have implications for nursing in rural areas. There is a greater concentration of people with low incomes and the uninsured in rural areas. Rural dwellers live longer, which contributes to the fact that rural populations have a greater percentage of the elderly than urban populations, 18% versus 15%, respectively (Dansky, Brannon, Shea, et al., 1998). Geographic distance and inadequate transportation are typical barriers to health care access. Consequently, rural dwellers are more likely to have complex and chronic health care problems (Gariola, 1997). Access is also limited because of geographic maldistribution of health care providers. Whereas 20% of Americans live in nonmetropolitan counties, only 11% of patient care physicians practise in those counties (Crittenden & Myers, 1997).

Unfortunately, changes initiated by the Balanced Budget Act of 1997 have significant potential for altering the structure of the rural health delivery system (Mueller & McBride, 1999). These changes could result in increased rural hospital closings, reduction of home health services, and increased maldistribution of the health work force. In most rural communities, nurses are the foundation and, in some cases, the sole source of health care.

Rural Nursing Theory

As a framework for building partnerships with rural populations, it is useful to consider the rural nursing theory development work of Long and Weinert (1989). They identified the following key characteristics of rural populations that affect nursing services:

1. Work beliefs and health
2. Isolation and distance
3. Self-reliance
4. Lack of anonymity
5. Insider/outsider and old-timer/newcomer designation

Work Beliefs and Health

Rural dwellers define health in terms of ability to work. A logger in a rural logging town probably considers himself in good health as long as he is able to work. He will try home remedies and neighbourly advice before he seeks professional help. Only when the remedies and advice fail will the logger consult a clinician. Treatment that will get him back to work is his dominant medical care expectation. Nichols (1989) described rural residents' health care orientation as present-time and crisis oriented. As such, these work/health beliefs make rural dwellers only minimally interested in health maintenance and disease prevention activities (Muldoon, Schootman, & Morton, 1996; Parrot, Steiner, & Goldenhar, 1996). Infrequent participation in smoking-cessation programs, tobacco chewing, obesity, and disregard for regular exercise are common.

Isolation and Distance

Residents accept and adapt to isolation and distance. Distance is integrated into everyday life. Residents anticipate and even relish shopping trips that require a 1- to 3-hour drive each way. With little hesitation, a neighbour may devote a day to driving the distance required for a sick friend's specialty doctor appointment. However, even with significant adaptive strategies, distance is a barrier that increases the likelihood of deferring health care until one is very ill. Furthermore, recovery times and optimal rehabilitation are compromised by inadequate and untimely treatment.

Self-Reliance

For survival, isolation and distance require the development of strong, self-reliant attitudes. The high value placed on self-reliance is readily observed both in individuals and the community as a whole. For example, a rural community's aspiration to develop a regional medical centre—and make the necessary financial commitment to support it—are consistent with the community's desire to take care of itself. Individual self-reliance is also typical. Take, for example, rural Rosebud resident Mr. Kane's response to his elderly wife's immobility. Rather than place his wife in a skilled-care setting, Mr. Kane fed her, bathed her, and changed her decubitus dressing as best he could. He maintained this exhausting care regimen until he developed pneumonia and had to be admitted to the hospital.

Lack of Anonymity

Rural communities are "fishbowls." Everyone knows about everyone. It is all too true that "You know you are in rural America when you find out the results of your daughter-in-law's pregnancy test before she does." Each person is observed and judged equally on his or her personal life and professional ability. A health care provider is known throughout the community, and privacy is limited. In the grocery store, school, or church, the provider is expected to deal with health care issues. Because people with advanced education or leadership skills are so often away, lured to larger cities, the role of the health care provider in a rural community frequently includes expectations of leadership. This additional visibility magnifies the fact that a rural nurse's credibility, trust, and effectiveness as an agent of change in partnership building depend on the community's judgment of the person as a whole.

Insider/Outsider and Old-Timer/ Newcomer Designation

Rural community residents tend to be less mobile than their urban counterparts. Several generations live within close proximity, and friends grow up and remain together for a lifetime. People are identified in the context of their relationships: "You know her. She's Mr. Gray's daughter-in-law." If one's grandfather was the town drunk, one is always known as the grandchild of the town drunk. This is often expressed in comments such as "Jill has done well in spite of the fact she's old man Jones's granddaughter." In a similar vein, it is easy to learn who is an insider and who is an outsider by listening to comments like "Make sure you include Mr. Wallis on your invitation list. He's on every money-raising committee in town," or "Why are you inviting Mrs. Leroy? She's never been involved in this kind of meeting before." In fact, newcomers may not join the ranks of old-timers for as long as 15 to 20 years. Mrs. Taylor came to one rural community when she was first married and was referred to as "the lady from Missouri" until her grandchildren were born. Lenz and Edwards (1992) stated that these distinctions usually produce more favourable considerations for insiders and old-timers. However, the outsider position is sometimes advantageous when issues of confidentiality arise and emotional distance is preferred. Acceptance of a rural nurse and his or her community role is influenced by the insider/outsider, old-timer/newcomer mind set.

Building a Partnership

With these five rural nursing theory concepts in mind, let us now consider how to develop a partnership with a rural community. We will include in the discussion examples from a rural community named Rosebud.

Assessment: Old-Timers and Insiders as Key Informants

In a rural community, nurses must pay special attention to personal contacts when implementing the community assessment strategies described earlier in this book. Before beginning the assessment process, or at least very early in the process, you should identify key informants in the community. If you are an outsider or a newcomer, an effective strategy is to have someone within the community "sponsor" you by introducing you to key informants, and you may want to refer to your "sponsor" when you make the contact with others. Discuss with the key informants your assessment goals and their perception of community health assets and needs. Also, ask them to identify other important contacts. Rural communities are self-reliant and may resist activity they perceive as interference from outside. By engaging community old-timers and insiders early in the process, you can build a network that will help assess, plan, and implement strategies to meet community-identified health needs. This network of community informants can identify resources, overcome barriers, and help to find solutions to problems that reflect the community's perspective.

The most important concept to keep in mind is that the rural community's perception of their community health needs defines the reality of those needs. Many rural communities will accept help identifying their community needs. A reliable, comprehensive assessment is essential in securing resources for a rural community, but the resources to accomplish an assessment are frequently limited. Some communities may have strong public opinion regarding community health needs, with or without the benefits of a formal needs assessment. However, if a community places high priority on a health risk that you consider less critical than others, the community's perspective is the priority. To attempt to address the greater health risk without the community's support would be to invite failure from the beginning. By empowering the community and thereby contributing to "healthy community" behaviour, you will offer a greater service. Often, when you help the community address the lesser risk, you build community awareness of the greater risk.

In rural Rosebud, several citizens were concerned about tobacco use by high school students. Our comprehensive community assessment revealed a high incidence of lung cancer in the community and no public activities to address the issue. We also identified as an asset the well-attended county fair, which contributes to Rosebud's economic health and civic pride. Utilizing both the community's identified need and the empirical evidence of an existing health risk, we make the community diagnosis: high prevalence of lung cancer related to long-term tobacco use.

Planning: Designing by the Community for the Community

The community needs information in a usable form about the results of the assessment process. An informed community can participate in effective planning. Key informants will again be excellent resources in suggesting a dissemination process for the assessment results. It takes time and energy to engage the community in the planning, but this "engagement" is the part of the process that builds the community's strength and ability to address its own needs. This empowerment is an important component of a community's "health."

Involving the community at every step is part of the partnership, whether you engage in a whole town meeting or an informal committee planning process with a few key informants. The plan should be achievable and appropriate for the rural culture. For instance, health promotion activities need to be threaded into the everyday activities of rural residents. A rural resident may not come to town just to participate in a free cholesterol screening session at the health clinic, but if the screening session was held at the grocery store on Saturday morning, he or she might take advantage of the opportunity. The action plan should include (1) clear objectives and action steps; (2) identification of resources needed, including people, budget, and materials; (3) identification of available sources such as grants, other funding, and volunteer time; (4) a timeline; and (5) an evaluation process.

In Rosebud, we posted the results of our community assessment, Rosebud's Top Ten Health Concerns, at the grocery store and the feed store as well as in the *Rambling Rose*, the weekly newspaper. Then, we convened five key Rosebud insiders to address the high prevalence of lung cancer related to long-term tobacco use. The informal group leader was a high school student's mother who was very concerned about smoking among her child's friends. By defining the goal, brainstorming, selecting interventions, and prioritizing the activities, we developed a project action plan. The plan included enlisting high school students to help us develop a "Health-Wise" booth at the county fair to promote antitobacco use behaviours and other health promotion activities.

Implementation: One Person Can Make the Difference

It is beneficial in the implementation process to enlist help from a community person who is energetic and enthusiastic about the project. Ideally, this person would have participated in the needs assessment and planning phases. Because of the "fishbowl" phenomenon in a rural community, a project's success may be linked to the person or people perceived as leading the project. That person may not be a "formal leader" of the community, but he or she must be able to influence others to participate in the intervention. One person does make a difference in rural settings. Furthermore, communities and community leaders need encouragement. Mark the milestones. Create opportunities to acknowledge publicly each incremental success. Develop effective relationships with news media. Signs in stores, newspaper articles, and radio and TV interviews are all effective strategies for maintaining the commitment and energy level of the community.

In Rosebud, when Ms. Carpenter, a local doctor's wife and community activist, learned of our "Health-Wise" booth project, she got excited and brought in all kinds of help. She was able to influence high school teachers to include research assignments about effective ways to prevent and change young people's tobacco-use habits. Students helped design materials and activities for the booth. Mrs. Carpenter's neighbour, the high school principal, allowed the students and other adults to use the wood shop to build the booth. Other project team members solicited donations for materials and coordinated work schedules. The newspaper editor wrote a small grant to the regional Lumber Industry Foundation to purchase sets of "Mr. Yuk Mouth," a bad-breathed, ugly-teethed model designed as a visual disincentive for tobacco use that targeted young people. We posted thank-you signs for every contribution. The local "investigative" reporter wrote a series of articles about youth and tobacco use and feature activities relating to the "Health-Wise" booth project.

Evaluation: Process and Outcomes

Rural community health needs rarely develop overnight. They are more often complex, chronic, and insidious problems. Evaluation strategies for community health interventions should include measures of anticipated long-term outcomes. In addition, assess the community's perception of the success of the project with respect to more short-range outcomes such as (1) partnership building and partnership strengthening, (2) numbers of individuals and groups involved, (3) quantity and quality of services provided, and (4) the impact of the project on the community diagnosis. Some of the outcomes may be new initiatives to address the problem or related problems. Acknowledgment of community assets is a healthy outcome. A community empowered to address its own needs is one of the most powerful outcomes possible. Finally, quantitative measures about behavioural changes and changes in health indicator trends should be reviewed in appropriate time frames. The results of the evaluation should be shared with the community.

In Rosebud, a feature article on the front page of the *Rambling Rose,* titled "Health-Wise Smoking Success," touted the community project's success. We received positive results from team members, including the high school students, who evaluated each action step and the overall project. The mayor acknowledged success of the project at the city council meeting. A new project was started in the elementary school, and the local merchants agreed to improve their strategies for preventing the sale of tobacco to minors. Another group began developing strategies to measure the actual tobacco use of children in their community. Although these outcomes were not anticipated in the original plan, they were legitimate and powerful project outcomes. Community empowerment was increased with this project, and Rosebud's self-image improved. It will be several years, if not decades, before the lung cancer rate health indicator may be affected, but Rosebud is proud of the changes that have already occurred.

Summary

Rural communities are wonderful places to live and work. Understanding the rural dweller's work and health beliefs, the challenges of isolation and distance, the concepts of self-reliance, lack of anonymity, and insider/outsider and old-timer/newcomer designations will increase our effectiveness in developing partnerships with rural populations. Throughout the nursing process, we can improve the strength of the partnership and healthy community behaviour by engaging the rural community in each step of the process. One of the most rewarding aspects of developing partnerships with rural populations is the realization that "one person can make a difference" in the whole community. Perhaps you are the one nurse who has or will make the difference in your rural community.

References

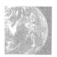

Baer, L., Johnson-Webb, K., & Gesler, W. (1997). What is rural? A focus on urban influence codes. *Journal of Rural Health, 13*(4), 329–333.

Crittenden, B., & Myers, W. (1997). Can Medicare medical education policies better address rural provider shortages? *Rural Policy Brief, 1*(3). Available at www.rupri.org/brief/PB97-3/index.html.

Dansky, K., Brannon, D., Shea, D., Vasey, J., & Dirani, R. (1998). Profiles of hospital, physician, and home health service use by older persons in rural areas. *The Gerontologist, 38,* 320-330.

Engelken, J. (1997). A wakeup call for rural health. *Rural Health FYI, 19*(1), 42.

Gariola, G. (1997). Developing rural interdisciplinary geriatrics teams in a changing health care environment. *Journal of Allied Health,* Winter, 27–29.

Lenz, C. L., & Edwards, J. (1992). Nurse-managed primary care. Tapping the rural community power base. *Journal of Nursing Administration, 22*(9), 57–61.

Long, K., & Weinert, C. (1989). Rural nursing; Developing the theory base. *Scholarly Inquiry for Nursing Practice: An International Journal, 3*(2), 113–127.

Mueller, K. & McBride, T. (1999). Taking Medicare into the 21st century: Realities of a post BBA world and implications for rural health care. Rural Policy Research Institute, Rural Health Panel Publication (pp 1–17), 2/10/99 P99–2.

Muldoon, J., Schootman, M., & Morton, R. (1996). Utilization of cancer early detection services among farm and rural nonfarm adults in Iowa. *Journal of Rural Health, 12*(4), 321–331.

Nichols, E. (1989). Response to rural nursing: Developing the theory base. *Scholarly Inquiry for Nursing Practice: An International Journal, 3*(2), 129–132.

Parrott, R., Steiner, C., & Goldenhar, L. (1996). Georgia's harvesting healthy habits: A formative evaluation. *Journal of Rural Health, 12*(4), 291–300.

Internet Resources

National Rural Health Association: **www.nrharural.org/**. A national membership organization whose mission is to improve the health and health care of rural Americans and to provide leadership on rural issues through advocacy, communications, education and research.

National Rural Health Services Research Database: **www.muskie.usm.maine.edu /rhsr/default.asp**: This site provides a database of funded rural health services research projects that are under way in the United States.

Rural Health WebRing: **www.rural-health.org.au/**. This is an Australian site dedicated to rural health issues. It includes government, educational, and hospital sites that contain information relevant to rural health.

Canadian Resources

Brandon University Rural Development Institute:
   http://rhrg.brandonu.ca/research_webpage.htm
Government of British Columbia: **http://www.healthservices.gov.bc.ca/rural/index.html**
Health Canada Rural Health Office: **http://www.hc-sc.gc.ca/english/ruralhealth/**
Laurentian University Centre for Rural and Northern Health Research:
   http://laurentian.ca/cranhr/
Nursing BC: **http://www.rnabc.bc.ca/pdf/rural.pdf**
University of Lethbridge: **http://staffweb.uleth.ca/news/display.asp?ID=3902**
University of Saskatchewan rural nursing: **http://www.usask.ca/nursing/rurnur/**

23

Promoting Healthy Partnerships With the Chronically Ill

PAMELA SCHULTZ

OBJECTIVES

After studying this chapter, you should be able to:

◆ Discuss the characteristics of chronic health conditions

◆ Describe health promotion strategies for the chronically ill

◆ Implement a health promotion plan for persons with a chronic health condition using strategies from other chapters

Introduction

Typically, illness is viewed as a condition in which optimal health is not achieved. An acute illness is one in which the illness resolves as a result of an intervention or the lapsing of time. A chronic illness is one in which there is no resolution of the disease process. The implication is that the person will have this illness until death; there is no cure. Because people frequently live long and productive lives with chronic illnesses, should they be labeled "ill"? Perhaps a more appropriate designation is chronic health condition. Many people in any community will be living with a chronic health condition.

On the surface, it seems that identifying those people with a chronic health condition is simple. But, on reflection, this is a daunting task. How should "chronic health condition" be defined? What elements must be present to differentiate the acute health condition from the chronic condition? Can a health condition be both acute and chronic? Under what conditions?

The holistic approach to nursing care refrains from compartmentalizing the individual. The holistic approach emphasizes the interconnectedness of the person. When taken literally, this approach can be used to describe a person with a chronic health condition. The health of the person should not be compartmentalized, such as the diabetic, the person with cancer, the schizophrenic, or the person with HIV infection. However, the nurse is bombarded by the health care system's approach to label and categorize the person's health. So, to discuss the chronically ill, an attempt is made to describe this population in the broadest of terms.

Characteristics of Chronic Health Conditions

Progressive: The health condition worsens or becomes more severe over time. The time period may be over an entire life span or major portions of time. There may be periods of quiescence followed by periods of exacerbation or there is a slowly evolving deterioration. Examples of progressive health conditions are certain types of slow-growing cancers that are not curable and there is an inevitability of dying of the cancer. Chronic obstructive pulmonary disease characteristically is a slowly evolving deterioration of lung capacity. Congestive heart failure has periods of quiescence and control with patterns of acute bouts of heart failure. Diabetes mellitus, especially insulin-dependent types, becomes progressively more difficult to regulate.

Irreversible: The condition is not curable. The chronic health condition takes a toll on the individual. Damage that cannot be corrected occurs. Examples include some cancers such as those of the pancreas, which destroy the organ's ability to produce enzymes for digestion, which leads to nutritional deficits. Several types of kidney diseases eventually result in complete renal failure, which damages other major systems such as the central nervous system and the cardiovascular system. Chronic obstructive pulmonary disease causes a loss of pulmonary function, which is not reversible. Schizophrenia and bipolar disease are not curable but can be controlled; however, a long history of these conditions produces impairments in judgment, social skills, and activities of daily living.

Complex: The chronic condition may involve multiple systems. The impacts of chronic health conditions reach beyond the arena in which they begin. People with asthma not only have physical manifestations of the process, but they frequently restrict their activities in such a way as to cause isolation, which affects their mental health and their recreation. Depression is a frequent sequelae of chronic health conditions (Davidson & Meltzer-Brody, 1999). The treatment of a chronic condition may have side effects, such as pain and nutritional deficits, that become a part of the condition. Diabetes mellitus can result in neuropathies, retinopathy leading to blindness, and circulatory problems leading to amputation, commonly of the feet and legs. Hypertension can lead to heart disease, stroke, and renal failure.

Treatment aimed at symptom control: The purpose of treatment is not to cure but to control symptoms. This implies an unknown cause or the lack of technology to enable a cure. In some cases, the condition is considered acute and treatment is aimed at cure, and, when this is unachievable, the condition becomes chronic. Some cancers follow this path.

A family affair and chronic sorrow: Chronic health conditions always have an impact on the significant others of the individual. Depending on the culture and the interfamily dynamics, this manifests itself with great diversity. Chronic sorrow is a condition that may be experienced by the individual and the family. This is a lasting phenomenon that can continue past the death of the individual with the chronic health condition. It is a sadness without end and comprises an accumulation of ongoing losses over time (Krafft & Krafft, 1998).

Health Perception and Chronic Illness and Health Promotion

Every individual has a unique perception of the state of his health. This state fluctuates with various events, but usually a person has a static view of his health. People with terminal cancer may be heard to say that they are in good health if it were not for the cancer. People may maintain that they are in good health but be denied life insurance because of their medical history. People may perceive their health as being very poor but live well into their nineties.

How is the perception of one's health important? If people perceive their health as good, then it is likely they will consider their quality of life as good. Studies have shown that the association between health status and quality of life is not clear (Covinsky, Wu, & Landefeld, et al., 1999). Covinsky and associates (1999) have shown that generally, one's health status is a reasonable indicator of perceived quality of life; however, incongruency is not uncommon. A person's perception of her health may sometimes lag behind actual health status. A 65-year-old woman is told she has severe osteoporosis and is at risk for hip fracture. She feels well and considers herself in good health. Within a few moments, she is given information about her health status that labels her as having a chronic health condition.

How people perceive their health has a major impact on how they respond to health promotion strategies. If people see their health as good they may resist health promotion strategies. If they view their health as not good, they may also be resistant to these strategies out of a sense of fatalism. Generalizations cannot be made. People with chronic health conditions typically are very informed about their chronic condition. They may have little patience with strategies aimed at areas of their health that are not perceived as part of that condition. Conversely, some people may choose to focus on an aspect of their health that can be improved.

Implementation of Health Promotion Strategies

When planning to implement a health promotion program for people with chronic health conditions, several principles should be considered.

Identification of specific health care priorities: People with chronic health conditions have special needs. Any health promotion activities must be tailored to those needs individually. The nurse must be knowledgeable about the person's health status as it pertains to the chronic condition. This requires a strong basic knowledge in the health care sciences. For instance, the nurse may want to emphasize the importance of drinking 8 to 10 glasses of water a day. For a patient on renal dialysis, this might not be appropriate.

Continuity of rapport: Stanley (1999) has described a program in which patients with chronic medical and psychiatric problems are placed in addictive treatment programs. Normally, these people would not be allowed to participate in the addictive treatment programs because of their conflicting chronic problems. But, because their program is designed to enable the health care professionals to respond to a variety of other health care needs, these patients can successfully complete programs aimed at addictive disease. This type of program allows for continuity of rapport. This partnership opens the nurse to intervene at all levels. It enables the psychiatric nurse to intervene in health promotion practices as well as the treatment for chronic conditions. In the milieu of managed care, continuity of care may become fragmented. Continuity of rapport is not only valuable in chronic health conditions but also in health promotion activities.

Social support: Social support has been linked to health and longevity in many studies (Lepore, 1998). It has been shown that social support enhances health. Many people with chronic health conditions develop a life pattern of isolation, which leads to difficulty in expressing themselves and relating to others (Jonsdottir, 1998). Many people with chronic health conditions have access to therapy and support groups focussing on particular chronic conditions. There are cancer support groups, AIDS support groups, sexual abuse support groups, and so forth. These types of groups provide comfort and camaraderie among the participants. Since 1960, group therapy has been shown to be a valuable tool of the helping professions (Bednar & Lawlis, 1971; Dies, 1979, 1986; Kaul & Bednar, 1986; Orlinsky & Howard, 1986). These groups are fertile ground for health promotion by nurses. Many times, these groups are community sponsored. Support groups can be extended to family caregivers; this, too, increases the opportunities for health promotion, in some cases to the entire family (Ellgring, 1999).

Health professionals, particularly nurses, need to avail themselves of knowledge about the group process. This is not an unnecessary frill that exists on the periphery of medical and nursing practice or the private domain of a subspecialty (Sampson & Marthas, 1981). The skills required to work effectively with groups are not intuitive; they need to be learned.

Nurses state that providing support for their patients is a basic tenet of providing care. Support implies helping the patient make adjustments for the experience he or she lacks and problem solve to adapt to health care conditions (van Servellen, 1984). DeYoung and Dickey (1967) found that certain nursing behaviours expressed support defined by nurses. These included attention, presence, "thereness," acceptance, care, concern, interest, involvement, understanding, and empathy. van Servellen (1984) states that in the chronically disturbed family, the support provided by nurses takes many forms, such as restoration, facilitation of strengths, and resources that are present to maintain whatever level of wellness is possible.

Sampson and Marthas (1981) identify the roles of group process for health professionals. As we review the tasks of group process, it will become clear there is overlap in these group processes.

Human Growth and Development

Human beings learn how to be humans in groups. The early family is usually the most significant. As people grow, school and friends form other groups. As adults, these groups are changing and each person brings to each group situation a unique experience, which helps to further personal growth and development. People learn how to be human as children, teenagers, adults, the elderly, the disabled, the chronically ill, and the dying.

Behaviour Maintenance and Change

Humans can learn and see modelled new or different attitudes or habits that need to be changed for certain health conditions. Smoking cessation, substance abuse, and obesity groups are examples of groups that use the group process to change health-related attitudes and habits.

Health Promotion and Maintenance

Physical fitness, cancer care, and stress reduction are examples of health promotion or health maintenance tasks of groups. People learn through interaction with the group about the health condition common to all. Nurses uses this format to share their expertise and direct the group to share experiences concerning pertinent issues.

Team Practice

We are in an era of specialization, and groups of health professionals care for individuals as a team. This team functions as a group also. Each professional has different functions, and patient care is more effective when the team understands and uses good group process skills.

Family and Community Work

For example, cancer patients are not products of their disease alone. Interactions with their families and communities affect the disease process. Families are often caregivers; there are work and social concerns within the community that are critical for the care of that patient. The nurse can be instrumental, not only as a consultant, but may actually see a need and organize a specific group within the community.

Teaching, Training, and Supervision

Health promotion with a group is a vital role of community health nursing. Many examples are offered in other chapters on health promotion programs. As you work with groups that have a chronic illness, consider which of the health promotion strategies described in other chapters might be applicable. Here is an example of a support group for persons with cancer and their families.

Cancer Patient and Family Therapy Support Groups: A 6-Year Community Experience

This is the description of an ongoing support group that was begun in the community and is facilitated by two volunteer nurses with psychiatric and oncology experience. The basic purpose of the group was to provide support for cancer patients and their families. However, it became obvious that more than social support was needed as health promotion issues not related to cancer began to surface. The facilitators had to expand their knowledge base in the areas of exercise, nutrition, elder abuse, sexuality, heart disease, hypertension, postpolio syndrome, Parkinson disease, hip and knee replacements, renal dialysis, and many other areas. Priorities in health concerns are in constant flux according to the individual. This experience highlighted the need for a comprehensive health education and promotion program. These people with a chronic disease sought information about how to be healthy. They also wanted new coping skills and new problem-solving techniques for living with their chronic disease.

GROUP DESCRIPTION

The group meets monthly for 90 minutes. The group is open and attendance is not compulsory. The group meets in a local church, and the one rule is confidentiality. There is no structured agenda, and the group members identify their immediate needs and the agenda for the group.

GROUP DEMOGRAPHICS

The age range of the participants is 29 to 83 years of age; 67% percent are women. The length of time that members have attended the group is 1 week to 6 years. The majority are upper middle class; most are college graduates. The most common cancer diagnoses are breast and prostate cancer.

EVALUATION

Evaluating a group process is problematic. The success of the program is best measured by its longevity. Some of these people have been attending these groups for 6 years. The social support they receive is apparent in their continued attendance. Some of these people know as much about their chronic health condition as can be known, but they continue to attend for the social support and other health information that they receive for themselves and their families. Families with chronic health conditions need to be able to talk with health care providers about quality-of-life issues. In today's health care environment, there is little opportunity for this. Community nurses with the appropriate education and expertise can use their unique knowledge to provide this service in the community. The nurses have built a rapport with these people. They have formed a partnership with this community; they have become a part of it as well. They have brought to this experience their expertise, commitment, compassion, and, most importantly, themselves.

Summary

Unlike other chapters in this section of the textbook, there have been no specific health promotion programs offered in this chapter. This is because we hope you will review all the chapters and choose health promotion programs appropriate to the need of the chronically ill you encounter. Indeed, we hope you have enjoyed all the many strategies for promoting health partnerships. *Health to all.*

References

Bednar, R. L., & Lawlis, G. F. (1971). Empirical research in group psychotherapy. In A. Bergin & S. Garfield (Eds.), *Handbook of psychotherapy and behavior change: An empirical analysis.* New York: Wiley.

Covinsky, K. E., Wu, A. W., Landefeld, C. S., Connors, A. F. Jr., Phillips, R. S., Tsevat, J., Dawson, N. V., Lynn, J., & Fortinsky, R. H. (1999). Health status versus quality of life in older patients; does the distinction matter? *American Journal of Medicine, 106,* 435–440.

Davidson, J. R,. & Meltzer-Brody, S. E. (1999). The underrecognition and undertreatment of depression: What is the breadth and depth of the problem? *Journal of Clinical Psychiatry, 60*(suppl 7), 4–9.

DeYoung, C., & Dickey, B. (1967). Support-Its meaning for psychiatric nurses. *Journal of Psychiatric Nursing, 5,* 46–58.

Dies, R. R. (1979). Group psychotherapy: Reflections on three decades of research. *Journal of Applied Behavioral Science, 15,* 361–373.

Dies, R. R. (1986). Practical, theoretical, and empirical foundations for group psychotherapy. In A. J. Frances & R. E. Hales (Eds.), *The American Psychiatric Association annual review, volume 5.* Washington, DC: American Psychiatric Press.

Ellgring, J. H. (1999). Depression, psychosis, and dementia: Impact on the family. *Neurology, 52,* S17–S20.

Jonsdottir, H. (1998). Life patterns of people with chronic obstructive pulmonary disease: Isolation and being closed in. *Nursing Science Quarterly, 11,* 160–166.

Kaul, T. J., & Bednar, R. L. (1986). Experiential group research: Results, questions, and suggestions. In S. L. Garfield & A. E. Bergin (Eds.), *Handbook of psychotherapy and behavior change.* New York: Wiley.

Krafft, S. K., & Krafft, L. J. (1998). Chronic sorrow: Parents' lived experience. *Holistic Nursing Practice, 13,* 59-67.

Leopore, S. J. (1998). Problems and prospects for the social support-reactivity hypothesis. *Annals of Behavioral Medicine, 20,* 257–269.

Orlinsky, D. E., & Howard, K. I. (1986). Process and outcome in psychotherapy. In S. L. Garfield & A. E. Bergin (Eds.), *Handbook of psychotherapy and behavior change.* New York: Wiley.

Sampson, E. E., & Marthas, M. (1981). *Group process for the health professions.* New York: Wiley.

Stanley, A. H. (1999). Primary care and addiction treatment: Lessons learned from building bridges across traditions. *Journal of Addictive Diseases, 18,* 65–82.

van Servellen, G. M. (1984). *Group and family therapy: A model for psychotherapeutic nursing practice.* St. Louis, MO: Mosby.

Canadian Resources

Chronic Disease Prevention Alliance of Canada: **http://www.cdpac.ca/**

Health Canada Centre for Chronic Disease Prevention and Control: **http://www.hc-sc.gc.ca/pphb-dgspsp/centres_e.html#ccdpc**

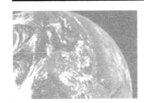

APPENDIX A

A Model Assessment Guide for Nursing in Industry

COMPONENTS	QUESTIONS TO ASK
The Company	
Historical development	How, why, and by whom was the company founded?
Organizational chart	What is the formal order of the system, and to whom are the health providers responsible?
Company policies	Is there a policy manual? Are the workers aware of the existence of the manual?
Length of the work week	How many days a week does the industry operate?
Length of the work time	Are there several shifts? How many breaks? Is there paid vacation?
Sick leave	Is there a clear policy, and do the workers know it?
Safety and fire provisions	Is management aware of situations or substances in the plant that represent a potential danger? Are there organized fire drills? (The *Federal Register* is the source of information for federal standards and serves as a helpful guide.)
Support services (benefits)	
Insurance programs	Is there a system for health insurance and life insurance, and is it compulsory? Does the company pay all or part? Who fills out the necessary forms?
Retirement program	Are the benefits realistic?
Educational support	Can the workers further their education? Will the company help financially?
Safety committee	If there is no committee, do certain people routinely handle emergencies? The Red Cross First Aid Course through programmed instruction is excellent (for information consult your local Red Cross).
Recreation committee	Do the workers have any communication with or interest in each other outside the work setting?
Employee relations	Are there problems in employee relations? (This is difficult information to get, but it is important to get a sense of how employees feel generally about management and vice versa.)

COMPONENTS	QUESTIONS TO ASK

The Plant

General physical setting	What is the overall appearance?
The construction	What is the size and general condition of buildings and grounds?
Parking facilities and public transportation stops	How far does the worker have to walk to get inside?
Entrances and exits	How many people must use them? How accessible are they?
Physical environment	What conditions exist in the physical environment? (Comment on heating, air-conditioning, lighting, glare, drafts, and so forth)
Communication facilities	Are there bulletin boards and newsletters?
Housekeeping	Is the physical setting maintained adequately?
Interior decoration	Are the surroundings conducive to work? Are they pleasing?
Work areas	
Space	Are workers isolated or crowded?
Heights: workplace and supply areas	Is there a chance of workers falling or being injured by falling objects? (Falls and falling objects are dangerous and costly to industry.)
Stimulation	Is the worker too bored to pay attention?
Safety signs and markings	Are dangerous areas well marked?
Standing and sitting facilities	Are chairs safe and comfortable? Are there platforms to stand on, especially for wet processes?
Safety equipment	Do the workers make use of hard hats, safety glasses, face masks, radiation badges, and so forth? Do they know the safety devices that the OSHA regulations require?
Nonwork areas	
Lockers	If the work is dirty, workers should be able to change clothes. Are they accidentally carrying toxic substances home on their clothes?
Hand-washing facilities	If facilities and supplies are available, do workers know how and when to wash their hands?
Rest rooms	How accessible are they, and what condition are they in?
Drinking water	Can workers leave their jobs long enough to get a drink of water when they want to?
Recreation and rest facilities	Can a worker who is not feeling well lie down? Do workers feel free to use the facilities?
Telephones	Can a worker receive or make a call? Does a working mother have to stay home for a call because she can't be reached at work?

COMPONENTS	QUESTIONS TO ASK
The Plant	
Ashtrays	Are people allowed to smoke in designated areas? Are they safe areas?
The Working Population: Include worker and management, but separate data for comparison.	
General characteristics	(Be as accurate as possible, but estimate when necessary.)
Total number of employees	(Usually, if an industry has 500 or more employees, full-time nursing services are necessary.)
General appearance	Are there records of heights, weights, cleanliness, and so forth? Ask to see them.
Age and sex distribution	What are the proportions of the different groups? (Certain screening programs are specific for young adults, whereas others are more for the elderly. Some programs are more for women; others are more for men.) Is there any difference between day and evening shift populations? Are the problems of the minority sex unattended?
Race distribution	Does one race predominate? How does this compare with the general community?
Socioeconomic distribution	Are there great differences in worker salaries? (This can sometimes cause problems.)
Religious distribution	Does one religion predominate? Are religious holidays observed?
Ethnic distribution	Is there a language barrier?
Marital status	What proportion of the workers are widowed, single, or divorced? (These groups often have different needs.)
Educational backgrounds	Can all teaching be done at approximately the same level?
Lifestyles practiced	Is there disapproval of certain lifestyles?
Types of employment offered	
Background necessary	What education level is required? Skilled versus unskilled?
Work demands on physical condition	What level of strength is needed? Is the work sedentary or active?
Work status	How many employees work full-time? Part-time? Is there overtime?
Absenteeism	Is there a record kept? By whom? Why?
Causes	What are the five most common reasons for absence?

COMPONENTS	QUESTIONS TO ASK

The Working Population: Include worker and management, but separate data for comparison.

Length	What are the patterns of absences? (Absenteeism is costly to the employer. There is some difference between one 10-day absence and 10 one-day absences by the same person.)
Physically handicapped	Does the company have a policy about hiring the handicapped?
Number employed	Where do they work? What do they do?
Extent of handicaps	Are they specially trained? Are they in a special program? Do they use prosthetic devices?
Personnel on medication	What medication does each of these employees take? Where does each person work?
Personnel with chronic illness	At what stage of illness is the employee? Where does the employee work? Will he or she be able to continue at this job?

The Industrial Process: What does the company produce and how?

Equipment used	Is the equipment portable or fixed? light or heavy?
General description of placement	Ask to have each piece of large equipment marked on a scale map.
Type of equipment	Fans, blowers, fast moving, wet, or dry?
Nature of the operation	Ask for a brief description of each stage of the process so that you can compare the needs and abilities of the worker with the needs of the job.
Raw materials used	What are they and how dangerous are they? Are they properly stored? Check the *Federal Register* for guidelines on storage.
Nature of the final product	Can the workers take pride in the final product or do they make parts?
Description of the jobs	Who does what? Where? (Label the map.)
Waste products produced	What is the system for waste disposal? Are the pollution-control devices in place and functioning?
Exposure to toxic substances	To which toxins are the workers exposed? What is the extent of exposure? (Include physical and emotional hazards. Remember that chronic effects of industrial exposure are subtle; a person often gets used to having mild symptoms and won't report them. The *Federal Register* contains specifications for exposure to toxins, and some states issue state standards.)

COMPONENTS	QUESTIONS TO ASK

The Health Program: Outline what is actually in existence as well as what employees perceive to be in existence.

Existing policies	Are there informal, unwritten policies?
Objectives of the program	Are they clear?
Preemployment physicals	Are they required? Are they paid for by the company? Is the information used to select?
First aid facilities	What is available? What is not available?
Standing orders	Is there a company physician who is responsible for first aid or emergency policy? (If so, work closely with him or her in planning nursing services.)
Job descriptions for health personnel	Are they in writing? (If there are no guidelines to be followed, write some.)
Existing facilities and resources	Sometimes an industry that denies having a health program has more of a system than it realizes.
Trained personnel	Who responds in an emergency?
Space	Where is the sick worker taken? Where is the emergency equipment kept?
Supplies	What are they? Where are they kept? (Make a list and describe the condition of each item.)
Records and reports	What exists? (The OSHA requires that employers keep three types of records: a log of occupational injuries and illnesses, a supplemental record of certain illnesses or injuries, and an annual summary [forms 100, 101, and 102 are provided under the act]. Good records provide data for good planning.)
Services rendered in the past year	Describe as specifically as possible.
Care needed	Chronic or acute? Why?
Screening done	Where? By whom? Why?
Referrals made	By whom? To whom? Why?
Counseling done	Formal or informal? (Often informal counseling goes unnoticed.)
Health education	What individual or group education was offered by the company?
Accidents in the past year	During working hours? After hours? (Include those that occur after work hours; some may be directly or indirectly work related.)
Reasons why employees sought health care	What are the five major reasons?

COMPONENTS	QUESTIONS TO ASK
Stressors	
As identified by employees	What pressures are felt on the job?
As identified by health providers	What problems do they perceive?

Adapted from Serafini, P. (1976). Nursing assessment in industry: A model. *American Journal of Public Health, 66*(8), 755–760.

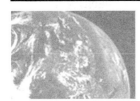

APPENDIX B

Assessment of an Industry

COMPONENTS	DESCRIPTION
The Company	
	The AAB Chemical Company
	Hampton Industrial Complex
	Located west of State Highway 519 and Loop 177
Historical development	The AAB Chemical Company separated from the AAB Refinery in 1957, and the present plant was completed in 1961. The parent company is a major oil company with headquarters in Chicago. The plant is today the most complex and versatile in the AAB system.
Organizational chart	A formal organizational chart was not available. However, by observation and interview, a structure consisting of a plant manager, with a supervisor in charge of each production area, safety, and maintenance was noted. There are overseers for each area of operation for each shift. The medical staff, which consists of one doctor and one nurse, are not hired by the plant personnel department but by the parent company in Chicago.
Company policies	The plant operations are never shut down. There are shifts around the clock for operators and craftspeople. Employees such as clerical, administrative, and medical staff work 8-hour days, 40-hour weeks. Breaks are provided during the work period. Employees are eligible for 2 weeks of paid vacation per year after working 1 year. This increases in 5-year increments. A 20-year employee is eligible for 5 weeks of vacation. Employees are eligible for sick leave after 6 months of service. Benefits vary with length of service. All benefits are published in an employee handbook, distributed to all employees.

COMPONENTS	DESCRIPTION

The Company

Company policies	Management is well aware of situations and substances that pose danger to the workers. The safety program, run by a safety supervisor and a safety engineer, is extensive. Organized fire drills are held frequently. Procedures for dealing with spills and other hazards are also well organized. Fire-fighting equipment and an ambulance are available on the plant site at all times. Certain employees are trained as firefighters. There are EMTs available inside the plant in addition to the nurse. Fire extinguishers are placed throughout the plant in strategic locations.
Support services	A comprehensive medical expense plan is compulsory for all employees. In addition, disability up to 40 weeks owing to occupational illness or injury is provided to all employees regardless of length of service. Term life insurance under a group plan is available at a low rate. A long-term disability plan is available to employees covered under the basic life insurance plan. A retirement plan is provided at complete cost to the company. A savings plan in which employees may invest in company stock and US Savings Bonds is also available.
	Employees are offered an educational assistance program and are encouraged to advance their careers. On-line-job training is provided to help employees advance.
Employee relations	The workers are affiliated with the Oil, Chemical and Atomic Workers International Union, a part of the AFL-CIO. It was difficult to perceive how management and labor relate to each other. However, several workers mentioned the family-like atmosphere among employees, and hopefully, this bridges the gap between labor and management. The last strike occurred approximately 2 years ago.

The Plant

General physical setting	The appearance of the plant is best described as an intimidating maze of pipes, towers, and vessels. The main building, in which the clinic is located, is modern and attractive, with well-tended grounds. Ample parking is available, with areas provided for the handicapped. The building is air conditioned, spacious, and clean, with a pleasing interior.

COMPONENTS	DESCRIPTION
The Plant	
General physical setting	The grounds and buildings inside the plant are also neat and well maintained. Scattered through the plant in strategic locations are eye-bubbling devices for flushing the eyes and showers for removing irritants from the skin. Danger areas are clearly marked with yellow paint and warning signs. Employees working in areas where hydrofluoric acid is used are provided with complete protective covering, and they shower immediately upon leaving the area. Earplugs and earmuffs are required in high-noise areas. Compliance in use of safety devices is good, and workers are aware of Occupational Safety and Health Administration (OSHA) regulations.
Work areas	Some work areas, especially where craftspeople are involved, are cramped and close, owing to the physical structure of the myriad pipes and lines. Some areas are also elevated in height. One problem noted by the plant nurse is occasional heat stress during summer months when employees are working in these areas on equipment that reflects heat. Another problem noted was the stress, manifested in muscle and joint discomfort, of working in cramped quarters, especially when employees work a lot of overtime. Occasionally employees are injured by falling objects, such as heavy wrenches. Burns are the most common type of injuries. Operators who work in the processing units and monitor the gauges and flow rates are in stressful jobs because a mistake could be costly and dangerous.
Nonwork areas	Each work area has a kitchen area, restrooms, and water fountains that are easily accessible. Lockers and showers are also available. Communication by phone is possible in all areas of the plant. Facilities are available in the clinic so that workers who are ill may lie down. However, in some areas, repeated visits to the clinic are discouraged. Employees are instructed regarding handwashing and prompt attention to small wounds by the nurse as part of new employee orientation. Smoking is permitted only in specifically designated parts of the fenced area of the plant, the docks, and warehouses.

COMPONENTS	DESCRIPTION

The Working Population

General characteristics	AAB Chemicals employs approximately 500 people. Age and sex distribution data were not available. However, the plant nurse stated that employees range in age from age 18 to retirement at age 65, and that male employees outnumber female employees. The nurse also stated that some women were moving into previously male-dominated jobs. Race distribution data were not available. By observation, the distribution appeared to be predominantly white, followed by black and then Hispanic employees, which is in line with the population distribution in the community. Data regarding religious and marital status were not available. Wages and salaries are commensurate with education, qualifications, and years of service. Educational backgrounds range from high school graduates to advanced degrees in engineering and the sciences. Therefore, health teaching must be geared to match the educational level of the group being instructed.
Type of employment offered	Types of employment include skilled craftspeople, operators, lab analysts, chemists, engineers, clerical and administrative personnel, and a nurse and a physician. The background required for each area varies with the complexity and nature of the job. Most employees are full-time and work overtime as required.
Absenteeism	Records of absences are kept in the employee's work unit. The nurse keeps records on illness- or injury-related absences. An employee who has been absent owing to an extended or serious illness, an injury, or surgery must report to the medical department before returning to work and must supply a statement from a doctor regarding the nature of his or her disability and the limitations, if any, on permissible work. The medical department then determines the physical condition of the employee and notifies his or her supervisor regarding the employee's return to work. Strict record keeping also is done for OSHA requirements. According to the nurse, the most common reasons for absence are not occupationally related. They are most often for upper-respiratory infections and other common health problems or for accidents that occurred away from the plant.

COMPONENTS	DESCRIPTION
The Working Population	
Physically handicapped	The AAB Company is an equal opportunity employer. Information regarding handicapped employees, the nature of their handicaps, and the jobs they fill was not available.
Personnel on medication Personnel with chronic illness	The nurse keeps records of employees on medication. This information is confidential. The confidentiality of employees' medical records is strictly enforced.
The Industrial Process	
Equipment used Nature of the plant operation	The basic job of the plant is to produce specialty chemicals and petrochemical intermediates for manufacture of products that range from boats and surfboards to carpets and furniture. Production of these chemicals involves moving raw materials (called "feedstock") from AAB's Hampton Refinery and another chemical plant and mixing them with xylenes and benzenes. Some of the chemicals produced are propylene, styrene, paraxylene, metazylene, aromatic solvents, oil-recovering chemicals, oil-producing chemicals, and polybutenes. The equipment used involves miles of pipes and many towers and vessels. Process units are designed to be energy efficient, and in many instances, energy-producing hydrocarbons are a by-product of a process. These are then recovered and used as fuel in other operations. Flammability and danger of explosion are major concerns when dealing with the above-named chemicals. Proper storage is essential and is carried out with care in this plant. The final product of the production process is barrels of chemicals. Workers take pride in turning out a certain number of barrels in a time period and in keeping the plant operating efficiently. The treatment of wastewater is through an effluent water-control system that is one of the most sophisticated in the industry. The facility handles wastewater not only from AAB Chemical but also from the AAB Refinery and another chemical plant in the area. Air-pollution control is done in two steps: first by eliminating potential contaminants whenever possible and then through the use of devices such as scrubbers, filters, cyclone separators, and a flare system to burn up the waste hydrocarbons.

COMPONENTS	DESCRIPTION

The Industrial Process

Exposure to toxic substances	The major substances of concern are benzene and xylene. Benzene is a colorless, flammable, volatile liquid. The major hazard with this chemical is chronic poisoning by inhalation of small amounts over a long time. It is one of the most dangerous organic solvents in common use. Benzene acts primarily on the blood-forming organs. Skin contact also is to be avoided. Benzene is suspected of being carcinogenic. Xylene resembles benzene in many chemical and physical properties but is not involved in causing chronic blood diseases. It has a narcotic effect and can cause dermatitis with repeated contact. Benzene screening is done on all employees on a yearly basis.

The Health Program

Existing policies	The objectives of the program are to monitor the status of each employee's health in order to pinpoint problems at an early stage and to provide prompt attention to accidents or emergencies as they occur at the worksite. The employees perceive the second objective more readily than the first. Many of them perceive the yearly physicals as a low priority.
	Preemployment physicals are done by the nurse and company doctor at no charge to the client and are used as a baseline for future reference.
	The ambulance kept at the plant is equipped for all emergencies. Injured or ill employees requiring more than initial first aid are taken immediately to Jefferson Memorial Hospital.
	There is a set of comprehensive standing orders, written through collaborative effort by the nurse and doctor. Yearly physicals include chest roentgenogram, blood work that includes benzene screening, urinalysis, vision and hearing assessments, and physical exams by the physician. Pregnant women are seen each month by the doctor in addition to their own private doctors. No screening programs alone are done, but they are incorporated into the yearly physical. Health teaching and informal counseling are done on an individual basis by the nurse and doctor.

COMPONENTS	DESCRIPTION
The Health Program	
Existing facilities and resources	CPR is taught to selected personnel throughout the plant by the nurse.
	The medical department consists of one full-time nurse and a physician who cover this plant and AAB's larger plant near Avina, as well as a part-time secretary. The facilities include the nurse's office, where all medical records are kept and where employees check in when visiting the clinic; a treatment room; a small lab and dispensary; a roentgenogram room; an exam room; and the physician's office. First aid facilities are extensive and well supplied. ECG equipment also is available. The nurse sees between 12 and 15 clients per day in the clinic. The major reasons employees seek health care are non–occupationally related sicknesses or accidents, stress-related complaints, and minor accidents on the job.
Stressors	
Employees	Job pressure, as with operators who control the process units
	Overtime hours, when worked frequently
	Knowledge of potential fire or explosion
	Shift work that may not be in sync with normal body rhythms
	Strikes or layoffs
Health care providers	Problems with role definition. Nurse wishes to do more health teaching but feels Safety Department has taken over many of her functions. Feels powerless to change the situation. Feels that physician also perceives her role as limited to specific, traditional areas.

Index

Note: Page numbers followed by f, t, and b indicate figures, tables, and boxed material, respectively.